"It is not the strongest of the species that survives, nor the most intelligent. It is the one that is most adaptable to change." - Charles Darwin (attributed)

"You try to plant something in the concrete, y'know what I mean? If it grow, and the rose petal got all kind of scratches and marks, you not gonna say, 'Damn, look at all the scratches and marks on the rose that grew from concrete'; you gonna be like, 'Damn! A rose grew from the concrete?!'" – Tupac Shakur

The

Kitchen Sink Farming

Series

The Complete Set, Volumes 1-4

Publisher:

Stone Soup Publications

Portland, OR 97239

publisher@KitchenSinkFarming.org

©2016 Jean-Pierre Parent

No part of this book may be reproduced or transmitted in any form or by any means, electronic or mechanical, including photocopying or recording or by any information storage or retrieval systems without prior permission in writing from Stone Soup Publications or Jean-Pierre Parent.

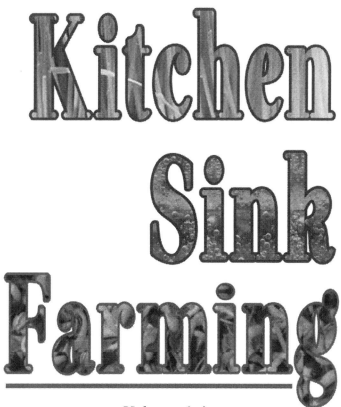

Kitchen Sink Farming

Volumes 1-4
Easily and Cheaply Grow, Sprout, and Ferment Your
Own Food for a Healthir Now and a Greener Future
and Homegrown Living Recipes
What to Do with Your Sprouts and Krauts

By Jean-Pierre Parent

In humble gratitude to the trees that grew to make the paper
recycled to make this book. I've tried to use you wisely

- Preface 13
- The "Why?" 17
  - A Deeper Reason to Take Control of Our Food: Truly Empty Calories 23
  - A History of Agri-Tech 24
  - Burger & a Side of Flies: Genetic Modification of Food 25
  - When Organic Isn't (It's too easy being green) 34
  - Collapse, the Future of Food 39
  - Peak Oil Pioneers 41
  - Easter Island's Last Lumberjack 46
  - Everyone but the Kitchen Sink: Modernization, McDonald's, and Hyper-Maturation 50
  - Using the Brain for a Change 54
- Sprouting: The "How?" 63
  - Hit the Ground Sprouting 63
  - Enzyme Inhibitors 67
  - Enzymes 68
  - Quantity 70
  - Sprouting in a nutshell 70
  - Clean, but don't get crazy… 71
  - Air Supply 74
  - The Jar Method 76
  - The Bag Method 77
  - The Basket Method 79

Robo-Sprouting (the Automatic Sprouter), for negligent parents 80

Specialty Sprouts 81

    The Clay Method 81

    Bean-Sprouting 82

The Dirt on Grass - Tray Sprouting 82

Grid-Iron Chef – The Moveable Farm 84

Growing for Your Pet 88

Appendix A: The Wide World of Sprouts - Sprouting Seeds 89

Appendix B: Sprouting Table 168

Fermenting - The "How?" 177

A Brief History of Slime 178

DNA Sluts and Your Guts: *Genetic Promiscuity* and its effect on human evolution and happiness 179

Public Enemy #1: The War on Bugs 181

Your First Fermentation: Probiotic Water 184

Local Flora - Sauerkrauts and Other Fermented Veggies 188

    Sterilization 194

    Seed Cheese and Yogurt 197

    Simple Seed Cheese 197

    "Advanced" Cheese Making: A 2-Day Degree 200

    Coconut Cream Cheese 201

    Vinegar 203

    Specialty Vinegars 208

- Mead and Ginger Beer 210
- Ginger Beer 217
- Fermented Bread 221

Cultivated Flora 226
- Kombucha 226
- Health Benefits of Kombucha 234
- Jun 238
- Kefir (Dairy) 240
- Tibicos (Juice Kefir) 250
- Fermenting Fats – Butter and Oil 252
- Raw Fats and Unrefined Oils for Weight-Loss and Well-Being 257

The "How?" - 263

Growing 263
- Sprouts and Greens 263
- Grass and Micro-Greens 263
- Why Grow Grass? 264
- Why Cleansing is Important 272
- How to Grow and Enjoy Grasses 274
- Dirt 275
- H, P, and That Sneaky Little O: Hydrogen Peroxide 289
- How to Juice Grass 293

Micro-Lettuces, Shoots and Greens 294
- Choosing your plants 295
- Shoots 297

Sunflower Lettuce.. 298
Container Gardening 300
　　Outdoor Growing.. 300
　　Light... 301
　　Choosing Crops 306
　　Indoor Growing 308
　　Self-Watering Containers 308
　　Simple Self-Watering Devices: "the spike" and "the holey bottle" 309
　　The Watering Spike 309
　　The Self-Watering Bucket 310
　　The Self-Watering Garden................................. 313
　　Fertilizing.. 314
Hooked on 'Ponics: Hydroponic and Aeroponic Gardening 315
The Plans: Hydroponics 318
　　Small-Scale Set-Up.. 321
　　Large-Scale Hydro Set-up 326
　　The Growing Wall 332
　　Barrel and Drum Gardening 342
DIY Aeroponics 346
　　The Aero-Tote 346
　　Composting and Worm-iculture 354
　　DIY Tumbling Composter................................. 361
　　Worm-i-culture 364
Appendix A - Plant Nutritional Deficiencies 372

Recipes - Why Living Foods?... 377
On Measuring:.. 386
The Blessing of Bad Food.. 388
Helpful Tools for Preparing These Recipes 390
Routine 397
Drinks and Smoothies.. 399
Vit-Ali Baba 399
Grape-Nuts Milk 400
Jamaican "A" Lemonade.................................... 401
Delhi Milk 401
Raw Honey 403
Chaach 405
Kefir Creamsicle 406
Vampire Juice... 407
Lentil-ade 409
Seed/Nut Milk 411
Basic Nut Milk 412
Cocktails.. 412
Basil-Grape Mojito... 412
Kefir Ginger Ale.. 413
Time to Make the Coconuts 414
Mains, Sides, Apps 417
Raw Portobello Mushroom Pizza......................... 417
Zucchini Hummus and Veggie Chips 420
Dolmas 424

Pasta	425
Making Noodles	426
Red Lentil Marinara	427
Pesto	429
Cooking with Science	431
Foamification	431
Gelification	433
Steps (presented here: Arugula Spaghetti, pictured)	433
Spherification	435
Steps (presented here: Balsamic Caviar, pictured)	436
Salads and Dressings	438
All-Cylinders Creamy Dressing:	442
Mellifluous Honey-Mustard	443
Cilantro Dried-Tomato Ranch	443
Sesame-Garlic Aioli	445
Strawberry-Poppy Seed Vin	446
Salt-free Asian Vin	446
Cucumber-Clover Vin	447
Raw Slaw	449
Sprout Salads	450
Apple Pie-laf	450
Other Salads:	452
Tantric Kale Salad	452
Quinoa-Kimchi Salad	454
Kashmiri Karrots	454

Bachelor Pad Thai 455

Mung-Cardamom Sundal 456

Sammies and Wraps.. 457

Burawtos.. 457

Garden Wrap 458

Inside-Out Tacos 461

Smoky-Maple Zucchini Bacon...................................... 463

Plymouth Rock and Rolls.. 465

Coconut Tortillas... 467

Asian Veggie Nori Wrap.. 468

Raw Pickled Ginger 470

Avocado ponzu.. 470

Soups and Stews 471

All-American Chowder 471

Cream of Mushroom 473

Goulash.. 474

Buddha Belly Soup.. 475

Coconut Corner! 476

Carrot Coconut Soup with Ginger................................. 476

Chilled Mango Soup with Lime-Macadamia Cream and Coconut Noodles 477

Coconut Noodles:.. 478

Lime-Macadamia Cream:.. 478

Clover Curry.. 479

Snacks and Condiments 480

Gomasio 480

- Living Parm 481
- Spicy Seed Mix 482
- Fall-nuts 484
- Cultured Kimchi 485
- Asian Dip 486
- Summer Sauer Slaw 487
- Strawberry Ambrosia Leather 488

Cheeses, Dips, and Spreads 492

Breads 495
- Basic Sprouted Bread 495
- Easy Crackers 500

Breakfasts! 506
- Simple Cereal 506
- Spanish Scramble 506

Desserts 508
- Banana Ice Cream 511
- Oatmeal-Raisin Cookies 512
- Chocolate Peanut Butter Tarts 513
- Smoky Apple Butter Bars 514
- Strawberry-Tomato Ice Cream 516
- Banana-Hemp Cookies 517
- Tahini Halava with Candied Cherry Frosting 518
- Macaroons 519
- Hemp Cacao-Nut Macaroons 520
- Berry Tart with Almond Crust and Sweet Kefir Cream
  521

Putting It All Together 524
Recommended Reading.. 527
Resources: 529
Index.. 530

Preface

This book is the result of a serious personality flaw.

Somehow, from a very early age, I've rarely been satisfied with anything. Or, more accurately, I'm only satisfied with perfection, that acutely rare and delicate moment when the stars align; the air is just so, filling the lungs with sweet fortitude and the project before you sparkles with temporal rightness…

This eternal dissatisfaction with the lack of perfection pervades every aspect of my life: my athleticism, health, relationships, even conversations. I practiced them beforehand, and I think about them afterwards, re-working them in my mind until my responses are the most thoughtful, compassionate, wise, and considerate statements possible. When I was a little kid playing with my Atari, I probably hit the reset button on the console more often than the one on the controller, starting the game over and over if I did something that wasn't *quite* right, so that I could have a chance to do it again, and this time, perfectly. At the time, I think I expected all of life could be like that.

But I think I really hit my "always-satisfied-with-the-best" stride with food. If I was eating something (and that happened quite often in those days), I would wonder "what's the best possible form of this food?" So I cut out junk food and soda (I think I was nine at this time), after experiencing how I felt after eating a fast food hamburger before a soccer game. Didn't make that mistake again. I soon came to learn about vegetarian, then vegan, then organic, then raw food. The quest didn't stop there though, because of the widely varying ideas of raw vs. living food, organic standards, and genetic modification of food. Recently, the world's largest chain of natural food grocery stores was caught selling frozen vegetables as organic that were actually grown in China with little respect for chemical-free farming, and the "independent" organic certifiers that permitted the labeling are owned by the store (more on pg 30). So it's a constant question about who's trustworthy, and "how long will they be?" (See chapter "Truly Empty Calories", subchapter "When Organic Isn't (It's Too Easy Being Green)" for more on this particular paranoia).

And then there is the immeasurable question of taste. All this wholesome, nutritious food (like the bland and boring natural choices when I was a kid and 90% of them today) might be good for the body but unless it can create sublime waves of closed-eye, tilted-headed moaning pleasure, it does little for the soul. And therefore leaves something to be desired. Incomplete. Imperfect.

These days, my slightly mellowed aspirations for perfection have made me an experimenter, a scientist, a chef, a do-it-yourself-er. Before sitting down to write this (at a desk that I built so I could be the perfect height, with a pillow that I cut from the perfect density of memory foam mattress, on which I am sitting in a yoga position called siddhasana, or perfect pose) I noticed that some pumpkin seeds I sprouted and put in my dehydrator for a crunchy snack were sticking together. Makes sense, if you've ever lobotomized a pumpkin for a jack-o-lantern, scooping out its slimy stuck-together seeds. I thought that natural cohesion might be a good start to a flatbread, maybe mixed with super-sticky flax. So, did I make *a* pumpkinseed-flax flatbread? No... I made about 2 dozen. Equal parts flax and pumpkin. Double one, and double the other. Each one of those split in thirds, one part put on the counter to ferment, one in the oven at a low temp, and the rest in the dehydrator at a lower temp.

> "I have simple tastes. I am always satisfied with the best."
> – Oscar Wilde

Each of *those* split in half again, dry or with some oil. One in each category blended with some sprouted spelt, to see if they'd be better a little cake-ier. All labeled and catalogued. You get the idea.

Some may think that this level precision is boring, rigid, anal-retentive, or obsessive, and I might agree if it was focused on a less important subject. But I think nourishment is just too important to be satisfied with anything less than utterly thorough knowledge, which until recently we've had to mostly figure by our lonesomes. I think that this mindset is an integral part of being able to draw the measure of life's awesomeness and maybe the best way to experience the most happiness, fun, health, contentedness, and eventual freedom, because I will *know* what the best choice is for me today. With certainty. That's the goal, anyways. And then I'm happy, because the mundane turns into magic when it's dove into with attentive and receptive enthusiasm.

This book is the result of my decades-long experiment that asks the question: what's the best food possible, to fuel the best life possible? I think I've found glimmers of the answer, and I'm so pleased to be able share them with you.

This is what led me to eating whole, organic, living foods: wanting to get as much out of my food as possible. Your reasons might be totally different. Starting with pure ingredients is a life-saver for someone with food allergies – the only way to take control of what goes into your body. Even someone lactose intolerant can enjoy the bowel-healing properties of milk (as raw kefir,), butter (as ghee), or cheeses of many kinds (all in Kitchen Sink Farming Volume 2: Fermenting). Cancer patients find remission through fermented foods. The environmental benefits of enough home growers and sprouters will have a major global impact. A network of neighbors that each specialize in a different product could build community like nothing else – focused around the most primal and fundamental cement of society. And as I'll mention time and again, it's also the cheapest way to eat what is possibly the very best food in the world.

The "Why?"

The world's best foods aren't available in stores. You can't get them from the home shopping network, either. It's a good thing, too, because then people would buy them and miss out on the particular satisfaction of eating something they grew themselves, acutely aware of the life cycle of and organic rhythms of nature in their current mouthful. It's also a good thing because they're really cheap and nearly really easy to make, and once you try it, it'd be laughable to pay someone else to do it. This book is based on the firm fact that anyone, anywhere, at any time, can be enjoying a bounty of fresh, living, incredibly nutritious food with very little work and expense.

Once you've enjoyed a delicious and vibrant lunch made from sprouted seeds, grains, or nuts bursting with taste and life, you won't need any convincing. You'll know by that point how easy, cheap, and fun it is to grow sweet strawberries, succulent micro greens, and juicy tomatoes with shocking depth of flavor in your seventh-story apartment kitchen, washing them down with home-brewed, wild-yeasted ginger ale or sparkling kombucha tea. In the meantime, though, before you figure all that out for yourself, it's supportive to know exactly why you're doing what you're doing. Maybe you're interested in increasing the amount of fresh, organic food you're eating (and

> "A great revolution in just one single individual will help achieve a *change* in the destiny of a society and, further, will enable a *change* in in the destiny of humankind."
> *Daisaku Ikeda*

there's no fresher food than something grown 5 feet away from your table and "picked" when you take your first chew!) and dramatically improving your health, energy, and immune system. Maybe you want to save money on groceries or have less of an impact on the earth, casting a vote against industrialized, destructive modern farming methods. Or maybe girls (and guys) just wanna have fun in the kitchen. Whatever your reason, learning about the myriad benefits of sprouting, indoor gardening, and fermenting at home will only encourage and inspire. And it just might make you able to explain to your mom why the dinner peas have leaves.

Nutrients and enzymes don't take kindly to cooking, canning, or sitting on shelves. Even fresh, organic produce loses valuable benefits every hour it's wilting away under the grocery store lights. In Los Angeles, it's hard to walk a few blocks and not pass a Whole Foods or organic restaurant. But even there, in the city with perhaps the greatest access to all things health, sprouted peanut butter, Kamut grass juice (wheat's superior ancestor), unpasteurized sauerkraut, enzymatically-active hot soups, and raw goat milk kefir are not for sale or else have to be painstakingly and expensively tracked down, even though these examples of the most healthful versions of common foods require very little knowledge, no expensive equipment, and less than a minute a day to make. When I was learning the things in this book, even though my efforts usually required a lot of trial and error, I kept coming back to the same eureka feeling: "It *can't* be this easy." But it is. A short and hopefully fun learning adventure will have you eating better than ever before, saving money, and feeling amazing. Maybe one day your local Piggly Wiggly will have a nut butter cafe, where they'll grind the freshly sprouted nuts of your choice, which you can spread on the apple a polite and well-groomed apron-clad deli worker just picked in front of you. If and when we get there through the slow and painstaking process of transforming consumer opinion and convincing the huge conglomerates that it's cost-effective to service us in this way, they'll surely charge an arm and a snout for it. No. The only way to eat living, vital, delicious food is to grow and prepare it yourself.

Nature is a hard-working and dedicated employee. Hire her to work for you and then sit back and relax. Nobody fertilizes or irrigates the forest. It's a complete system that does these things on its own. Make a "food forest" in your apartment, home, or patio, and your main effort is to pick the food. You put in some effort at the very beginning, but once the system is established, you work a lot less. You could call kitchen sink farming "lazy agriculture", because you're working *with* nature, and not against it. You're using the laws of nature, forces that apply equally on a rainforest floor, a Brooklyn backyard, or a Tokyo high-rise to grow your lunch. Sprouting, fermenting, and growing your own food are plain and simple the best foods you can get. They're the least amount of energy to digest, the most nutrition, the least impact on the environment, resources, and humanity for the longest, most disease and discomfort-free life. And wouldn't you know it: it's the cheapest and easiest way to create food, too. Anyone in the world can apply at least one principal in this

> **Nerd Corner!**
>
> Sprouting seeds increases their nutrient availability by 50-2000%, with an average of about 500%. See table on pages 14-15 to see the effects on specific nutrients after sprouting mung beans (not the most common spout, but possibly the most fun to say).

book, and the more you work into your own everyday life, the better off that life will be for it.

Sprouting: Why Mess with a Perfectly Good Seed?

1) Sprouting activates enzymes.

> "Intelligence is the ability to adapt to change."
> Stephen Hawking

Sprouts have an average of 7 times the enzymes needed to digest them, enzymes that can go to work digesting other foods, repairing and regenerating the body. See page 62 for more on enzymes.

2) Sprouting Increases Nutrition

Sprouted seeds supply nutrients in a predigested form – food is broken down into its simplest and easiest-to-digest components. During sprouting, much of the starch is broken down into simple sugars such as glucose and sucrose by the action of the enzyme 'amylase'. Proteins are converted into amino acids and amides. Fats and oils are converted into more simple fatty acids by the enzyme lipase. Sprouts are also high in fiber, so that along with their water helps digestion even more.

3) Sprouting removes "Enzyme Inhibitors"

Enzyme Inhibitors keep seeds from sprouting at the wrong time, and keep nutrients locked up. Sprouting seeds makes them easier to digest and more nutritious for this reason as well, and actually makes everything you eat before and after more nutritious too. (see pg 62 for more)

Table 1: Effects of Sprouting on Mung Beans

Protein	Increases 30%	The increase in protein availability is an indicator of the overall enhancement of nutritional value of a sprouted seed.
Carbohydrates	Decreases 15%	The simultaneous reduction in carbohydrate and caloric content indicates that many carbohydrate molecules are broken down during sprouting to allow absorption of atmospheric nitrogen to reform it into amino acids. The resulting protein is the most easily digestible of all proteins.
Calcium	Increases 30%	
Potassium	Increases 80%	
Sodium	Increases 690%	The skyrocketing sodium content is a good indication that

		foods are much more easily digestible in the sprouted form, as sodium is essential to the digestive process, particularly in the intestines, and also to the elimination of carbon dioxide. The building blocks of both nutrition and digestibility peak simultaneously.
Iron	Increases 40%	
Vitamin A	Increases 285%	
Vitamin B1 (Thiamine)	Increases 208%	
Vitamin B2 (Riboflavin)	Increases 515%	
Vitamin B3 (Niacin)	Increases 256%	
Vitamin C	Infinite Increase	Dry seeds don't show a measurable amount of Vitamin C, but it skyrockets when they're

		sprouted. Vitamin C is important in the metabolization of proteins, which also increase in sprouted seeds.

A Deeper Reason to Take Control of Our Food: Truly Empty Calories

Food that's not organically grown by traditional, natural methods (paradoxically called "conventionally-grown"), is fairly devoid of nutrients. Large-scale commercial farmers discovered in the 1940's that three nutrients are required to grow and produce normal-looking crops: nitrogen, phosphorus, and potassium, or NPK, but plants, like us, require over 100 minerals to be at their best, and if it's not in the soil, it's not on your plate. Plants grown "conventionally" don't have the nutrients they need to develop healthy immune systems, requiring farmers to spray them down with a heavy coat of pesticides, herbicides, and fungicides. When we eat the fruit and vegetables that comes off of nutrient-deficient, chemical pesticide-laden plants, we suffer in two ways: very little nutrition and a dose of cancer-causing chemicals. When I'm travelling and can't get organic produce, I feel as if I'm eating photographs of food. The apples look like apples, they're red and round, but they're tasteless and my body feels a lifeless chunk of food in my belly as if I've been chewing on paper. My body is waiting for the flood of nourished happiness that it's used to, but doesn't come.

> "The nation that destroys its soil destroys itself." – F.D.Roosevelt

It gets worse. Turns out this disconnect is the well-planned stratagem of big business, who can almost always be counted on to put profits before people. Consumers are starting to become aware of a decades-old curtain of misinformation and propaganda drawn between grocery store shoppers and the contents of their carts by massive agribusiness and their bigger, cheaper, faster business model. But it wasn't always this way.

A History of Agri-Tech

Before World War II, people farmed the way they always have: fertilizing their fields with nutrient-dense organic matter or growing where rivers overflow and deposit the year's worth of mineral-rich silt. They rotated crops so that plants that take certain nutrients from the soil are supported by a season of plants that put those nutrients back. They relied on the strength of the crops' own immunity to fight off pests. Rainbows glittered over every dew-speckled family-farmed field of organic heirloom veggies… Ok, not really, but food *was* more nutritious and less carcinogenic.

> "Humanity consumed 120% of the earth's sustainable resource capacity in 1999" - National Academy of Sciences, June

World War II inspired many advances in industrial science, from napalm and synthetic rubber to the atomic bomb. When it was over, huge stocks of nitrates from ammunition building, organophosphates for making nerve gas, and other chemicals had accumulated. Nitrates contain nitrogen, one component of the NPK triad, and an enterprising chemical company re-labeled them "fertilizer". Nerve agents like mustard gas, shown to block communication between the brain and organs in both humans and insects alike, were called "pesticides", and both of these were sold to post-war farms. These chemicals, with only slight variations are still used today, and over 1.5 million pounds of organophosphates are sprayed every year on California farms alone.

The huge demand placed on modern farmers to feed more and more people on less and less space is creating an unparalleled desperation. In an attempt to keep up with demand, farmers have fired nature and are courting the promise of a dangerous and only partially-understood technology.

Burger & a Side of Flies: Genetic Modification of Food

Pick a single-ingredient food off the supermarket shelves and you have a 70% chance of grabbing a genetically modified organism, or GMO. This is the volatile and very scary process of splicing a fruit, veggie, or grain's DNA with genes from another organism, always part bacteria, often animal and sometimes even insect, human, or virus. Choose something with corn (or a derivative like corn syrup, dextrose, baking powder, caramel and caramel coloring, mono and diglycerides, modified food starch, vegetable anything: broth, oil, protein, shortening, and the many other ways industrious food scientists have found to pump the most heavily-subsidized and therefore most commonly-grown crop in the US into our diets) or a food with more than a few ingredients and unless it's organic or specifically labeled "non-GMO" your chances go up to around 100%. The ancient process of plant breeding is this: put two plants with traits you like next to each other and hope they'll cross-pollinate and the next generation will be an even better plant.

This wasn't precise or fast enough for modern agri-business. GMO was born out of the desire to achieve total dominion over crops, under the guise of lowering costs and increasing yields. But as with the attempt to control most things in nature, the outcome was not the expected one. Genetic modification has actually cost agriculture more, after recalls on untamable seeds, the inability of GM plants to access nutrients in the soil, puzzlingly lower yields in drought conditions and increased needs for more powerful pesticides with the consequence of mutant super-weeds. None of these issues have impeded cell-invasive technology's expansion, however, as the planting of BT crops went from zero acres in 1988 to 3.7 million in 1996 to 100 million in 2003. Most of the financial burden has fallen not on the slick-talking companies, however, but on the farmers who were taken in by their glimmering promises. It becomes a deadly gamble when, like between 2001 and 2005, 32,000 Indian farmers committed suicide underneath the avalanche of debt an Indian subsidiary of the Monsanto Corporation pawned off onto them when their GM cotton fields were ravaged by a disease that affected only GM plants. Ironically, at least one of the farmers killed himself, at 25 years old, by drinking a liter of pesticide.

Monsanto is one of the companies that is single-handedly destroying the traditional methods of farming in favor of a near-fascist domination of farmers and the very DNA of the seeds they plant, and along with it the worlds' food supply. Monsanto, whose first success was Agent Orange, the forest defoliant used in the Vietnam are and has since been found guilty in Federal courts of falsifying their earnings statements (<u>Foreign Corrupt Practices Act</u> (15 U.S.C. § 78dd-1)), bribing government officials around the globe (15 U.S.C § 78m(b)(2) & (5)), knowingly polluting the small town of Anniston, Alabama, with dangerous levels of polychlorinated biphenyls (PCBs) resulting in over 3.500 cases of cancer and other degenerative diseases, mislabeling pesticides to minimize their dangers (*Monsanto guilty of chemical poisoning in France,* Reuters Feb 13,

2012) and countless other crimes against humankind and nature. In the year 2000, it was estimated that 10 new people everyday are diagnosed with cancer due to exposure to dioxin produced by Monsanto (US Environmental Protection Agency's (EPA) draft reassessment on dioxin) and as of this writing, Monsanto is being taken to court by a group of Argentinean tobacco farmers who say that the biotech giant knowingly poisoned them with herbicides and pesticides and subsequently caused "devastating birth defects" in their children.

But the *really* scary part of this whole mess is that these "Franken-foods" reproduce in unexpected and uncontrollable ways. Bizarre monstrosities of barely recognizable plants discovered in fields. 1000-generational heirloom corn farms contaminated by invading mutant DNA. Monsanto's BT corn, cotton, and soy are *themselves* registered as pesticides. The process of genetically modifying foods is not only unethical and disgusting, but we're messing with forces we don't understand and the current results are hinting at world-wide epidemics of sci-fi horror film proportions. For example, in 1989 there was an outbreak of a new disease in the US, traced back to a batch of an L-tryptophan food supplement produced with GMO bacteria. Though it contained less than .1% of the highly

> "A molecular study conducted by Mexican, American and Dutch researchers demonstrates the presence of genes from genetically modified organisms (GMO) among the varieties of traditional corn cultivated in the remote regions of Oaxaca State in the southern part of the country, even though the Mexican government has always maintained a moratorium on the use of transgenic seed." - from "GMO Contamination in Mexico's Cradle of Corn" *Le Monde*, December 11 2008

toxic compound, 37 people died that year and 1,500 were left with permanent disabilities.

The Food and Drug Administration declared that it was not gene modification that was at fault but a failure in the purification process. However, the company concerned, Showa Denko, admitted that the low-level purification process had been used without ill effect in non-GM batches. Scientists at Showa Denko blame the GM process for producing traces of a potent new toxin, and this new toxin had never been found in non-GM versions of the product. In May 2008, new findings by the Physicians and Scientists for Responsible Application of Science and Technology (PSRAST) caused them to state "Most importantly, the poison considered most important in the tryptophan was closely similar to tryptophan (a dimer), but never found in natural bacteria. This indicates that disturbed tryptophan metabolism generated the poison. Moreover, the inserted genes were directed at altering the metabolism (so as to increase tryptophan production).

> "Typically, if something is to be considered Generally Recognized as Safe (G.R.A.S.) it needs lots of peer-reviewed published studies and an overwhelming consensus among the scientific community. With GM crops, they had neither." – Jeffrey Smith, author, *Seeds of Deception*

Our conclusion is that the only plausible explanation for the appearance of this poison is disturbances of the natural metabolic processes due to genetic engineering."

This is just one example of the dangers of genetic manipulation. It's easy to imagine that every instance of genetic modification has its own tale, or will. In fact, children have more adverse reactions to GMOs than adults, and it's hard to not picture a future without horrible consequences from freely fucking with nature. The idea hits home even harder when a public official in Japan,

> From news footage of Vice President George Bush Sr. at the Monsanto factory in 1987:
>
> Monsanto Executive: "We have no complaint about the way the USDA is handling it; they're going through an orderly process… Now if we're waiting til September and we don't have our authorization we may say something different!"
>
> Bush: "Call me. We're in the de-reg [de-regulation] business. Maybe we can help."

where GM foods are outlawed stated their plan to "watch US children for the next ten years" before they determine their next course of action, according to the documentary "The Future of Food" (Deborah Koons Garcia, Lily Films, 2004).

Bio-engineered foods don't have, and were never designed, to provide any benefit to the consumer. No attempt has been made to make more nutritious wheat or better-tasting spinach. Instead, the GM industry's only goal is profit (of everyone but the farmer), so the scam has been sold to the American consumer as a way to provide food for the masses of overpopulated future generations. One problem with this logic is that the nearly 1 billion malnourished people (10,000 of which die every day from starvation) don't do so because of a lack of food. Many of these people used to be farmers, but were kicked off their land when their respective governments accepted huge loans from multi-national banks, and subsistence farming wasn't a workable way to pay them back. Forced off their farms and into the slums of industrializing third-world cities, they have gone from being food independent to food-dependant. The calamitous issue of world hunger is not a problem of production; it's a crisis of access, which is strange when one considers that the average piece of food travels 1500 miles from the farm to the supermarket. The other argument with this propaganda is Monsanto's plan to include in all seeds they produce a "terminator gene", a self-destructing abomination that creates a plant with sterile progeny. That means that if you buy a seed from Monsanto and plant it, instead of being able to harvest the seeds from your plants for next year, you will have to buy more seeds. This is clear proof that the biotech industry has no interest in "feeding the world", as their propaganda states. In the same way that GMO seeds have mysteriously found their way into native plant genes (see quote below), the danger of this terminator gene out-crossing into the plants that make up the world's food supply, effectively ending traditional,

> "AG Biotech will find a supporter occupying the White House next year, regardless of which candidate wins the election in November."
> – Monsanto In-House Newsletter, Oct 6 2000, in reference to the multiple White House officials that are also board members of Monsanto.

sustainable farming, must have gone unnoticed by the company's scientists and members of the USDA who both approved the use of the gene and co-own it. No one can be that evil.

But who is responsible if terminator genes cross-contaminate unsuspecting food supplies? By past precedent, it's not the seed company that's to blame but the farmer, and courts have told farmers that by not protecting their fields properly from seeds blowing in (an absolutely ludicrous idea), they have unwittingly signed a contract with the biotech company that's patented that specific invading gene. Is it possible that one day the world's entire food supply will be controlled by the company that brought us PCB's (which are present in the cells of every man, woman, and child on Earth), DDT, bovine growth hormone, and dioxins, and who has bribed government officials to look the other way while illegally dumping 50 tons of mercury into one Alabama river, stating "We cannot afford to lose one dollar of business" in an internal memo (a leaked copy of which is readily available online) when this criminal polluting was exposed?

Monsanto does, however, have most of America's, and soon the world's, farmers completely dependent on them each planting season. And their wrath is swift and brutal against farmers even suspected of saving viable seeds. Even farmers with neighboring fields that have had these manipulated genes carried by the wind into their crops, which then cross into the genes of the new plants, are pressured with debilitating lawsuits to either go out-of-business or sign a contract and enter into the cycle of dependence and perversion.

> "We received over 44,000 pages from the FDA's own files and they revealed that the FDA has been lying to the world since 1992, if not before. But they continue to lie, they're still lying, they claim that there's an overwhelming consensus in the scientific community that genetically engineered foods are as safe as their conventionally produced counterparts and they claim that there has been sufficient data to back up this consensus. [Based on the FDA files] both of those claims are blatant lies." Steven Druker, lawyer for the Alliance for Bio-Integrity, who forced the FDA to declassify its internal files on GMOs.

Not surprisingly, by current FDA regulations, GMO foods aren't allowed to be labeled as such.

And back to the history… After WWII, famers began growing just one crop on a field, requiring more and more chemical support as the malnourished plants weakened. In fact, according to the National Resources Defense Council, pesticide use since the 1940's has gone up 10 times, but crop loss due to insects has doubled, and in the meantime the Environmental Protection Agency

> "This [genetic modification of food] is the largest biological experiment humanity has ever entered into." – Dr. Ignacio Chapel, Microbial Biologist, UC Berkeley

estimates that there are pesticide residuals in the tissues of every American. Our current agricultural system now relies on toxic fertilizers to keep the land producing food, as the precious topsoil that took thousands of years to develop is being washed away at an alarming rate. In fact, in the last 50 years, America has lost over 75% of its fertile soil. It takes 200 to 1000 years to create just one inch of topsoil; no modern technology can make it faster than that. Add to that the fact that the world's main food-producing countries like the US, China, India, Australia and Spain have or are about to reach their water resource limits, and you have an unsustainable agricultural system that can't go on this way much longer. Our dependence on chemical agriculture is a slippery slope. Like hard drugs, we need more and more to get the same affects. Something's gotta give, or soon there will be no seeds to sow, no topsoil to sow them in, no water to water them with, and certainly no way to protect them from the very gentlest of bugs. The only way out is for you and me to take responsibility for what we're putting into our bodies by growing it ourselves, not just voting for change but passionately and peacefully dissenting against an untenable system by planting or sprouting a seed and eating it with delight.

There is hope that the US will follow the example of Europe and Japan who, not beholden to the rebates, subsidies and political and collegiate contributions of the biotech industries, have outlawed all GM foods. A federal judge recently invalidated the patent on a gene that is known to cause breast cancer, owned by Myriad Genetics in association with the University of Utah, who charged exorbitant fees to research facilities using the gene to research breast cancer prevention. This ruling casts doubt on the motives of the companies holding gene patents and raises important ethical questions about the ability to patent life.

When Organic Isn't (It's too easy being green)

Obviously, it's better to buy organic food over conventional. It's a vote for the health of your family, your community, and the environment. Unfortunately, just choosing produce with an organic sticker isn't enough. I want to believe the strict and stringent guidelines for organic certification are followed by participating farms with enthusiasm and far-sighted wisdom, but I know too much about the funding the certifiers receive from the corporations whose goal it is to relax the laws for the betterment of their immediate profits. I hear too many stories from friends in the biz who are told to slap an organic sticker on every fifth crate of asparagus they're packing and call it a day. In 2005 in the UK, the wide-spread epidemic of fraudulently labeling meat as organic was a scandal that required a major government crackdown. The USDA, America's main certification agency who both makes the rules and sells organic certification, is heavily funded by Monsanto and other biotech conglomerates. It's companies like these that are fighting for (and paying for) more lenient rules within an increasingly lucrative market.

"If we're still dragging our feet in 2015, it really becomes almost impossible for the world to avert a degree of climate change that we simply will not be able to manage", John Holdren, Professor of Environmental Policy, Harvard University, and Director of the White House Office of Science

And it's working: a 2006 amendment created a list of 38 synthetic ingredients allowed in products that can still be called organic. This allowed Anheuser-Busch in 2007 to have its "Wild Hop Lager" certified organic even though it uses hops grown with chemical fertilizers and sprayed with pesticides. Advocacy groups fear that, since almost all organic foods are now sold through high-volume distribution channels like Target and Wal-Mart (the #1 retailer of organics in the US), the laws will change to support the massive producers, and the small farms that pioneered traditional methods of farming will be squeezed out. While they wait for the laws to change, Wal-mart continually pressures their suppliers to cut corners, if not to break laws outright. In 2007, Aurora Organic Dairy, Wal-mart's main supplier of organic dairy products, was found to be in violation of 14 organic regulations and would have lost their certification if it weren't for some unusual leniency on the part of the FDA. The truth is, the organic label can be bought, and is at best a vague indication of standards practiced in fields and facilities. On the other side of the coin, many small farms that operate according to organic guidelines and beyond aren't certified simply because they can't afford to be.

The simple truth is that big business cannot be trusted to do the right thing when millions or billions of dollars are at stake. Advertisers use buzz words like "fresh", "family-owned", "natural", "local" not in an effort to accurately describe, but to sell with little interest in the truth. It's gotten quite out of hand how advertisers can say absolutely anything and we, in our nose-to-the-grindstone haste to feel better, or check "good for us" off of our grocery lists, let ourselves be unthinkingly swayed.

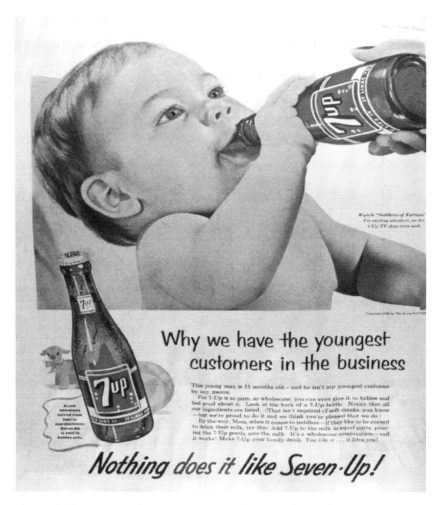

A would-be-funny-if-it-wasn't-so-sad example of deceptive 1955 advertising. Will we look back in 50 years with an equally ironic sophistication to Wendy's "You Know When It's Real" campaign, Nestle's "eco-shaped bottled water", and the other 98% of products world-wide tested in 2009 (by TerraChoice, who runs the Environmental Choice Program *for the Canadian government) whose labels were found to be misleadingly green-washed?*

Recently, the world's largest chain of natural food grocery stores, came under fire for misrepresenting the quality of their store-brand frozen organic vegetables. Turns out the "Organic California Blend", as well snap peas, spinach, and some others, were produced in China, and the store misleadingly and illegally put "USDA Organic" and "QAI" (Quality Assurance International) stamps on the foods, though neither organization had inspected the farms or food. They have, however, inspected hundreds of tons of food grown in China that were contaminated with chemicals and/or pathogens.

These stories shed light on the dark corners of the entire organic movement, which retailers like Whole Foods have ridden to massive financial success. Agriculture giants like Gerber's, Heinz, Dole, ConAgra and ADM, who have no problem poisoning workers, consumers, and the Earth with toxic chemical practices have jumped on the bandwagon with Earthy-friendly sounding organic subsidiaries. It takes little common sense to realize that massive conglomerates, who commonly purchase pesticides that have been outlawed in the US to use in their South American plants before shipping them back to American consumers (a bizarre loophole in the law), can't be trusted to make ethical decisions about my food when one simple lie can net them millions of dollars. Same goes for Target, recently sued for mislabeling natural products like rice milk and tofu as organic. Or that, though "organic farm" and "small family farm" are interchangeable in most consumer's minds,

> "If people let government decide what foods they eat, their bodies will soon be in as sorry a state as are the souls of those who live under tyranny." –Thomas Jefferson

almost all the organic food produced in America comes from California, where 5 or 6 huge operations dominate the market. 80% of US beef is produced by 4 companies[1]. The vast majority of the seeds planted by the world's farmers come from 4 conglomerations of companies. Food retailers are also on a consolidation track, and by some estimates, in the next ten years all of the retail food in the world will be controlled by 6 companies, only one of which will be American, Wal-Mart. Represent! This means that the selection and labeling of products on your grocery store shelves will be decided by a broker, potentially on another continent, based on what will return the largest profit.

If you sprout and grow your own food, you know it's organic. If you buy it, you only hope it is.

Home growing, sprouting, and fermenting is one of the best way to take responsibility for your own health and impact on the environment, and creates a haven from the conspiracy of corporate greed and consumer manipulation that plays like a Hollywood movie. The few seconds it takes to rinse our sprouts can re-establish our primordial bond to the land, the elements, and the moment-to-moment birth, maturation, and transformation of the pulsating forces of life around us. Even 100 glass and steel stories above the cement, life presses powerfully on. All this from an unused square-foot spot on a kitchen counter or closet shelf that would otherwise be collecting dust or worse, historical spoons from eBay.

---

[1] Nebraska and S Dakota passed constitutional amendments banning all farms not family-owned. Corporate agri-business didn't like that one bit, but state constitutions (and government in general) are in fact of, by, and for the people. Oops.

Collapse, the Future of Food

> "A living planet is a much more complex metaphor for deity than just a bigger father with a bigger fist. If an omniscient, all-powerful Dad ignores your prayers, it's taken personally. Hear only silence long enough, and you start wondering about his power. His fairness. His very existence. But if a world mother doesn't reply, Her excuse is simple. She never claimed conceited omnipotence. She has countless others clinging to her apron strings, including myriad species unable to speak for themselves. To Her elder offspring She says – 'Go raid the fridge. Go play outside. Go get a job. Or, better yet, lend me a hand. I have no time for idle whining.'" - David Brin, physicist and sci-fi writer

At a certain point, the rate of global extraction of crude petroleum products is reached, after which the rate of production enters a terminal decline. This is called "Peak Oil", and is another reason to become self-sustainable sooner than later. This is to say that there will come a day when our oil use will surpass the oil that's left in the ground, heading us towards the inevitable moment when there's no more left to power our cars and homes, our electric plants, to make our fertilizers and pesticides, or to run our farm equipment or the trucks that bring us the food.

Let's talk again about how commercial farms work. A field is fertilized, and all commercial fertilizers are made from ammonium nitrate, which is made from natural gas. This is sprayed onto the fields by an oil-powered machine. Another oil-powered machine ploughs, and another comes by and plants. The fields are irrigated with pumps powered by electricity, which comes from coal or, you guessed it: natural gas. But wait, there's more - oil-powered crop dusters spray oil-derived pesticides, once, twice, thrice. Then, when it's time to harvest, one oil-powered machine cuts, another loads, and another takes it to where it'll be processed by electric contraptions, and it's wrapped in plastic (made of oil) and trucked to a distribution center, then to the store. You can take it from there. There are 10 calories of hydrocarbon energy in every one calorie of food produced this way. Imagine that there's a finite amount of oil in the world and you'll soon realize that this would be a blatantly unsustainable system. Unfortunately, we'll soon be forced to see the end of this strategy.

Oil is made from the fossilized bodies of microorganisms, a process that takes millions of years. As of this writing, half of all the oil in the world has been used. The remaining half is of increasingly lower quality, and will require more and more energy to extract and refine. Oil is finite. Natural gas is finite, coal, uranium; all non-renewable energy sources are finite. There will be a peak for all of them. We're using, in a few decades, energy resources that took the planet millions of years to produce. Right now we are consuming 5 barrels of oil for every 1 barrel discovered.

> "Our agriculture system is almost wholly dependent on cheap fuel. Tremendous amounts of diesel fuel that are used in planting, and harvesting, and then, moving the stuff all these vast distances." - James Howard Kunstler *The Long Emergency*

For as long as I can remember, just about everyone I knew consumed like there was no tomorrow. My family threw away more food than many families in developing countries had. Now, when some of us in the West are just beginning to wake up to the realities of our wasteful lifestyle choices, those that have looked on hungrily for decades are starting to be able to enjoy the ease and luxury of modern life. In 1993, China had three quarters of a million cars on the road. At the start of 2004 they had 6 million, and in now (2010) they have 24 million. They idea behind a "developing" country is that one day they'll be able to consume like a first world country; they'll be able to live like the people in the movies. But this is clearly impossible. Even Americans in the near future won't be able to consume like Americans today.

Most of us have our heads in the sand about this to one degree or another; we know there's a problem looming but we're hoping that if we bring our own bags to the supermarket it'll go away. But the average person in a developed country can't really be blamed; with the demands of modern life, most people are happy with just a few minutes a day to relax and enjoy the life they're working so hard for. We've never had a peak in resources before and we have blinders on about it. Like statistics about climate change or overpopulation on a piece of paper, it's not an idea we can easily digest. We need new role models.

Peak Oil Pioneers

From 1950 to 1990, Cuba lived comfortably under Soviet communist care. Then, with little warning in 1991, the Soviet Union collapsed and Cuba's access to oil dropped to less than 25%. Everything changed in a matter of weeks. Suddenly, malnourished children, anemic pregnant women, and underweight babies became commonplace. The impact on food production and availability was disastrous. The average Cuban lost 20 pounds. Massive blackouts made refrigeration difficult so the little food that was available would often spoil. Cubans had to wait 3 to 4 hours for a bus to take them to school or work, and when it came it was often full, so they'd have to wait another 3 to 4 for the next one. And when they finally got to work, there might be no power, or no materials for them to do their jobs.

Then in 1992, the 30-year-old American embargo of Cuba was tightened. Before, companies were prohibited from doing business with both communist Cuba and the freedom-defending USA. Now, any ship even docking in a Cuban port was denied access to the US for 6 months afterwards. Almost overnight 750 million dollars worth of food and medical supplies pulled up anchor and sailed away. Then in 1996, the stranglehold was intensified. Cuba abruptly found itself with almost no access to foreign resources. The American dollar was worth 150 pesos, and the average daily salary was 20 pesos. Cubans was making about 4 dollars a month, so money was no longer a commodity that could be used to acquire the basics of life. A recently comfortable society abruptly found themselves cut-off, destitute, and hungry.

> "So we had now been like an experiment, with controlled conditions… Nothing, or very little… could get in from the outside, so everything had to happen from the inside. " - Roberto Perez, Cuban permaculturist and educator, from documentary film *The Power of Community*

Every aspect of Cuban life was affected, but none more potently than farming. Before the collapse, Cuba's agriculture was more industrialized than any other Latin American country. It used a massive amount of fossil fuel for fertilizer, pesticides, farm machinery, and transportation - 2 or 3 times more than any other Latin American country, and acre for acre it surpassed the US in fertilizer consumption. Their farms had high yields, but these were in huge single-crop operations like tobacco, sugarcane, and citrus, which were exported while the basics were imported. The system wasn't set up to feed the people.

So the people: doctors, engineers, and lawyers, started sowing seeds in open places, without knowing how, because they were starving and there was no end in sight. The older generation, those that remembered how to operate a plough, how to tell if soil was acidic or alkaline by rolling it around in their mouths, were suddenly a valuable resource. A movement to use every arable piece of local land for growing food began. Every park, front yard, school, and vacant lot in Havana became a garden or orchard because there was no gas to transport food. And because there were no fossil fuels to produce chemical pesticides and fertilizers, over the months and seasons the fledgling farmers learned to use natural, organic pesticides like bugs and companion plants. Organic fertilizers like manure and compost were all they had.

They found ways to replenish the depleted soil with cheap and available resources, and to do their farming without the use of machinery. They used worms to turn sandy, dead soil into lush and nutrient-rich fertile ground. They found that they could extend the growing season by putting a fiber mesh between the plants and the sun, which would also control pests and was easily replaceable during hurricane season. As time went on, Cuban urban farmers found infinite small solutions to improve their lives. They dealt with the myriad complex problems that come with a new kind of agronomy by trial and error, and thrived. Formerly larger farms were divided up and leased to citizens for free by the government and the 2.2 million residents of Havana fed themselves from these rooftop gardens, schoolyard nurseries, and small farms within a few kilometers from the city.

Today, urban gardens in small Cuban cities and towns are even more productive, providing 80-100% of the residents' food, and over 80% of Cuba's food production is organic. In the 1980's Cuba used 21,000 tons of chemical pesticides per year; now they use less than 1000. Good for the soil, good for the environment, good for the economy, and great for the people.

Now, apartment-dwellers with a well laid-out porch, rooftop, or patio garden improve their lives by both cutting back on their food spending and selling their produce or homemade products like wine. Cuba's 140,000 urban farmers aren't the poorest people in society, as they are in many countries, like America, where farmers are constantly forced to cut corners and take the chemical way out. They are among the highest-paid professionals in the country, and are even exporting their natural pesticides, fertilizers, and knowledge to other countries. This rewarding occupation attracts people from all walks of life who don't want to be dependent on others for their sustenance. They have the respect of their communities and dignity of working in what has become one of the noblest professions.

The country as a whole is enjoying a slew of fringe benefits as well. They developed bio-organic farming methods because at the time they had no other choice. But now, with less than 2% of the population of Latin America, Cuba has 11% of its scientists. At the start of the

> "It wasn't the *Exxon Valdez* captain's driving that caused the Alaskan oil spill. It was yours." - Greenpeace advertisement, 1990

"Special Period", the name for Cuba's quiet revolution starting with the collapse of the Soviet Union, Cuba had 3 universities. It now has about 50, with 7 in Havana alone. Cuba's urban farmers produce much more from the same amount of land as their corporate counterparts and many of them donate a portion of their crops to the elderly, day-care centers and schools, orphanages, and pregnant women. They do this for free with no government involvement, because they want their community to thrive. Small farmers form co-ops, if they wish, to buy in bulk and share machinery. In many cities in richer countries, we don't even *know* our neighbors.

 Cuba has roughly the same life expectancy and infant mortality rate as the US, though the average citizen uses 1/8th the energy and resources of the average American. They were once forced to be frugal with their energy consumption, using the sun to pre-heat cooking water, for example, but now it's a way of life. Why do most American homes have their hot-water heaters in cold closets and basements, requiring more fossil fuels to heat them, instead of outside in the sun? Sugar mills, which produce gas when the fibers are heated, are used as power plants, which now provide the country with 30% of its energy during harvest seasons. Increased walking and biking improved Cubans' fitness and drastically reduced diabetes (51% less deaths attributed to diabetes since before the Soviet collapse), heart disease (35% less), and strokes (20% less, and 18% less deaths overall). Cuba trains more doctors than they need, more than double the number of physician-to-citizen ration as America, and sends the surplus to developing countries around the world. Urban planners from all over the world study Havana as a model of livability. 85% of Cubans own their own home. The countryside, which has been called the last romantic place on earth, looks like a science-fiction comic book come alive with solar cells home-spun shacks, country school and rural hospitals. Cuba has reclaimed its health, its communities, its ethos, and its future.

The fact that Cuba is still looking for oil off their shores may surprise some. But unlike the vampires in developed countries that will start wars and enslave weaker nations for the life-blood of their consumer culture, they don't use what they find. If Cuba does hit upon the Texas tea, they sell it to wealthier countries at a premium, because they how to get by without it. We can wait until our own energy crisis to enact sustainable practices, and certainly the GOP government and their "head in the sand" policy-making will wait until it's too late. Or we can make changes now while we have some breathing room?

The concept of peak oil brings up another, much bigger question: what will happen to us when the greasy lubricant of our society becomes too expensive to be a viable means of energy?

Easter Island's Last Lumberjack

Easter Island is a remote dot of earth about 1500 miles off the coast of Chile. It's so small you can walk around the whole thing in a day. It's also the hauntingly desolate remains of a once-thriving civilization that numbered over 10,000 people.

When Easter Island was settled by 20 or 30 Polynesians halfway through the first millennium, it was a

> "There is a sufficiency in the world for man's need but not for man's greed." – Mahatma Gandhi

lush forest. The sweet potatoes and other crops the settlers brought with them thrived in the rich soil, living was easy, and the Easter Islanders found themselves with lots of free time. In about 1000 years, they swelled to a burgeoning society, and one of the most technologically advanced in the ancient world. Crops were protected by complex rock formations, and by some accounts every rock on the island was moved at least 3 or 4 times. The island's famous 600 stone statues, many of which were in sophisticated astronomical alignment, weighed tens of tons and were transported by human force, often for several miles over forested, hilly terrain. Each monument was laboriously carved from different color rock from quarries all over the island so the leaders of the clans could ask for favors from the Gods, and for a while it seemed to be working. But when European explorers reached the island in 1722, they found an arid grassland with less than 2000 malnourished people, many of whom had become cannibals, living in squalid reed huts and constant warfare. The explorers couldn't fathom how such a primitive society could be responsible for the socially and technologically advanced monuments, and because the island was now a barren prairie, the transportation of behemoth idols seemed impossible. When asked how the 20-foot-high stone gods had gotten there, the inhabitants, wholly disconnected from their history, replied simply, "They walked".

Actually, the statues were pushed along rolling roads made of the island's trees, chopped down in huge swathes to make way for the huge stone carvings and laid side-by-side through miles of forest. The trees, which provided shelter, canoes for fishing, and fuel, were so abundant at the time that they could be used without fear of running out. But as the population continued to swell, and more and more clans were formed with more leaders, all needed their own statues lest their dependants miss out on their slice of the divine benevolence pie and the ability to live as well as their neighbors. Competition for resources between clans grew fierce, and then someone, one day, cut down the last tree on the island. No more boats for fishing. No more fuel for heat, cooking, or transporting statues. The topsoil eroded at a breakneck pace and the gravely land couldn't hold in moisture or nutrients. Hundreds of great stone deities were abandoned, unfinished, in quarries around the islands. The gods were not happy. With no logs for buildings, people began living in caves and flimsy reed huts, fiercely protecting their meager assets. Cannibalism became a reasonable means of dealing with both enemies and hunger. Like the Romans, Byzantines, Vikings, and Mayans before them, the Easter Islanders didn't think total collapse happen to them, and lived recklessly until it did.

The pattern is clear. When civilizations over-consume, they cut off the legs of their own life-support systems and begin to fight each other over what little is left.

> "We never know the worth of water till the well is dry." - Thomas Fuller, *Gnomologia*, 1732

Then they either starve or leave. Our current problems are global: climate change, overpopulation, peak oil, genetically manipulated genes out-crossing into the DNA of the world's food supply; so there's nowhere to go, just like boatless Easter Islanders on a remote island in the middle of the Pacific. We can't abandon our planet and set off for a new Eden. We're here, and we have only two choices: cut down the last tree, or take an objective look at the dilemmas facing our species as a whole, and find another way to live.

A very early action of the Bush administration upon assuming office in 2001 was to lobby for the replacement of the chairman of the official United Nations Intergovernmental Panel on Climate Change (IPCC). This was done at the request of Exxon, who felt the sitting chairman, Dr. Watson, was too "aggressive" in pursuing action on the issue of global warming. As a result of actions taken by the administration, Dr. Watson was replaced ("at the request of the US") by the industry-friendly Dr. Rajendra Pachauri, hand-picked by the administration, and referred to by former vice-president Al Gore as the "let's drag our feet" candidate. Four years later, Dr. Pachauri issued the strongest warning yet in regard to global climate change, and a most urgent call for immediate action. His report stated that there is not a moment to lose, and added that we are risking the ability of the human race to survive. He called for "very deep" cuts in current pollution levels, stating that the point of no return was rapidly approaching.

> "The American way of life is non-negotiable" - Dick Cheney

Sometimes big change comes through a big effort. But more often, revolution is the result of very small actions repeated over time. For a while, maybe for several generations, the results of our efforts are almost unnoticeable, but then there comes a "tipping point" where the slow incremental change has completely reshaped society. It's like driving. Turn the wheel dramatically and you find yourself on the beginning of a different road, or in a ditch. But turn the wheel just 5 degrees, and for a while it seems like nothing's different. Then, after enough miles, the car is in a completely different place, a totally different course. This is the way to lasting change, to guaranteed metamorphosis. When someone wants a major turn-around in their health, for example, I always recommend making one small change a day. In a year, they'll have made 365 little improvements, which adds up to a big difference. And they'll have made new habits and the stamina to maintain them, encouraged by the changes they notice in their life, how they feel, etc. I encourage treating anything important as a marathon, not a sprint, and digging in for the long haul.

It's true that massive change is overdue: in the way we treat each other, our world, and ourselves. But I don't have the dynamite nor a flair for drama. Instead, I just make one improvement at a time, stabilize it, and then see where I'm at. I've gotten

> "Greater than the tread of mighty armies is *an idea whose time has come*." - Victor Hugo

excited and gung-ho about a lot of things in my life, but I've noticed that permanent and powerful transformation has come about from a sustained 5% turn of the wheel. If you're different, that's awesome, together I hope we can make something really magical happen.

Everyone but the Kitchen Sink: Modernization, McDonald's, and Hyper-Maturation

I'd like to make it clear that this book is for absolutely everyone. The ways of making and preparing food in here aren't just for already-organic urban yoga hipster families; they're for the low-income families that can't afford fresh vegetables, communities and aid-workers in developing countries, and the one-third of American kids that eat fast food every day.

Evolution is slow; it certainly can't keep up with the modernization of our diets. Our Paleolithic hunter-gatherer ancestors lived on hundreds of different wild plant sources, some meat (in the few climates where killing a creature that was running or fighting for its life was less effort than foraging for edible plants), and thereby guaranteed themselves a vast array of potent, living nutrients. Just to put it in perspective, of the food crops grown in 1900, 97% were extinct in 2000, just a hundred years later. And we're talking about the vast changes in lifestyle over the course of half a million years, while our basic biology has stayed the same. In the prehistoric world, starch, fat, and salt were rare commodities that our brains were programmed to seek out with the fervor of junkies. Now, they are available on every street corner in the developed world, and the fast food "restaurants" that offer them claim different characteristics and even different cultures, starch, fat, and salt are found in almost every case in the precise proportions that mirror the cravings imprinted in our very genes, with lab-concocted cocktails of smells pumped into the air to lure our Paleolithic minds in the door.

Ten thousand years ago (a time frame too short to cause many genetic changes, though one exception is the continued production of lactase, the milk enzyme, in about 25% of post-nursing humans), our ancestors went from a wild food diet totally free of grains to an agricultural lifestyle, in a move that author and UCLA Professor of Physiology Dr. Jared Diamond calls "The Worst Mistake in the History of the Human Race" in his essay of the same name. Our forefathers began growing not the crops that would protect the delicate balance of their health and longevity, but the ones that were the easiest to cultivate, harvest, and store: wheat, rice, and corn began providing the most calories to humanity. The average lifespan promptly dropped seven years[2].

It's no surprise that we're not cut out for the amount of starch, salt and particularly fat in our diet, as it's quickly

---

[2] Pia Bennike, *Paleopathology of Danish Skeletons* [Copenhagen: Almquist and Wiskell, 1985]; and N-G Gejvall, *Westerhu: Medeviel Populations and Church in the Light of Skeletal Remains* [Lund: Hakan Ohlssons Boktryckeri, 1960]

killing us; heart disease, diabetes, and cancer are all linked to a diet too high in these foods. McDonalds lost two CEOs in a single year to diet-related diseases (2004): heart attack and colon cancer[3]. The majority of Americans are on at least one prescription drug to treat type-2 diabetes, cholesterol, and high blood pressure, all of which are directly related to starch, fat, or salt.

Less lethal but just as alarming are the effects of diets high in trans- and saturated fats on children. The number of overweight children has tripled in the last three decades. Kid's menus at sit-down restaurants are usually much worse than the adults'. Our schools are "7-11's with books" (Yale diet expert Kelly Brownell). Shortened and less happy lives will be the obvious result, but there are more nefarious effects as well. Throughout most of our species' history, female sexual maturity was reached at 17 ½ to 18 years old. In 1900, the age had dropped to 15 ½ in developed countries, and now the average age that girls reach puberty is 11, while many girls mature sexually at 9 or 10. Many researchers originally believed this accelerating change was due to ingesting the hormones given to milk cows and meat animals to speed *their* maturation and growth, but recent studies show that the single greatest cause is the estrogenic effect of additional fat cells in the girls' bodies. Boys show a much less dramatic change, putting them far out of sync with the girls, with the exception of the most overweight boys whose puberty is actually slowed down by the increased estrogen in their body fat. One result of living out of harmony with our biology.

---

[3] I'd like to add, however, that the second CEO, Australian Charile Bell, perhaps prompted by the release of the documentary film Super Size Me criticizing the health of McDonald's food, led efforts to add healthier choices to the McDonald's menu and offered parents the option to substitute juice and apple slices for fries and soft drinks for their children. The "Supersize" option was also eliminated.

Cultural awareness of the alarming health problems has been steadily growing over the past decade. Ten years ago the public acknowledged that we were in the throes of a losing battle with obesity and heart disease. Two-thirds of Americans were overweight. Obesity-related illnesses killed a third of a million people every year, crippling millions, and costing our health care system almost a hundred billion dollars annually. Overwhelmingly, people singled out their excess weight as the thing they most disliked about their bodies.

In the past ten years, Americans have made a number of choices about their diet and health. The average America has eaten 50% *more* fast food meals and 5 more pounds of sugar per year. Hospital bills related to obesity have risen to $117 billion, and it's estimated that 8 out of 10 Americans are or will become overweight.

In 2004, the World Health Organization proposed dietary guidelines to reduce fat and sugar consumption. The US delegation, which represents the fattest nation in the world, protested these changes, on behalf of the food industry, as "scientifically unproven". While the WHO guidelines call on governments to reduce the unhealthy food advertising aimed at children and use fiscal incentives to limit the availability of junk food and amount of trans fats in the diet, the US Department of Health and Human Services responded that it would be best to use tactics like "better data and surveillance, and the promotion of sustainable strategies that focus on energy balance," hollow and meaningless expressions with just enough buzzwords to dupe the most foolish into thinking that something was being done.

Former senator Peter Fitzgerald noted that putting the USDA, whose first job it is to sell agricultural products, in charge of our dietary guidelines was like "putting a fox in charge of the hen house". The USDA subsidizes farmers to grow high-calorie, low nutrition crops for $19 billion annually, making white flour, corn syrup, hydrogenated margarine, and white rice cost sometimes less than nothing to produce. It becomes these foods that are the most heavily-advertised and make up the bulk of ingredients of fast food, junk food, and school lunches. And while the current administration is offering small subsidies to farms that convert to organic methods, an initiative spearheaded by Mrs. Obama (who is taking much of the ill-placed heat from farmers losing their hard-won handouts), still not a penny goes towards large-scale vegetable farming. I've gone into such detail in these last few paragraphs to illuminate the fact that the very government agencies we've put in place to protect our health and well-being can't be counted on to do that very thing. It is, once again, up to us to take responsibility for our own health.

But it's difficult to choose fresh food when $5 feeds a busy family at McDonald's. Fast and junk food are designed to maximize the cheapest ingredients, and grocery stores can rarely compete. Add to that the time it takes to shop for and prepare dinner and it becomes a daunting task for haggard parents. But an even less expensive meal, both in money and in medical bills, can be had with a deep breath, a few minutes' forethought, and the application of the methods in this book, in even less time than it takes to round up the kids and drive to the transfat pusher on the corner with a winning goatee and bowtie or cute red pigtails. While the dangers of not making a change in our families' diets could be their own encyclopedia, the benefits of doing so are simple: turning our children into vivacious young people with strong immune systems, increased focus and learning - the kids they were meant to be. It's my fervent desire that the mostly unoriginal ideas presented in these books will spread not only to the families that can most easily implement them, but to the ones that need them most.

Using the Brain for a Change

Changing Food Habits

I doubt that the previous section is enough to shock people into changing their diets. We all know what to do to be healthier: eat more vegetables and less crap, exercise. It's usually not the why nor the what that holds us up, but the how. Willpower or self-talk alone isn't enough to make lasting changes for most people, and just like the force that drives us to continue eating the ice cream our conscious minds know we've had enough of, the reason is our wiring.

The human brain is "an organ so complex we may never fully understand it", says Colin Blakemore, <u>British</u> neurobiologist. There are 100 billion nerve cells in the brain, with ten thousand times as many connections between them. On average, our brains make one million data transfers every second, for the entirety of our lifetimes. Recent studies have found brain cells previously thought to exist only inside our skulls are actually dispersed throughout our entire bodies, amplifying the previous number by orders of magnitude.

In addition to being the miraculous instrument of human achievement, according to David Linden, a professor of neuroscience at Johns Hopkins University the brain is a "cobbled-together mess… quirky, inefficient and bizarre ... a weird agglomeration of ad hoc solutions that have accumulated throughout millions of years of evolutionary history," he states in his book, "The Accidental Mind," from Harvard University Press. Interestingly, when new kingdoms of species evolved: reptiles to mammals, lower mammals to humans, the brain didn't actually evolve. The entire reptilian brain stayed almost as is, and a new brain was added on top. That means that we're all carrying around the brains of a flatworm, a snake and a primate right next to our advanced thinking capabilities.

The reptilian area of the brain governs habits and emotions and will always choose the easy route if left to its own, literally subconscious, devices. Specifically, the basal ganglia (BG) is a loosely grouped collection of nerve cells located deep within the reptilian part of each cerebral hemisphere. It's responsible for rage, fear, love, lust, contentment, and automatic behaviors like slamming on the brakes, smashing a vase against a wall in startling anger, or opening the fridge to grab the cheesecake before you even know you're doing it. The pre-frontal cortex (PFC) is the newest addition to the human brain, situated right behind the forehead and is in charge of the things that make us human: personality and executive functions: goal-setting, understanding consequences, and differentiating between conflicting thoughts to choose (hopefully) the most enlightened course of action. Basically, it's considered to be the conscious conductor in the orchestration of thoughts and actions in accordance with internal goals. The BG pushes for habitual behavior, while the PFC considers whether or not that deed is going to bring us what we want in the long run. An over-simplified example of this is the drug-addicted brain, which tells the owner in increasingly creative ways that more drugs are needed. We know as observers that the best course of action is to re-shape the desires of the BG by stopping the drug use and consequently changing the messages being sent to the PFC, but just like an addict's brain invents evidence to show that more drug use is the best course of action, within the individual an entirely different story is told.

An iguana or python doesn't respond to coaxing, cajoling, or bargaining; it changes its habits based on repetition, pure and simple. The ritualistic nature of this organ leaves no room for complex emotions (my apologies to the shirtless-under-their-leather-vests guys at the beach with their scaly loved ones.) The time it takes to change a habit depends on how ingrained it is. It's a simple formula. When a wagon wheel goes over the same road, in the same way, an ever-deepening rut results. If the wheel happens to find new ground, all it takes is a little push in the same old direction and the wheel teeters then returns to the rut. But push in a new direction everyday and the wheel will in no time make a new groove, soon becoming deeper than the first and the wheel will easily stay into it, propelling the cart effortlessly in a new direction. Absolutely any habit can change from a rut to a groove, given enough pushes. Research states that simple habits take 21 days to break, and while we're dealing with more complicated lifestyle changes, 3 weeks of daily action and at least the beginnings of changes are guaranteed. If it's a worthwhile goal, these incremental encouragements may, like signposts on the proverbial road, be all that's needed to propel you towards lasting change. It all starts with one action, today.

The pleasure mechanism in the human brain is *extremely* flexible. It will attach to whatever is introduced, whether unconsciously, like heroin or Big Macs, or consciously like whole living foods. We can quite literally re-engineer our evolution, rewire our brains. The brain of someone who has made a habit of a simple sprout salad with homemade vinaigrette will release just as much dopamine, the "pleasure chemical", as a steak and potatoes guy will get from his 20-oz rib eye. The satisfaction of improving our health and the self-esteem that results is enough to pull back the veil of denial that results in actions that destroy ourselves, other creatures, and the planet, and we will soon have a network of habits and beliefs that will make it easy for us to make better choices.

I know from personal experience. As I slowly started eating more and more whole, living, simple foods, I was surprised to find myself craving whole, living, simple foods. If you've never jonesed after raw baby spinach, it is a pretty wonderful feeling. Processed food started looking like wax fruit, (e.g. - not food), and non-organic food had an unmistakably flat and empty taste. When I travel, I try to sprout as much food as possible and I obviously lean towards authentic and clean cuisines, especially in places like Germany where GMOs are outlawed and almost all the food is grown with traditional organic methods. It's not always possible or polite to eat this way, however and after a month or two of bratwurst, potato salad, and strudel and the impulses coming from my BG have become quite distorted. It takes just a few meals to start affecting unconstructive change, and about 3-4 times as long to re-position positive habits in the BG. I don't know why negative transformation seems to have more pull than the other direction, but when I get back home I'm bolstered by the fact that the challenging choices I face will soon become effortless, and because of the nature of the basal ganglia-pre-frontal cortex connection, dramatic changes in behavior can make it even easier. Humans have the largest PFC of any animal. Let's put it to use for a better life now and a brighter future for the planet.

Transitioning to a Living Diet

When we're used to cooked food, we usually look for one thing out of our meals, besides the immediate taste sensations: a "feeling of fullness". Living foods nourish our bodies in a completely different, and much more thorough way. This become clear to me during a recent dinner I prepared for some friends and family where one person refused to eat the meal, worrying that they were sure they "wouldn't get filled up from it". That relation grabbed a sandwich from a nearby convenience store and scarfed the fistful of spongy white bread and deli meats while the rest of us enjoyed a living meal. Afterwards, I noticed the general ebullience of the family and the heavy, lethargic quality of that individual. Granted, their food choice may have been healthier if they hadn't had to scrounge for dinner after being ambushed by an alfalfa-wielding hippie, but it's an interesting dichotomy. The "fill your belly", "stick to your ribs" mentality is quite the opposite of being fed on a cellular level, really nourished down to the nerve, where the energy that used to go into digestion and assimilation are already in the food and don't need to be stolen from the body's other processes. It's a different kind of satiation with living food when you're used to heavy meats and caramelized starches, but in time you will adjust, if you choose to go that route.

Table 2: Seed/Nut Digestibility Chart

How	What	Why
Toasted	Starches (usually the main component) are caramelized and impossible to utilize. Most vitamins and minerals diminished or gone. Enzymes gone. Some oils are toxic.	Enzymes are destroyed over 108 degrees; most nutrients are destroyed at high temperatures. Heating some oils past 170 degrees creates free radicals and other toxins.1
Raw, right outta the bag	The most difficult to digest and assimilate; heating does destroy (denature the molecular bonds and render inert) some EI's.	Nutrients are in a dormant state and bound with EI's; these rob the body of its own enzymes and more effort than necessary is put into digestion, while less energy than possible is gotten out in nutrition. The living enzymes of the seed are dormant and unusable.
Soaked in	Easier to handle, but	Soaking starts the

water	not at peak nutrition.	germination process, breaking down the EI's so they can be rinsed away, but enzymes aren't fully activated, nor are nutrients levels substantially increased, but you're on the right track...
Fermented (in probiotic water, miso, or seed cheese, for example)	Partial probiotic pre-digestion makes protein, healthy fats, vitamins, minerals, and starches present in dormant seed more available.	Beneficial microorganisms go to work on the starches and long-chain proteins, turning them into more easily-digestible simple sugars and amino acids, and thereby taking some of the strain off of the human. Blending with probiotic water releases EI's which are removed by bacteria.
Sprouted	Nutrient levels are at their peak, enzymes	

	fully active. Provides the body with the building blocks of health and an abundance of energy with which to use them.	
Sprouted and Fermented	Bacteria make immunity-supporting compounds you can't get anywhere else. Peak nutrition and complex components broken down into easily-assimilable forms. The benefits of the seed's inherent nutrition and life force, the short-term benevolent action of friendly bacteria on the seed and the long-term advantages to the digestive system as probiotics settle in and prepare to convert everything that comes their way into a greater you.	Plus it tastes freaking awesome.

Sprouting: The "How?"

This is the simplest section of the book, and possibly the most important, because it's the easiest to get started doing and might have the most dramatic effect on your health. There are no microbial cultures to lure into your home with sweets, no artificial lighting to buy, nothing to build, plug in, or even measure, but the benefits of following these simple and straight-forward directions are many. "Sprouting" just means: getting a seed, nut, or grain wet, and keeping it wet, until it grows into a tiny plant. No farm needed, no garden, no dirt. Just some water and something to hold it in – that's it. But the benefits of sprouting are pretty monumental…

- Dramatically improved digestibility - *gives* energy to digestion instead of *taking* it away like most foods.
- Increased nutrition - vital nutrients increase, sometimes thousands of times.
- More food - the mass of the already inexpensive seed you're sprouting increases by a few to a few thousand times.
- Unlocks a world of fresh and vivid flavor, and all of this is available in the dead of winter, while travelling or anytime, with just a couple of days' to a weeks' notice.

…all for about 60 seconds of work a day. Sound worth it?

Hit the Ground Sprouting

Sunflowers are most definitely my favorite sprout, so let's start with those. They can be sprouted in less than a day with just a minute or two of effort. They're ridiculously nutritious: full of calcium and the co-factors needed to use it, just a quarter cup provides the RDA of skin-nourishing, cancer-fighting vitamin E, they're rich in healthy unsaturated fats and fiber, and are 33% protein (more on pg 153). They blend up smooth and their mellow nutty-flowery flavor makes them great for use in virtually any culinary application, from creamy seed milk and nut butter to soups, salads and dressings, desserts and snacks. I'm actually eating some as I write this, with diced golden delicious apples, coconut butter, cinnamon, vanilla and a little raw honey, though they're great just by themselves. Sunflower seeds with the shell on can also be grown in trays with or without dirt into sunflower "micro-lettuce", which is a delicious salad green.

To sprout sunflower seeds, we're going to soak them and drain them. In a glass, jar, bowl, or gumball machine put some hulled (no shell) sunflower seeds. Then cover the seeds with pure water, leaving a little room for the seeds to expand as they drink. Leave them soaking for about 6-8 hours (overnight is good), then dump them into a colander to drain the water, or use your hand to hold them in the glass while the water pours out, then dump them out onto a kitchen towel. We just want to make sure they're not sitting in water. Let them hang out for another 8 hours and you will notice the pointy end of the seed get pointier. This is the beginning of a root system emanating from the seed, and if you continued to rinse them, it would keep lengthening in a curious quest for nutrients. But we don't need to let it go any further and in fact they will start to get a little bitter after a couple of days' growth, as they enter the teenage stage between seed and plant.

That's it. You have in your paws: sunflower sprouts. In 16 hours the seed fats have converted to essential fatty acids, the enzymes have been activated, the carbohydrates have converted to simple sugars and the proteins to usable amino acids, the vitamin and mineral content has increased substantially, and the life force has increased deliciously. Yes, it is that easy. Bon appétit.

Any seed, grain, or nut can be sprouted (grains and nuts are also seeds), as long as it hasn't been cooked, toasted or sterilized in some way. The life's purpose of each sunflower seed is to grow into a big, beautiful sunflower. Each little peanut has the potential to germinate, mature, and reproduce itself into thousands of other peanuts. When you sprout, you make use of that naturally built-in power. There are four reasons sprouted is better than un-sprouted: nutrition, digestibility, quantity and enzymes – let's go into each of them in a little more detail.

Digestibility

Seeds are naturally protected by enzyme inhibitors, or EIs, which keep them from sprouting on top of the ground, or on your counter, or in a bag at the baseball stadium. I'd love to see some burly, body-painted Yankee fan reach into his bag of peanuts and find the green and tangled mass of a peanut shrub growing from his sack of salty snacks. EIs are what keep seeds in a dormant state, able to withstand the high heat of baking in the sun or sitting in a warehouse for 20 Arizona summers, and still able to grow into a vigorous plant when the opportunity presents itself. They also keep us from digesting the seeds very well, and in fact many nut allergies are exacerbated by the presence of these natural chemicals. So getting rid of EIs is very important and makes seeds much better for us. The good news is that nothing could be easier. It's as simple as soaking the seed for a while in water, which makes it think it's time to let down its guard and germinate, and the water will often become cloudy and bubbly - visual evidence that our food is transforming. After the EIs are soaked away, the seed can sprout freely, and all of its resources go into getting ready to shoot up into the sky. As a result, the nutrients become much more available to us. For example, mung beans, which you may have seen in Chinese food as "bean sprouts", have trace amounts of vitamin C normally, but a couple of days of sprouting and there's at least 600 times more. Just soaking seeds and grains before they're cooked will improve their nutritional value a lot, so if you're going to be cooking beans or quinoa or whatever, soak them overnight, drain the water, then cook them. You'll be pleasantly surprised at how this simple step will improve your food. But soaking is just a small step towards unlocking the full potential of a seed.

The simple process of sprouting will, by making digestion easier and more effective, increase energy, immunity, mental functioning, and well-being. When I say that something is more digestible than something else, I'm talking about two things: 1) that it requires less energy by your digestive system to process, leaving more energy for other things, like growing beautiful hair, detoxification, or choosing a great Halloween costume, and 2) that its nutrients are more plentiful and easier to get at. It's not some magical, "take my word for it" kind of thing, it should be obvious to all by having more energy and feeling lighter and happier immediately after eating, no gas, eliminating better, waking up feeling refreshed, and myriad other benefits in the slightly longer run. Everyone is different, and while it's fun and delicious for everyone to play with making nut cheese and yogurt, some may not be able to digest cashews, for example, any other way than soaking and/or sprouting and/or fermenting them. It's a good idea to eat nuts and seeds as far down the Seed/Nut Digestibility Chart on page 69 as possible, but it takes diff'rent strokes. If you're one of these "stomach of iron" people, you may need to plan ahead a little less than the rest of us, though in the long run it sems to all even out: people that overtax their healthy genes or strong consitituations tend to have more problems in those areas as they age than those those who learn healthy habits earlier in life.

Enzyme Inhibitors

Seeds and nuts contain something called "enzyme inhibitors", or EI's, which prevent them from sprouting somewhere that's not a good place to become a plant, like when a seed drops from a tree onto the surface of a rock. Enzyme inhibitors inhibit our enzymes, too, the things in us that not only break up food and grab its nutrients but also heal cuts, get rid of damaged cells, repair and rebuild skin, bones, and organs. EI's keep your own cleansing and healing power under lock and key. The key is water.

One enzyme inhibitor, phytic acid, binds with B vitamins, calcium, zinc, copper, and iron in the digestive tract and can lead to a deficiency in these nutrients. In the recent past, all grains were soaked and/or fermented to improve their nutrition and digestibility. More recently, store-bought oats had soaking instructions printed on the label, but in an apparent effort to be attractive in a world of ever-decreasing attention spans that vital information was replaced with mazes and facts about leopards, leading to a measurable increase in nutrient deficiencies and its symptoms like bone loss and ADD. See a connection? Or were you thinking about leopards lol?

When nuts and seeds are fermented into cheese or yogurt, bacteria go to work on the starches and long-chain proteins, turning them into more easily-digestible simple sugars and amino acids and thereby taking some of the strain off the human. When they're both sprouted *and* fermented it's like your digestive system is in a hammock in Mexico, simultaneously getting a week's worth of office work done every hour… it just doesn't get any better than that.

Enzymes

These are the catalysts of life, the tiny biochemical machines that make it all happen. From blinking an eye to healing a cut, from growing hair to breaking down food into usable parts, enzymes are the superstars. There are three types of enzymes: food, digestive, and metabolic. The first, food enzymes, is the only one we can take in[4]. We have to make digestive enzymes, mostly in the saliva, stomach, pancreas, and other places in the body. Metabolic enzymes are also produced in the body, and the term applies to a wide range of substances that carry out a variety of functions, like cleansing toxins and rebuilding cells, the two basic functions of life. As we age, our ability to produce metabolic enzymes diminishes, and the elderly are increasingly deficient, leading to both the aging process and the rapid deterioration of health after a certain age.

The good news is that these little critters are interchangeable, so if you have leftover enzymes from your

---

[4] if you don't count eating pig pancreas and gleaning some of their digestive enzymes, which is what most bottled enzymes are.

lunch, the surplus will get to work on purifying and rejuvenating your body. The *great* news is that there is an abundance of food enzymes in all raw produce, and especially sprouts. Freshly sprouted seeds, wiggling their little tails and all ready to shoot up into a full-grown plant, have many times more enzymes than are needed to digest them, so eating sprouted seeds, nuts, and grains will not only take the burden of enzyme production *off* of your body, it will also *supply* lots of extra horsepower to rebuilding your age- or stress-weakened systems, supporting your immunity, and making you happy. Eat a meal full of food enzymes, and your organs need to make less or no digestive enzymes. Free nutrients = happy organs. Extra food enzymes convert to metabolic enzymes; free energy for life = happy you.

Joy, enthusiasm, contentment and deep peace are the default emotions of our physiology. Take away the things keeping us un-centered and happiness is ours, consistently and continually. The *really really* great news is that our bodies are so intelligent, that all we need to give them is the extra enzymes and it knows exactly where to apply that energy for our ultimate long-term well-being. So studying how this particular nutrient is for this or that purpose, this food that's supposed to have this certain effect, these things are important, especially if you're combating a specific symptom or ailment, but it's far more important to supply the stimulating tonic of living enzymes to the body and let ancient cellular wisdom figure out what's best done with it.

Quantity

On top of sprouted seeds being the healthiest food on the planet that can be eaten in quantity, they're also cheap nutrition. A couple of bucks per pound for the highest quality organic heirloom lentil seeds – sprout them and the price per pound goes down to 25 cents. Plant a few of these sprouts, grow them into plants and harvet their seeds, and you have real wealth, all from a few lentils or whatever. The same seeds that might have been cooked and eaten in one bite become "seed factories", and can sustain countless people and is a much more effective means of feeding people. Sprouting is an utterly sustainable system of growing food that will not only save you money, but can also provide under-nourished, impoverished populations with an abundance of fresh, revitalizing nourishment.

Sprouting in a nutshell

Sprouting a seed, nut, or grain just means that we wake it up so that it starts the process that ends in a plant. Whether it's a tree, shrub, bush, or grass doesn't matter, because it's not going to make it that far (sorry). All we care about is the prodigious nutritional force being awoken in the thing while the tiny root or stalk is starting to grow out. Anything that's sprout-able is actually a seed or part of one; it has the ability to grow into the entire plant. So we'll call them seeds from now on, whether they're rightly or wrongly called nuts, like almonds, pistachios, or peanuts (which are actually more closely related to peas, and are the underground-growing fruits of the plant. I'm just sayin'), grains like wheat, rye, or quinoa, or beans like pinto, adzuki, or garbanzos. All of these will sprout in exactly the same way. Some very slight modification in techniques and growing times will bring out the best in the different seeds, but the fundamental process is the same.

Here it is:

The Soak: submerge the seeds in clean water overnight (8 hours or so), and then drain them.

The Twice-A-Day Rinse: keep 'em slightly damp and let air get to them for a day or few.

Then… that's it. Nature has made it easy for us to enjoy this super-fresh, vibrantly living and nutrient-packed food. Now let's look at these steps in a little more detail.

Soaking a seed is the big wake-up call it needs to begin germination. Seeds that are sitting on the ground, or the supermarket shelves, are in a state of dormancy or hibernation. They wouldn't want to start sprouting yet, because their chances of growing into a healthy plant wouldn't be very good. They need to be underground, for starters, and have access to plenty of fresh water and nutrients. So unless they get flooded with water, all their nutrients are going to stay locked up. So while water is the key, the lock is the enzyme inhibitors. The nutritional effects of these biochemical padlocks have been discussed, but now you know the botanical reason these exist, the reason they evolved in the first place. Soaking tricks the seed into thinking it's in the ideal conditions to wake up and come back to life.

Clean, but don't get crazy…

The purity of the water is, as you can imagine, pretty important. The cleaner the water the more enzyme inhibitors are removed, which you can sometimes see as a brown foam on the surface as they're pulled out of the seed. During the soaking, the seeds also begin to take in water and minerals to fuel the sprouting process, so for seeds with a lot of EIs, changing the water, as needed, will ensure that the future little plants have the best molecular building blocks possible for their healthy growth. There are vastly different opinions on the actual type of water that's best for sprouting, whether distilled, reverse osmosis, filtered, tap, etc, but in classic kitchen sink farmer tradition, the simplest is usually the best.

Using distilled water, that is – water that's been removed from any impurities by turning it into steam, then collecting the pure H20, by some accounts is actually too clean. Because nature strives for balance, it may actually pull nutrients *out* of whatever it's in contact with, whether a helpless little sprout, or you. Yes, distilled water will extract minerals from your body, particularly your teeth, like microscopic vacuums. Filtered water like reverse osmosis is best for drinking, but the minerals that filtration removes, that are too concentrated for human bodies, are actually good for plants. It works like this: minerals in the soil (tiny rocks in this case) are drawn up the roots of a plant and utilized for growth, fruiting, seeding, etc. Meanwhile, the plant is converting the minerals into forms that animals and humans can use (called chelating, or organically-binding minerals). These chelated minerals eventually return to the soil, whether through compost, manure, or the bodies of the animals who ate them. Then, soil bacteria digest these organically-bound minerals and break the bonds that make them accessible to us, turning them back into little rocks, when they can again be used by new plants. Pretty cool system. The short answer is: we don't use minerals the same way as plants, so go ahead and use tap water with the chlorine (which kills everything) removed[5].

With the exception of chlorine and its relations, those pesky minerals that your drinking water should be without are genrally good for your sprouts. A whole-house chlorine filter is best, filtering your sink water is good, but the cheapest and simplest method is to fill a jar or pot with tap water then let it sit. In about 24 hours, all the chlorine (a gas that's lighter than air) will have "floated" out. The water can then be put into a bottle for future use and another "batch" started. It's much easier to be able to fill soak jars and rinse sprouts from the sink as opposed to a jar or bottle of water, but you do what you have to do. I do my sprouting in the shower, because it's a nice humid area with good air flow and low light, but mostly

> All living matter (on this planet, at least) is based on the element carbon. Most people would assume that the increasing carbon in a growing tree comes from the soil, but in fact in comes from the air – carbon dioxide, or $CO2$, is breathed in by the plant, the $O2$ is split off and the C, carbon, sticks around to make more tree. Another reason free access to fresh air is important for your sprouts to grow up big and juicy.

---

[5] More on how to do that in a bit. The first step is to start getting sprouts into you asap. Fine-tuning production and culinary details come after, and maybe go on forever, so don't get stuck in the trap of thinking you need to know everything before you do anything. The seed knows. Just let it do its thing. Start today.

because I don't have room anywhere else. I have a corner shower caddy that holds my jars and bags, but the key is my hand-held chlorine-filtering shower head. I can easily bring in my trays of grasses and spray everything twice a day. The most work in this method is finding a place to put everything when I actually take a shower, so I try to keep that to a minimum. Just kidding, but if someone doesn't eat things that putrefy in the body like meat and dairy products, junk food, and white sugar and the diet is full of fresh, cleansing green foods, there's no such thing as body odor, even after a week of manual labor or camping.[6]

Air Supply

Like us, sprouts need to breathe. We both take in nutrients and expel wastes through respiration, so good air circulation is key. It's also important for plants for another reason: unfriendly microorganisms thrive in stagnant conditions. This could be still water in a puddle after a rain, our intestines clogged with slow-moving red meat and dairy, or a jar of wet alfalfa sprouts without proper drainage and air flow. In all of these conditions, tough and resourceful microbes - ones we haven't formed a mutually-beneficial relationship with - will move in and there goes the neighborhood. It's an interesting fact that, almost exclusively, "good", or probiotic bacteria, those that live in our digestive system and benefit us in countless ways (see Kitchen Sink Farming Volume 2: Fermenting), thrive in the presence of oxygen, or aerobically, and the "bad" bacteria, the disease- and poor digestion-causing ones are weakened or killed by oxygen (anaerobic). Oxygen-loving

---

[6] Other communities, like mine (Portland, Oregon) use chemicals other than chlorine (chloramine here) for disinfectant, which may not evaporate in the same way as chlorine.

microorganisms are the ones that ferment our many brews and cultures, and excellent health seems to have been made readily available to us by the universal principals of organic chemistry. The perfection of our relationship with aerobic and anaerobic bacteria (along with the profile of available enzymes in living foods being the exact ones we need to digest them) is one of the clearest signs I know of that there's an intelligence and benevolence behind creation. Anyways, we can avoid the infestation of "bad" bacteria – those that will rot our sprouts - by making sure our plants have adequate air flow and good drainage. We can further help oxygenate our crops with the generous use of hydrogen peroxide – an atom of oxygen loosely carried around by water. More about hydrogen peroxide in Kitchen Sink Farming Volume 2: Fermenting Sprouting Methods.

There are a few different ways to sprout seeds, and if you become a virtuoso you may eventually start using them all, as you find this nut is best sprouted this way, and this grain another. For now, though it doesn't get much easier than the vague description above, the following list goes from cheapest to easiest. In true kitchen sink farmer fashion, I recommend you start at the beginning and go down the list until you're comfortable with the time/money ratio.

Remember, each of these techniques does basically the same thing: soak and germinate the seeds, then rinse them periodically to keep them moist and clean off any toxins that may have come to the surface. They vary in ease and application. For example, if you have lots of places to hang bags and not much counter space, you may gravitate toward the bag method. If you have a huge dish draining area and no other room, the jar method is for you. If you need to produce a ridiculous amount of sprouts for a school, for example, and have only the floor in the corner of a room (and power, and are under-budget from the last tax levies), go automatic.

The Jar Method

Get some half gallon canning jars (mason, ball, or some lovely antique ones with colored glass), with 2-part lids, and some porous material that won't corrode or decompose. My favorite is fiberglass window screen, cut into squares plenty big enough, though panty hose or a piece of coarse natural fabric may work too. Take off the lid, put the screen over top the jar, then screw down just the ring part of the lid. Ya got yerself a sprouter, partner.

There are many free alternatives if you need to save cash, or you're the type to serve a loaf of delicious sprouted bread with the question, "Know how much that cost me? Nuthin'. Sprouted the wheat in my sock, ground it with my boot heel and baked it on the manifold of my truck." If so, I'd be proud to be your guest. However, these big jars are very cheap (around a buck each) and are super convenient for a great many things. In fact, I have about a dozen half gallon and a dozen quart mason jars, and use them for everything: drinking and transporting water (there *are* other options than ocean-polluting, land-fill-clogging, sometimes toxic-BPA-containing, not-really-recycling, plastic water bottles), food and bulk grain storage, fermenting, microwaving water to heat and/or sterilize it, and of course sprouting. The quart sized jars are even cheaper, and are available with normal and wide mouths. The wide mouths are the same size as the half gallon mouths, if you choose these you'll only have one size lid in your kitchen. Plus, you may be able to reach your hand in to clean them or pull stuff out. Very convenient.

Note: If you'll be storing prepared food or dry grains, nuts, or fruit in your canning jars (and why wouldn't you?), I recommend a "Pump N Seal", available online for less than $30. Just as you may have guessed, this device allows you to remove the air from your jar, keeping it fresh for longer. If you've been lucky enough to find fresh grains, flours, and nuts, vacuum-sealing them will help preserve their delicate oils, nutrients and flavors. In fact, most flours purchased from the store, whether organic or not, are already rancid, as grains that are milled no longer have the protection of the bran and germ, and the precious oils and oil-soluble vitamins like A and E are lost. Unfortunately, spoiled flour doesn't smell or taste any different, but has a profound effect on nutrition and digestibility. In fact, this rancidity is a common perpetrator in the indigestibility that then is misdiagnosed as a wheat allergy. Grinding flours at home is the best (and cheapest – surprise!) way to preserve their nutrition and taste.

The Bag Method

A few companies, such as Pure Joy Planet and Sproutman sell drawstring sacks that are great for allowing an abundance of oxygen to your teeming progeny. But mesh produce bags work just as well (except on the tiny seeds like amaranth) and cost about $1/10^{th}$ as much. They're also convenient for storing onions and garlic, and are helpful when soaking seeds with shells, which like to float. Put them first in the bag, then in a bowl or jar full of water, and weight them down with a clean rock or other heavy thing. Same with making sauerkraut and other fermentations, when you want to keep everything submerged under the protective surface of salt water. They can also be used to strain nut milks or "blender juice"; throw a bunch of veggies in your high-speed blender with some water and pour the resulting sludge into a sprout bag over a bowl or wide-mouthed glass. Squeeze out the liquid and you have a pulp-free juice, and though the left over pulp will be wetter than if you'd used a top-of-the-line juicer, I think it's worth saving $400 on a juicer, the room in my kitchen, and it's *much* easier to clean. Just dump the pulp out, turn the bag inside out, slide a hand in like a mitten and proceed to wash your hands. The pulp, just as if it came from a juicer, can add dietary fiber to recipes or be fantastic compost or worm food (see Kitchen Sink Farming Volume 3: Growing for more on vermiculture, worm farming). Sprout bags can also be used as tea bags, saving about 90%, by buying loose tea instead of bagged and measuring it into the bag. A very handy, space-saving, and durable piece of kitchen equipment.

A resourceful soul can find a yard of nylon or hemp and sew them up themselves. Or, lay out a square of material, put the seeds in the middle, bunch up the edges and secure it with a rubber band. I also don't see what would stop someone from using nylon panty hose. Or just hold your sprouting seeds in your hand, sit in a field for a few days, and *really* connect with the lifecycle. Not really, but free options abound. Whatever you use, the bag shape lets in air from all directions and limits mold growth, a definite advantage over the jar method. They're also a snap to rinse, especially if you have a chlorine-filtering, hand held sink sprayer or shower head. I hang my bags from a shower caddy, and in less than 5 seconds I've sprayed pounds of food in several mesh bags.

The Basket Method

This system is best for sprouting leafy greens, such as alfalfa, clover, broccoli, and onion. The process is scientifically the same, of course, that is: soaking the seeds and then keeping them moist and breathing, but the basket gives the plants' roots something to grab onto, and they grow straight up, looking for light with their gracefully unfurling green leaflets. Because of the open top of a basket, more chlorophyll can develop than if you were to sprout these tiny seeds as a jumbled mass in a bag or jar. The square plastic boxes of sprouts that you find in the grocery store (what most people associate with the term "sprouts") are grown this way, in the boxes.

There is a cheap and an even cheaper method to grow delicious alfalfa, wild-tasting clover, vegetal broccoli and spicy radish. The first is to buy a basket or vertical sprouter, usually around $30 and consisting of a few baskets made of plastic with many tiny holes in the bottom for drainage and footholds for roots, and covers/soaking containers. Put a thin layer of seeds on the bottom of the basket and submerge it in the dish full of water. When they're done soaking, lift the basket out, dump the water, flip the dish over and it's now a drain board for the basket. Gently rinse a couple of times a day, making sure not to dislodge the sprouts and their delicate grasp on the textured surface, and in a few days you'll have tall and slender plants, opening pairs of leaves to the sun. You'll want to keep them covered and out of the light for the first couple of days (the soaking dish inverted on top works), then give them time in the sun or artificial light so they'll develop chlorophyll and turn green.

The cheaper method is to use circular natural-fiber baskets and large bowls. Make sure the baskets have a tight enough weave that your little seeds don't fall through, and are untreated. These baskets won't last as long as plastic ones, but in my local Chinatown they can be had for less than a dollar each. You can also use the bamboo steamer baskets that every kitchen seems to have hiding in the back of a cabinet.

Robo-Sprouting (the Automatic Sprouter), for negligent parents

Automatic sprouters are usually large, expensive appliances that make sprouting slightly easier by doing the rinsing for you. When I first looked into them, I expected to find a tube to hook up to a water source and another to run to a drain so I could turn it on and come back a week later to perfect sprouts, but thus far that important feature seems unavailable. The machine still needs to be drained of the used water and refilled by hand daily, which saves a 30-60 second rinse per day. Worth a couple hundred bucks? Not to me it isn't.

There is one product, however, the Easy Green Automatic Sprouter, which is a fairly simple little machine that both sprays the sprouts and drains into a tube, run wherever you like. It saves having to drain the machine by hand which, in my opinion, justifies not doing the whole thing oneself. They're also pretty cheap at $175 and have room for quite a lot of sprouts - about 2 square feet – and also do wheatgrass, so the price could be justified when you're eating all those sprouts you might not otherwise have time to grow. I got mine on ebay for around $90.

Specialty Sprouts

The Clay Method

An exceptionally easy, albeit specialty, sprouting method. The (don't get turned off by the name) "mucilages" (flax, chia, psyllium, and some mustard seeds, to list some of my favorites) are by far the lowest-maintenance sprouts, and some of the most rewarding. These seeds are protected by not just a shell (insoluble fiber), but also by a slippery gel when wet (soluble fiber) which keeps them hydrated, nourished, and oxygenated, like the albumen of an egg does a baby chick. This means that if you try to sprout them using a jar or bag you'll end up with a slimey mess, but if you just cover them with water in a bowl, they'll sprout beautifully. Make sure to put in plenty of water, as they soak up 2-4 times their size. Mucilaginous seeds can also be grown into leafy nano-greens with similar ease – sprinkle a layer onto the bottom of a sterilized, unglazed clay saucer (the kind kept under houseplant pots) and cover them with plenty of water. Keep them covered with water over the next week, put them in the sun when leaves develop, and you'll soon have tall green sprouts. Pull them up by the roots if you can (which will have attached quite securely to the clay) to get all the benefits of the fiber and essential fatty acidss. An even easier way to do this is float the tray on top of a bowl filled with water. The porous clay will soak up the water in just the right amount to keep the sprouts hydrated. Neat trick.

Bean-Sprouting

Thick, crunchy bean sprouts are common in Asian cuisines, and require a little pressure to take their distinctive shape. Sprout mung or adzuki beans with the bag method and adding a little twist: between rinsings put the sprouting bag in a colander with a weighed bowl on top of it. A rock or full jar with the lid screwed on will work fine. Keep them in a dark place, and in 3 or 4 days you'll have long, fat sprouts to use in salads with an umeboshi-ginger-wasabi dressing, or soy-sauce marinated eggplant sandwiches.

The Dirt on Grass - Tray Sprouting

Some sprouts have more to offer when they're given the chance at a longer life cycle. So far we've been taking sprouts from embyo (seeds) to infancy (small sprouts) and sometimes, in the case of leafy green sprouts, early childhood. "Planting" the baby sprouts and letting them grow into teen grasses and micro-lettuces is a whole new world of nutrition, life force, and culinary application, and requires a slightly larger skill-set. In the section on growing grasses, such as wheatgrass and sunflower greens, we'll be spreading sprouted seeds onto a thin layer of soil or a fabric-like growing medium, or sometimes nothing at all, as the roots of some seeds will act as their own support structure. By continuing twice-daily rinsings (now called "watering"), you'll have tray-bound fields of 4-8 inch plants that you'll harvest with a serrated knife and eat with a smile. Wheatgrass juice is one of the healthiest and most cleansing foods on the planet, and a salad made of home-grown sunflower greens, piquant mizuna nano-greens, mustard micro-greens, or baby oak leaf lettuce, is a crisp and delicious treat. A tray of greens is also a portable oxygen factory, a handy thing to have in an urban setting. At bedtime, I carry a flat of wheatgrass to my bed like it's a teddy bear. Tray growing is covered thoroughly in Kitchen Sink Farming Volume 3: Growing.

Check out Apendix A: The Wide World of Sprouts - Sprouting Seeds, pg 93 - pg 157, for detailed information about most seeds appropriate for sprouting. Flip through, pick some that sound familiar or fun and get started!

Grid-Iron Chef – The Moveable Farm

Eating well while travelling is surprisingly easy as the forces of nature are the same everywhere on earth. We can employ the natural laws of germination and sprouting anywhere on the seeds we find, buy, or bring to supplement the local cuisine. In places where food is expensive, sprouting your own meals can be a fantastic way to save some green while feeling a lot better than a $25 crepe would make you feel. Your friends will certainly make fun, but when you leave their exhausted selves in a park while you detour to new sights a few times, they'll magically change their tune and start getting inquisitive about the jumble of green hanging in the hotel or host's bathroom, especially as their money exits their wallets and purses as if it had wings.

If you're staying put in one place for a few days and have an adequate supply of water, sprouting is a no-brainer. Bring a few sprout bags and doubled plastic bags full of your favorite seeds on your trip; then soak your seeds in the sprouting bag in a sink or a bowl and then hang it up over one of those or in the shower. The routine of rinsing sprouts twice a day can be disrupted by the stresses and excitements of travel; I do it when I wake up and go to bed just like at home, as consistently as is convenient. If you're growing sprouts that can develop chlorophyll hang them in a sunny window, if possible, when they're ready to green up. The leafy green clover, radish, and alfalfa are among my favorites to grow when away from home because they increase in size a lot and I have to pack less seeds for the same amount of food. They can be eaten at any stage of sprouting for a week and a half or more, and their extra enzymes help with the digestion of new and unusual foods.

I also rock sunflower seeds, of course, because of their quick turn around, high protein and incredible nutrition, as well as for my daily flax.

> "Travel is fatal to prejudice, bigotry, and narrow-mindedness" – Mark Twain

If you're backpacking, sleeping on trains, or otherwise nomadic, you'll have to put a little more thought into it. Fill sprouting bags with seeds inside a Ziploc gallon bag and fill it with water from bottles or, when necessary, sinks or drinking fountains. Then seal the plastic bag, put it inside of another one in case of a leak, and put the whole thing in with your dirty laundry as a last line of defense against gnarly enzyme-inhibitor water. Long flights are the perfect time to start sprouts, when you're already through security you can start them in the airport bathroom sink while waiting for your plane, then drain and rinse them when you land 6-10 hours later. I like to start with sunflower sprouts because they're quick and full of protein. Then I get a few-day mix of peas, lentils, and some flavoring herb seeds going as well as a leafy mix, both of which I rinse and drain for a week, snacking on them the whole time. A mix of fennel, fenugreek, and cardamom are a great after-restaurant supplement, aiding digestion in a variation of the Indian tradition. As much as I love quinoa, needing to be rinsed more than other sprouts means that it may not be the best choice for travelling, when clean water might be scarce or expensive.

Even grasses can be enjoyed on the road for those with no problem with glutens: germinate and sprout a combination of kamut, rye, barley, or your favorite grass grains in a sprout bag, and instead of planting them in soil, soak the whole mess for 10-20 minutes, two or three times a day in a bowl filled with fertilizer water, in a kind of manual hydroponic system. Fertilizers are diluted with water anywhere from 100 – 700 times, so a couple of ounces of concentrate can last for months, especially if the water is re-used a few times. As explained in Kitchen Sink Farming Volume 3: Growing, soil has two purposes: to hold roots and supply nutrients (including moisture and oxygen), so as the air-bound roots of your grains matte together, all that's really needed is the nutrients. The grasses will grow up towards the top of the bag as it hangs, but won't be accessible to scissors like when they're grown in a tray. Instead, pull an entire chunk of root, seed, and grass off the mass and blend it with water if you have the capability, or just take bites and chew it up. The sweet-sticky grain will mask the intensely nutritive flavor of the grass. The residual fertilizer, if you're using the recommendation of kelp or ocean-based, is perfectly edible. There will be gluten in wheat seeds, whereas there is none in the grass, so if you're sensitive be aware of that.

With the new climates, water sources, foods, and "experiences" you'll be enjoying on your journeys (I pretty much mean drinking), bringing probiotics along with you is also a good idea. Kefir and kombucha can be blended with berries or citrus and sprouted

> "The world is a book and those who do not travel read only one page." – St. Augustine

hemp, sunflower, flax and oats, and dehydrated at 108° in leathers, cookies, bars and wraps, and in their dry state take up very little room in your pack. It's actually quite feasible to carry a month's worth of home-grown friendly bacteria in a quart-size Ziploc. With a little bit of planning you can easily enjoy the best food in the world, wherever in the world you are.

Probiotic water (Kitchen Sink Farming Volume 2: Fermenting) can be made on the go as well, sprouting your grain of choice then fermenting whenever you're stopped. Try fermenting in a nalgene wide-mouthed bottle, using a sprouting bag for a breathable cover. Screw the lid on when you're on the move, and take it off when you stop for the night or several hours. Your fermentation will continue whenever there's oxygen, supplying your immune system with vitality-boosting local wild yeasts, kind of like getting vouched for in the microbial community and enjoying VIP status wherever you go.

Growing for Your Pet

Did you ever notice that dog food sits for months or years on unrefrigerated shelves, and it doesn't go bad? Bacteria, with their incredibly resourceful digestion that can literally utilize cyanide for food, want no part of dry pet food. How well do you think your pets will be able to break it down and extract its nutrition for a vibrant life? And for that matter, how different is it from ancient bagged gas-station snacks covered in an orange powder so virulent it can permanently stain clothes? Any and all of the methods in this book are applicable to your pets as well as yourself. Sprinkle sprouts on your cats' wet food. Make dog biscuits by skipping the sweetener in a raw cookie and drying it until it's hard. Sprouted whole hemp seeds are a super food for your parrot.

I'm toying with dehydrating Kombucha SCOBYs as dog chews ("SCOBY Snacks" – credit my best friend from childhood Buell Davidson), the dogs I've experimented on didn't seem to enjoy the unflavored chews (kind of vinegary. Yes, I chew them, too) but did carry them around for a while. I'm considering marinating in peanut butter or another canine favorite, and supplementing the chew with EFAs like sprouted flax seed.

> "All animals except for man know that the principal business of life is to enjoy it." – Samuel Butler

Appendix A: The Wide World of Sprouts - Sprouting Seeds

The following is an alphabetical list of the sprouting seeds in my kitchen, with a few more that I don't use but am very opinionated about. See if you can pick those out.

The symbol is next to my favorite seeds.

Adzuki

A medium-sized red bean, adzukis are poplar in Asian cuisine, made into everything from thick and crunchy bean sprouts to desserts and ice cream. They're high in protein, calcium, iron, phosphorus, potassium and vitamins A and C. One of the few beans that I recommend for sprouting because of their great flavor, digestibility, and nutrition, one still has to be careful with them because invariably a small percentage of them will not sprout; be careful when you're chewing, as a small percentage of them might stay hard and pebble-like. Add them to an Asian-themed sprout mix like mung grown into thick bean sprouts with mustard and poppy (or any mix that begs for a firm, slightly sweet, bright red constituent).

Method: Jar or Bag

Alfalfa

Alfalfa is the sprout most people think of first because they're abundantly available in grocery stores across the world. There's much fuss made over this little guy in the natural and raw food communities and even its name is suffused with fanfare: al-fal-fa, from the Arabic, meaning "Father of All Foods". It's true that alfalfa is abundantly rich in hard-to-find minerals, probably because its roots can reach 100 feet down through the soil with its ravenous appetite for moisture and nutrients. And because it's a leafy green sprout, it also has an even higher abundance of extra enzymes than most, and because of its mild flavor is extremely versatile in food prep, equally at home in salads, wraps, sandwiches, soups, the juicer and the blender. Personally, I think that there are much more interesting, nutritious and flavorful leafy sprouts out there like clover, radish, daikon, and broccoli, but it might just be my inherent need to stay ahead of the curve.

Alfalfa sprouts come into their full glory in about a week with the basket method, but I usually throw sprouts of this type in bags of salad mixes and let them grow for a few days. I am probably lazier than you, however, and when I put in the small effort to grow armfuls of leafy sprouts *en baskette* my digestion is always happier for it. Because they grow so rapidly, they are voracious for air and generate a higher-than-average amount of heat, so are much happier in a bag than a jar.

Some other leafy green sprouts are pretty spicy – radish, clover, celery – and the addition of alfala can help mellow them out.

Method: Basket (preferred) or Bag

Almonds

See "Nuts", pgs 174-184

Amaranth

Amaranth is a tiny South American seed that grows by the thousands in tight cones on a medium-sized red shrub. Popular with both the ancient Aztecs and the Himalayan cultures, this hearty plant can thrive in weak light, poor soil, arid climates and drought conditions.

15-20% protein, which is more than most meats, amaranth also contains the amino acids lysine and methonine, which are necessary for the assimilation of protein but are rarely found in other grains. Amaranth has more calcium than milk and plentiful magnesium and silicon, cofactors necessary for the digestion of calcium which milk does not have.

Amaranth is a deliciously nutty and malty sprout which takes a day to reach its peak and because of its teeny size is best sprouted in a fine mesh bag. Amaranth doesn't require soaking. If you sprout it with anything else, like for "Aztec Bread" (see "Kitchen Sink Farming Volume 4: Homegrown Living Recipes - What to Do with Your Sprouts and Krauts"), it will sink to the bottom of the mixture and hold a lot of moisture so make sure to shake up the bag after every watering. I don't recommend letting it go longer than 2 days after germination, because it will get especially bitter.

Method: Bag

Black Beans

Beans have a diversified portfolio of starches, and it takes a well-educated digestive system to smoothly cash in on their dividends. More often than not, the body has to spend more resources breaking them down and eliminating them than actually assimilating their nutrients. Sprouting (and fermenting) these difficult foods can make them much easier to deal with. I always recommend sprouting everything possible before they're boiled, steamed, baked, or whatever, but I even more passionately advocate sticking with foods that are easily turned into fuel for a vibrant life, namely, those that are still alive themselves. If a food has to be cooked to make it digestible, that food loses the enzymatic life force that inspired me to want to eat it in the first place.

Anyways, black, or turtle, beans are an oval bean with a black skin, cream-colored flesh, and a sweet flavor. Black beans have long been popular in Mexico, Central and South America, the Caribbean and the southern United States. This is not the same bean (fermented black beans) used in oriental cuisines. When sprouting them, let their tails grow as long as the beans themselves, indicating that they've reached the peak of nutrition and digestibility. Black beans are so beautiful and flavorful that I've used them very sparingly in pilafs and crackers, coarsely grinding them and running cold water over them to remove as much unbroken down starch as possible. Again, if you're going to be cooking black or any other beans, sprouting them will add a lot to their flavor and digestibility, especially if they're coarsely ground and rinsed first.

Method: Bag or Jar

Barley

Similar to wheat, barley must be sprouted in the shell and is best grown into a grass. Barley's slightly bitter flavor comes from a more diverse mineral portfolio than wheat, and as a grass is thought to contain more free-radical scavenging antioxidants than wheatgrass. Interestingly, before World War 2, the massive depletion of the soil because of growing one crop over and over again on the same plot of land (monoculture) required the introduction of chemical fertilizers and pesticides and for the first time, the dietary need for vitamin and mineral supplements. Barley grass was dried in tablet form and sold as a primitive multi-vitamin. Since barley grass doesn't have the sweetness of wheat, kamut or spelt grass, it can be grown with these if you're looking for a more nutritionally varied (or "vintage") green drink. "Insta-Grass".

Barely grass has 11 times the amount of calcium than cow's milk, 6.5 times as much carotene and nearly 5 times the iron content of spinach, close to seven times the vitamin C in oranges, four times the B1 in whole wheat flour, and an abundance of B12. It's very high in organic sodium, which dissolves calcium deposits in the joints and also replenishes the lining of the stomach, aiding digestion. People with arthritis routinely use celery juice because of the organic sodium it contains (28 mg per 100 grams), but barley grass contains almost 30 times more (775 mg per 100 grams). As a whole sprout, barley contains 45% protein, twice as much as wheat. It has 5 times the nutrients in the same amount of protein from meat, and in a much more bio-available format.

Method: Grass (preferred), or Bag or Jar

Buckwheat

A mild and delicate microgreen, buckwheat lettuce must be sprouted in the shell and grown in trays on soil, soilless mix, coconut mats, etc. All greens need a good amount of nitrogen, so if you're not using fresh soil with composted manure make sure you fertilize. Cow manure is the best with a little extra boost of nitrogen; chicken and bat guano is a bit too rich - some earthworm castings can be added to potting soil for a similar effect. Soaking the seeds with a little liquid kelp fertilizer should do the trick.

Originally from China and Tibet, buckwheat is a dark green and broad leafed, tender lettuce whose mild flavor is a delicious addition to a salad. It's also a good way to ease into grass juice; start with half buckwheat and half wheat for a milder juice.

Method: Micro-lettuce for salad or juice

Broccoli

A crucifer sprout like kale, cauliflower, and arugula, broccoli sprouts are leafy greens that taste like the full-grown plant and come with an entertaining story.

In 1992, a team of Johns Hopkins University scientists isolated two powerful cancer-fighting phytochemicals in broccoli, glucoraphanin and sulforaphane, which when chewed would combine to form a super molecule called sulforaphane glucosinolate, or SGS, which was particularly effective at fighting free radicals. A 1997 report followed, stating that SGS is in higher concentrations in 3 to 4 day-old broccoli sprouts, at least 20 times the concentration of full-grown broccoli. This discovery was written about in the *New York Times*, and a global shortage of broccoli seed came as a result of the sudden high demand. Then, a year later, John Hopkins University's hastily erected "Brassica Protection Products, Inc.", filed for and received a patent on the method they used to grow broccoli sprouts (to "...exploit the financial benefits of [their] findings" wrote Dr. Paul Talaby in his application), which, according to the lawyers of the sprout farmers that were then sued for infringement, is the same way everyone sprouts them, and the way they grow in nature. BPP formed a partnership with the hulking and deep-pocketed Sholl Group of Minnetonka, MN, a subsidiary of Green Giant Fresh Inc., and promptly started offering sprout farmers a choice: buy an expensive license, stop growing broccoli, or be sued.

"My complaint," said Greg Lynn, owner of Harmony Farms in Auburn, Washington and one of the defendants in the case, "is that Mother Nature should be the one getting the royalties here, and not some researchers milking the money-rich cancer research cow or some corporate opportunists extorting their way into sprout industry domination." Though broccoli sprouts account for only 5% of his revenues, Lynn planned on spending as much as 50% of his yearly sales to fight the suit.

Because the patents had already been issued, they were to be assumed valid by the court and the defendants must present "clear and convincing evidence" otherwise. In order for them to get a summary judgment, the five growers being sued needed to show an argument so compelling and persuasive that "no reasonable finder of fact could conclude otherwise". The sprouters presented this question to the court: "Can a plant, cultivated and eaten by humans for centuries, be patented merely on the basis of a recent realization that it has always had some recently uncovered, but naturally occurring, benefit?"

In the court brief accompanying his ruling, Judge Nickerson wrote, "The Plaintiffs... do not claim that their patents involve doing anything to alter or modify the natural seeds. They are simply germinated, harvested and eaten." He continued, "In construing the claims at issue here, the Court finds that they describe nothing more than germinating sprouts from certain cruciferous seeds and harvesting those sprouts as a food product... Phrases in the claims such as, 'rich in glucosinolates,' or 'containing high Phase 2 enzyme potential and non-toxic levels of indole glucosinolates and their breakdown products and goitrogenic hydroxybutenyl glucosinolates,' simply describe the inherent properties of certain cruciferous seeds. Plaintiffs attempted ... to argue that the claim language, 'identifying seeds which produce cruciferous sprouts ... containing [the desired properties]' introduces a new 'selection' step that was not a part of the prior art. All this step entails, however, is choosing to do something over another, in this case, choosing to grow broccoli instead of cauliflower sprouts instead of cabbage, cress, mustard or radish sprouts. Any process could be prefaced by a similar 'selection' step. Certainly, that one first chooses to perform a particular process cannot be enough to make the process 'new'. Thus, the Court finds that the patents in suit are invalid by anticipation." BPP appealed the case all the way to the Supreme Court, but the ruling was upheld. Five products containing broccoli sprouts are still sold by BPP in grocery stores, including "BroccoSprouts", which are not organically grown and therefore unequivocally cancer-*causing*, and described on their website as "The only product that guarantees a consistent level of sulphoraphane GS", an obviously misleading representation.

Stand up against corporate greed. Fight cancer. Grow and eat broccoli sprouts (which are also high in vitamins A, C, and E, and minerals calcium, phosphorus and magnesium, the cofactors needed to use calcium which are missing from milk.

Method: Basket (preferred) or Bag

Cabbage

The ancient ancestor of broccoli and cauliflower, most people know cabbage from Eastern European soups and the fermented condiments sauerkraut and kimchi. The sprout's distinctive flavor (a lot like cabbage, actually) may take a bit more of a stretch to include into the diet than alfalfa, but the many health benefits are certainly worth it.

Cabbage is rich in vitamin C and glutamine, an amino acid that has anti-inflammatory properties and speeds muscle recovery. Glucosinates, organic compounds consisting of glucose, amino acids, nitrogen and sulfur, are natural pesticides produced by plants in the brassica family, such as cabbage, mustard, kale, horseradish, broccoli and cauliflower, and while they have only a slightly bitter taste to humans, are intensely caustic to insects (taste like napalm). One might think that an organic pesticide might have negative effects on a non-bug, but in fact quite the opposite is true. Many varieties of these vegetables have been developed to remove this slightly bitter taste, but people that eat these cultivated foods are missing out on the anti-cancer benefits of glucosinates, which are being researched for their apparent carcinogen-blocking qualities. Additionally, cabbage is by far the number one vegetable to ferment, and it also has the most naturally-occurring beneficial bacteria of any vegetable. Co-incidence? I think not. I also speculatively theorize that it's the presence of glucosinates that allow these probiotics to thrive, namely lactobacillus, the family that the most common bottled probiotics, acidophilus and bifidus, are in, and have their own set of anti-cancer, anti-inflammatory, and anti-aging properties. Cato the Elder, the famed Roman historian, praised cabbage for its medicinal properties, declaring: "It is the cabbage that surpasses all other vegetables." Some question the universality of this statement (ok, just me), but it's definitely up there.

Cabbage seeds are tiny like alfalfa and clover, but with a slightly lower yield of 1 to 5, and sprout just as easily in a jar, bag, or basket. They taste just like cabbage, only a little milder, and are therefore a great garnish to warm tomato soups, or put them in place of sauerkraut in Rueben sandwiches or stadium-style hot dogs. I have yet to ferment them into sauerkraut sprouts, but one day, when I feel like eating something adorable...

Method: Basket (preferred), Bag, or Jar

Chia

Chia is a small mucilage seed from a desert plant closely related to mint, and is both black and white in color. In pre-Columbian times, chia was an important staple in both the Aztec and Mayan diets, and was the basic survival ration of Aztec warriors. It's been said that one tablespoon of the seeds could sustain a runner or scout for a full 24 hours. Banned by the Spanish government in the 16th century after a millennium of cultivation because of its close ties to the Aztec religion, chia is currently experiencing a cultural renaissance, which I hope is due in some small part to their incredible nutrition and not entirely the result of chia-pets and -presidents.

The highest plant source of Omega-3 EFAs (higher than even flax, but not quite as yummy), chia is rich in fiber (over 25%), has 3 times the antioxidants of blueberries, more calcium than milk, and more iron than spinach. Chia also contains high quantities of phosphorus, magnesium, manganese, copper, molybdenum, niacin, and zinc. The Aztecs used chia medicinally to relieve joint pain and sore skin, and I expect both of our cultures can respect the fact that it's so high in anti-oxidants that it will stay fresh for years longer than most seeds, especially as ours deals with a peak oil crisis. As a mucilage, the gel that forms when put in water helps slow down the breakdown and metabolization of carbohydrates and sugar, so it's the perfect thing to add to dessert to keep blood sugar from spiking. Now that modern society is noticing this mighty little seed again, it's being fed to laying hens to increase the omega-3 in their eggs, and chickens and cattle to increase the nutritive value of their meat. If I had to pick an "Official Seed of Societal Collapse", this would be it.

Method: Long Soak or Clay

Clover

Similar to alfalfa, and becoming as popular, clover sprouts have a bit more kick and texture than boring old alfalfa, and are just as versatile.

Method: Basket (preferred) or Bag

Flax

Flax might be one of the most important sprouts for health, as it contains six essential ingredients that are commonly missing from the modern diet. It is unparalleled as a source of essential fatty acids, both kinds of dietary fiber, antioxidant lignans, and is an easily-assimilable complete protein. And of course, enzymes when sprouted. It's also surpassingly easy to sprout and tastes wonderful. Everyone should slowly build up to eating a few tablespoons once or twice every day.

Flax seed is one-third oil and the rest is a combination of fiber, protein and soluble fiber or "mucilage", a gummy, slippery substance that makes jar or bag sprouting impossible. Flax must be sprouted with the long-soak or clay methods, which are actually the easiest ways to sprout; just put some flax seeds in a bowl, cover them with water, and in a day many of them will have broken their brown or golden seed coats and sprouted tiny tails. Flax oil is one of the best sources of the rare but essential fatty acid (EFA) omega-3, necessary for good brain function and higher intelligence, mood elevation, inflammation reduction, proper mental development in children, but most importantly (kidding), beautiful skin and hair. (more on EFAs on next page)

The protein in flax seeds is easily digested and contains all the amino acids needed for building and maintaining a strong body. Flax's insoluble fiber comes from the shell and acts like a broom, sweeping the colon of toxic material, impacted waste and dried mucus. Flax fiber is excellent nourishment for friendly bacteria in the intestine, which keep disease-causing organisms in check. Twelve percent of flax seeds is mucilage which makes it a gentle, non-irritating, natural laxative. Flax mucilage is perfect for those who have a sensitive stomach, acting as a buffer for excess stomach acids, soothing ulcers or irritable bowel disorders. Dry flax absorbs 20 times its volume in water and can seriously dehydrate a person and become lodged in the colon; sprouting flaxseeds is the best way to enjoy its host of benefits.

Flax is available in two varieties: brown, which is higher in omega-3s and has a harder shell, and golden, which is softer and has a sweeter and milder flavor. If you don't have a high-speed blender, use the golden seeds, because the brown need to be pretty well pulverized, otherwise they can pass through the digestive system intact.

In low-temp baking, the mucilaginous aspect of flax makes it a great substitute for sticky gluten in sprouted loaves. Lightly sprouted ground flax seeds make a light and creamy, mild flavored bread with a spongy quality which makes living tortillas or elastic Ethiopian Injera bread possible. Add a little or a lot of sprouted Kamut or spelt for a more sticky and dense loaf, which will require several times longer to cook. Include some to the pulp leftover from juicing and dehydrate it to make crackers, or add it to young coconut meat to make flexible, thin wraps more pliable than tortillas and nori.

Method: Long Soak or Clay Method

Essential Fatty Acids

Essential fatty acids, or EFAs, carry a slightly negative charge and spread out as a thin, even layer over surfaces. This makes cell membranes soft, fluid and flexible, allowing nutrients to flow in and wastes out. EFAs produce detectable bioelectrical currents, which make possible the vast number of chemical reactions in the body like nerve, muscle and membrane function. This living current is also a measurable difference between alive and dead tissue, and fact of interest in many fields of study, I would think.

EFAs absorb sunlight and attract oxygen; a plentiful supply of oxygen, carried by blood to our cells is fundamental for vitality, pain relief and healing - EFAs are able to hold onto this oxygen at the cells' boundaries, making a barrier against viruses and bacteria. Beneficial bacteria are great in our digestive systems, which aren't really considered to be inside our bodies, because they're not sterile - we don't want any bacteria crossing into our blood or cells, and because EFAs help prevent that they are vital for our immune systems. Because fats are the second most abundant substance in the body (water is first), high-quality EFAs are also important in countless and varied metabolic reactions in the body like fat burning, nutrient absorption, mental health and growth , making them especially

important for children. They can substantially shorten the time required for recovery of fatigued muscles after exercise or physical work. Eczema is a severe allergic inflammation, and through their partnership with oxygen, EFAs scavenge allergens from the blood, decreasing inflammation and bringing suppleness and a youthful appearance to the skin. Modern medicine is discovering more and more that many modern health problems are the result of inflammation, so an anti-inflammatory diet with plenty of EFAs is essential for health, especially as we age.

The absorption of sunlight is a curse, however, when the EFA is outside of the living seed. LNA (Alpha Linolenic Acid, an omega-3 EFA), for example, is about five times more reactive to light than LA (Linoleic Acid, an omega-6 EFA). Light increases LNA's ability to react with oxygen by a thousand times. The unsaturated fatty acids with more cis- bonds, like omega-3s, are extremely sensitive to light and will spoil rapidly when exposed to it. So the special nature of the EFAs that make them essential to life - the absorption of oxygen and transformation of solar energy - causes them to decompose when left exposed to air and light, like when seeds are ground and packaged as in the case of flours.

When EFAs and their highly unsaturated long-chain fatty acid cousins are open to the elements, free radical reactions start to take place. Just one photon of light can start a destructive game of telephone, breaking bonds down the line until it peters out around the 30,000 mark. The incomplete molecules join together forming new and toxic compounds. Nature to the rescue: protection from these free-radical toxins is supplied by the fat-soluble vitamins such as A and E, which trap these light-caused chain

reactions before they get out of control (and become denatured themselves). These powerful anti-oxidants are always found in concert with EFAs in whole seeds, the perfect container for what might be the body's most vital nutrients.

At best, the refining, bottling, cooking, shipping and storing of EFAs renders them unusable or non-existent, and they can quite easily become carcinogenic. By far the best way to include these vital nutrients in our diets is to sprout the troika of seeds high in EFAs: hemp, flax, and chia, which will offer them the 3-part protection of the seed's shell, free-radical scavengers, and living tissues. It's also (surprise, surprise) the cheapest way: 3 tablespoons of sprouted flaxseed contain 6 grams of omega-3s, the recommended daily allowance, for about 6 cents, in contrast to the 2 dollar shot of bottled EFAs from companies like Udo's Choice and Barleans. Chia provides even more, and of course, both are whole seeds and therefore supply countless other benefits.

All three kinds of EFAs (omegas 3, 6, and 9) are necessary, but special care must be taken to get enough 3. Omega 6 is quite plentiful, available pretty much wherever fats are sold, and we need very little of omega 9, so unless you're eating one bite of celery a day so you can be a prima ballerina, chances are you're fine. But as important as EFAs are to health, the really important thing is the *ratio* of

EFAs to each other. The optimal proportion of the 3 and 6 EFAs is 1 omega-3 to 4 omega-6s, 1:4, but the standard modern diet is more often a ratio of 1 to 20 or more. This imbalance causes the body to make fat-soluble hormones called prostaglandins to deal with the excess 6's, wasting valuable globular proteins and essentially creating toxins

out of unusable fats. Adult acne is usually created, or at least exacerbated, by this imbalance. This I know from experience, breaking out like crazy when I (as I slowly discovered) ate foods with an over-abundance of omega-6's, avocados and cashews especially. This is why I try to steer raw food chefs away from these ingredients, which seem to be in just about every dish on raw food menus - more like a crutch than an opportunity to feel amazing and alive. Cashews are in fact not raw, but more importantly have little nutritional benefit and a few major drawbacks, such as the toxins and allergens they contain. One of these, urushiol, is the same irritant found in poison ivy, a relative of cashews.

Whenever you eat anything with an excess of omega-6 EFAs (also called oleic or linoleic acids), like cashews, peanuts, olives and oil, almonds, or avocados, make sure to add some sprouted flax seed (or flax oil in a pinch) to the meal to balance out the fats in a healthier ratio.

Garbanzo

Best known as the basis of hummus, garbanzo beans, also called chick peas or chi chi beans, are actually legumes like peas and lentils. Starchy and fairly hard to digest on their own, sprouting simplifies their complex carbohydrates and turns them into a chewy treat in a salad mix; coarsely grinding and rinsing them will remove even more of the tough-to-digest starches. Sprout them alongside sesame seeds for a ready-to-go hummus – just add garlic and lemon and you've got a party in a jar. Large and light brown, these nutty seeds have more iron than any other legume and are a healthy source of saturated fat. They're also high in calcium, potassium and vitamin A.

Method: Bag or Jar, coarsely ground and rinsed after they've sprouted

Hemp-in' Around

Hemp, the male version of the cannabis plant, has none of the mind-altering chemicals that has made this family of weeds so controversial, and so popular with west coast hip-hop artists. It's unfortunate for the nutritional field, and therefore everyone that eats, that hemp has such a bad… rap? It's an inexpensive and fast-growing source of what may be the best protein found in any food, and certainly best vegetable source of EFAs like omega-3 and -6. Expensive, "essential", and very difficult to find in proper amounts for those that can't or choose not to eat deep-water fish daily because of a growing concern for our ocean's toxicity, ethics, preference, or because they're the 1.4 billion people in the world who live on less than $1 a day. Actually, I find it strange that anyone would want to eat an animal's liver, the organ that is full of fat-encased toxic substances so damaging that the body shut them away instead of risk putting them into the bloodstream to flush away. Fish, especially the ones not from the frigid waters of the arctic (though them too to a lesser degree), live their lives in constant contact with all sorts of toxins, from heavy metals and industrial waste to agricultural run-off and just plain garbage, one patch of which, in the Pacific, is the size of Texas. Plants are the best suppliers of vital EFAs (see pg 113) and lucky for us they're plentiful, cheap, pure, of unsurpassed quality, and quite tasty.

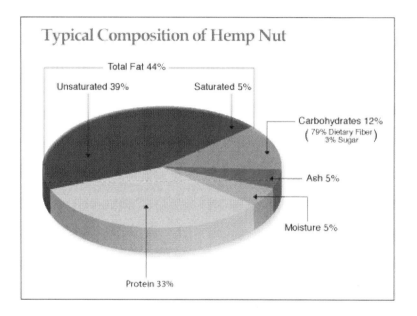

Hemp Protein

Hemp protein is the most complete and usable protein in both the vegetable and animal kingdoms. The reason for this is less about the amount than the *type* of protein offered by hemp. Hemp protein, comprising about 35% of its total mass, is a complete protein, containing all 8 essential amino acids needed by the body. It's also about 65% *globular* proteins, **the highest of any food** (this in relation to only about 20% usable protein in beef, and with it a host of problems, like being directly linked to cancer, heart disease, global food shortages and many of the top environmental problems). There are two kinds of proteins: fibrous (or structural) and biologically active (or globular). Fibrous protein builds tissues like muscles, organs, skin, and hooves. Globular proteins make hormones like insulin, hemoglobin and plasma, antibodies in the immune system (also called immunoglobulins – makes sense, huh?), and enzymes, and are therefore responsible for the hundreds of thousands of reactions occurring within each cell at every moment.

Though we can make globular proteins out of any protein we eat, it's much more efficient to take them in in a ready-to-use form. And while conversion of fibrous proteins to usable proteins is an energy-depleting task, globular proteins convert to structural tissue (like big biceps) quite easily as the body's intelligence deciding the best use of each molecule.

These factors make hemp one of the most important foods for overall health and unlike whey, dairy, soy, nut, grain, rice, and egg proteins, it's completely devoid of allergens,

> "Plasma, the fluid portion of blood which supplies nutrients to tissue, contains three protein types: serum albumen, serum globulin, and fibrinogen, which together compose about 80% of plasma solids." - Gray's Anatomy, 1978. Hemp protein closely resembles the globulin found in human blood plasma, which is vital to maintaining a healthy immune system.

making it great for anyone and everyone.

Hemp Oil

Hemp seed oil comprises 35% of the total seed weight. This oil has the lowest amount of saturated fatty acids at 8% (the ones found in animal products), no trans-fats (the worst ones), and the highest amount of polyunsaturated essential fatty acids at 80% (the good ones) total oil volume. Flax seed oil comes in second at 72% combined total essential fatty acids (though it and chia are higher in omega-3s, the harder to find EFAs). Hemp oil is the only whole food source of both the 'super' polyunsaturated fatty acids gamma-linolenic acid (GLA) and stearidonic acid (SDA), a combination that is required for proper immune system functioning. [7]

> "Qualitatively, it is considered desirable to secure amino acids similar to those of human tissues, both as to kinds and relative quantities of the various kinds." - From the "Textbook of Anatomy and Physiology", Kimber, Gray, Stackpole, 1943

Hemp is also high in:

- Inositol, which promotes hair growth, reduces cholesterol levels, prevents artery hardening, and is calming to the nervous system.

---

[7] ("Gamma-linolenic and stearidonic acids are required for basal immunity in Caenorhabditis elegans through their effects on p38 MAP kinase activity" Department of Genetics, Stanford University School of Medicine, Nandakumar M, Tan MW. Epub 2008 Nov 21)

- "Plant hormones", also called phytosterols or phytoestrogens, affect cholesterol absorption, hormone regulation, and cell metabolism.
- Potassium, which supports the nervous system and regular heart rhythm and, with the help of sodium, aids in the body's balance of water.
- Calcium is essential for a regular heartbeat, strong teeth and bones, and nerve impulses.
- Magnesium, a cofactor for calcium, is also needed to transmit the messages throughout the nervous and muscular systems.
- Sulfur helps the body resist bacterial invasion and protects it against toxic substances.
- Iron facilitates the production of red blood cells and energy.
- Zinc is important for a healthy reproductive system and the prostate gland. It speeds tissue regeneration and strengthens the immune system.
- Scientists are studying the use of hemp seed extracts to boost the immune systems of people suffering from immunosuppressive disorders such as AIDS and cancer.

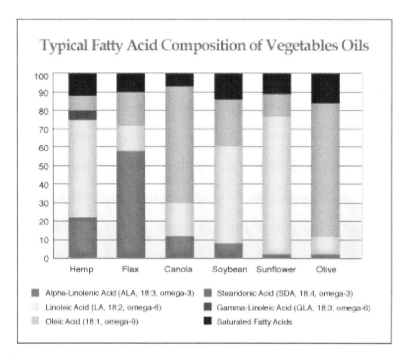

Graph, and previous, reprinted from Gero Leson and Petra Pless', "Hemp Foods and Oils for Health", 2002

- Edestin is a highly digestible and complete protein which comprises about 65% of hemp's total protein. This extremely vigorous globulin is so compatible with the human digestive system that in 1955 a Czechoslovakian Tuberculosis Nutrition Study found hemp seed to be the only food that successfully treated tuberculosis, a disease in which nutritive processes become impaired and the body wastes away. Edestin is such a perfect protein that *Science Magazine* complained in 1941, "the passage of the Marijuana Law of 1937 has placed restrictions on trade in hemp seed that, in effect, amounts to prohibition … It seems clear that the long and important career of the protein is coming to a close in the US."

Again, the use of hemp seeds has absolutely no correlation with marijuana in the body, and won't cause any adverse reactions in the body or come up on a drug test. Its astounding nutritional profile makes it an extremely important seed that should be a part of everyone's diet. For those in impoverished regions where malnutrition is the norm, the fact that hemp comes from a fast-growing and tenacious plant means that one day its widespread protein-rich nourishment could be possible.

Hemp is only legal today because in the 1930's, when the anti-hemp insanity began in the US, bird seed companies told congress that songbirds would stop singing without this addition to their seed mixes. The compromise was that hemp seeds would be sterilized with infrared heat, making minute cracks in the shell and rendering the seed only semi-viable, even though it's not possible to grow hemp into wacky tobaccy. What this means in the US is that whole organic hemp seeds are available as bird seed and slightly sproutable. The whole seed can be soaked and germinated, then sprouted for a day or two and many of the seeds will start to grow a tiny root. But without the protective integrity of a whole seed, they can start to mold soon after. Stick 'em in the fridge when you see the first tiny tails and enjoy their crunchy benevolence in a myriad of ways.

The seed is also available with the shell removed, called hulled hemp or hemp hearts, and it's automatically sterile. These seeds haven't been heated in any way and therefore all the wonderful oils are still fresh. Though most of the enzyme inhibitors will have been removed with the shell, these seeds also benefit from a two-hour soak. The available enzymes will be activated and in turn the vitamin and mineral content will increase. This is evidenced by the cloudy soak water and change in taste. Until I find a source of organic, unsterilized whole hemp seeds, I use hulled seeds, which I keep in the freezer to preserve the delicate EFAs. Hemp seeds are absolutely delicious, and even if they weren't ridiculously nourishing I would still eat them everyday on their fresh and nutty flavor and creamy texture alone. They're very small, soft, off-white disks, and sprinkled on salads or easily ground into a rich nut butter. Hemp's tastiness makes it easy to enjoy this powerhouse of nutrition and vital life force.

See the "Resources" section for sources of whole and hulled organic hemp seed.

Method:

Whole – Jar or Bag, refrigerate when sprouting begins

Hulled – Soak for 2 hours

Kamut

Kamut is the trademarked name of Khorasan wheat, an amber spring variety with a large, humpbacked kernel. It is an ancient, un-hybridized grain and its high lipid content gives it a buttery taste.

The story goes like this: a US airman in Egypt during World War II was at the bazaar one day when a man who had just finished robbing a pyramid sold him a handful of the 4000-year-old grains he had found there, 36 kernels to be exact, which were apparently the last of their kind. The airman sent the grains to his father, a wheat farmer in Montana, who began to cultivate this venerable and storied grain. County fairs were won, paper boys yelped, and the revival of this near-extinct grain began. Fun story, but unfortunately, at least partially a myth. Most scientists believe Kamut probably survived the years as an obscure grain kept alive by the diversity of crops common to small peasant farmers in Egypt or Asia Minor, and the story was spun by enterprising street vendors, looking to market an inexpensive local grain to wide-eyed US soldiers, one of whom had never before been out of Montana.

Tombs and exotic black market transactions aside, it somehow ended up in the hands of a wheat farmer who planted and harvested a small crop and displayed the grain as a novelty at the local fair in 1964. The legend that the giant grain was taken from an Egyptian tomb was further propagated at this time, and it was called "King Tut's Wheat". In a white flour and new-and-improved crazed America, the novelty of a rich, coarse heirloom grain quickly wore off and it was almost forgotten. Then, in 1977, the one remaining jar of King Tut's Wheat (see a pattern here?) was obtained by T. Mack Quinn, another Montana wheat farmer, who with his son Bob, a plant biochemistry graduate student at UC Davis, spent the next decade cultivating the seeds. The Quinns patented the seed and copyrighted the trade name "Kamut," an ancient Egyptian word for wheat which Egyptologists say comes from the root "Soul of the Earth". Whatever the origin of this special grain and the ethical consequences of patenting seeds, the protection the Quinns have given it has allowed Kamut to keep its heirloom genes unadulterated and it has always been grown organically.

Kamut is higher than wheat in eight out of nine minerals, contains up to 65% more amino acids, the building blocks of protein, and boasts more healthy fats and fatty acids. It's also an excellent source of magnesium, niacin, thiamine, and zinc. But perhaps the most impressive aspect of Kamut is its protein level - up to 40% higher than the national average for wheat. And while its nutritional profile is exciting, perhaps the coolest thing about Kamut is its accessibility to all, including those with wheat sensitivities, gluten allergies, and celiac disease. In a 1991 clinical trial, scientists and physicians tested two different wheat-sensitive populations - people with immediate immune responses and those with delayed responses. In the delayed immune response group, a remarkable 70% showed greater sensitivity to common wheat than Kamut; in the immediate immune response group (the severely allergic) 70% had no, or only minor, reaction to Kamut wheat and were able to continue eating it on a rotational basis. People with allergies should always seek the advice of a trusted health-care practitioner, however, the study concluded that "for most wheat sensitive people, Kamut can be an excellent substitute for common wheat", Elleen Yoder, Ph.D., President of the International Food Allergy Association and head of the team that conducted the study.

Kamut is the best variety of wheat to grow into grass, and alongside spelt, is far better than wheat in food preparation. It gives a rich, buttery flavor to sprouted breads, in contrast with spelt's light, slightly sweet flavor.

Method: Grass (preferred), Bag or Jar for sprouted bread

Lentil

A round, flat seed, like a tiny coin, lentils are commonly found green, yellow, brown and red, though in India over 50 different varieties of lentils are grown. One of the first cultivated plants in human history, lentil seeds have been found in the Egyptian pyramids. The Hunzas of the

Himalayas, known for their great physical endurance and long life ("as healthy as a Hunza" is an expression well-loved by many a great-grandparent) ate lentils in abundance. They're said to be one of the most sustaining of all natural foods; during the World Wars, one handful of cooked lentils was the daily ration for many European soldiers.

Soluble fiber increases 300% in 3-4 days in sprouted lentil seeds, which helps lower LDL cholesterol, blood pressure, blood sugar and regulates insulin levels. Fiber of this kind is also a "pre-biotic", feeding beneficial organisms in the digestive tract while simultaneously lubricating the intestines and colon. Lentils are 26% protein and high in calcium, magnesium, sulfur, potassium, phosphorus, and vitamins A, B, C, and E.

Lentils are a member of the pea family but are treated more like beans in food prep, though they're much easier to digest than beans. This gives people interested in maintaining the enzymatic integrity of their foods a hearty and richly-flavored legume to work with that they won't regret later. They sprout easily with the jar or bag method, cook more quickly than beans if you go that route, and give a sweetish, garden-fresh flavor to any dish they're in - brown have the heartiest flavor, green the spiciest, and red are the most mild and lovely to look at.

Method: Bag or Jar

Millet

Prehistoric evidence shows that millet was grown since the stone age in lake regions around Switzerland, and remained popular in Mesopotamia and ancient China. One of the very few alkaline "grains" (actually a seed, which is why it's sproutable and loved by kitchen sink farmers worldwide), millet can help bring our blood pH into balance. Very easy to digest, millet provides both serotonin (a hormone) and tryptophan (an essential amino acid) which are most beneficial when combined. These two nutrients combine to create a powerful team that has several vital functions that effect mood, appetite, sleep, muscle contraction, memory and learning. Millet is also rich in anti-oxidants, magnesium (can help reduce the affects of migraines and heart attacks), niacin (can help lower cholesterol), phosphorus (helps with fat metabolism, tissue repair and energy production) and nutrients that protect against diabetes, cancer and asthma.

Millet must be sprouted in the hull, which isn't how they're usually offered in stores. (See Appendix C, "Resources", pg 174) Hulled, they can be soaked and rinsed before cooking for increased nutrition and digestibility, but sprouting them will improve them in countless ways.

Method: Bag or Jar

"I don't think most hunter-gatherers farmed until they had to, and when they switched to farming they traded quality for quantity." – Mark Cohen, *Paleopathology at the Origins of Agriculture.*

Alkalinity

Alkalinity is on one end of the pH spectrum, and acidity is on the other. Alkaline foods aren't actually themselves alkaline, but based on their nutritional profile, help bring the body into a more alkaline state. This is the healthy, disease-free state that our nomadic, hunter-gatherer ancestors and animals in the wild enjoy. Acid-forming foods are meat, dairy, alcohol, sugar, saturated fats, and cooked foods, whose starches have caramelized, tissues are lifeless, and nutrients are bound in mostly unusable structures. You knew they were bad for you, now you know (very basically) why. In fact, skeletal records show that the average lifespan dropped by seven years when humans started raising and cooking crops and livestock.[8] Fresh veggies, low-sugar fruits, sprouted seeds, and fermented food and drinks (non-alcoholic, sorry) all contribute to an alkaline system.

The brain, which can't store fat, must get all of its energy from the blood flowing through it. It's hard to extract energy and nutrients in an acidic environment, which explains why energy and mood drops after the stimulating effects of sugar have worn off. Same goes for cigarettes, caffeine, and cocaine, powerful *alkaloids*, substances that artificially push the blood into an alkaline state. When these compounds lose their potency, the body swings back

---

[8] N-G Gejvall, *Westerhus: Medieval Population and Church in the Light of Skeletal Remains* (Lund: Hakan Ohlssons Boktryckeri, 1960); and Pia Bennike, *Paleopathology of Danish Skeletons* (Copenhagen: Almquist and Wilksell, 1985).

> into an increased acidity, creating an unhealthy, pendulous imbalance.
>
> Higher acidity in the blood also makes it stickier, not a good thing in a society whose leading cause of death is clogged arteries. When the diet converts to at least 80% alkalizing foods nutrients are more readily absorbed and cellular degeneration (aging) is slowed or reversed. Depression and illness are much less common because of the increase in vitalizing nourishment and energy.
>
> Our optimal pH is about 7.3-7.5, more alkaline than acid, and can be very simply tested by placing a pH strip on the tongue. The pH of saliva mirrors the alkalinity or acidity of the blood, lymph, and spinal fluid, so this cheap and easy test should be conducted regularly to monitor overall health, and changes in pH can be telling signs of increased well-being or impending disease.

Mung

A smallish bean with a beautiful sea-green color, mung beans are a member of the kidney bean family and are commonly sprouted into "bean sprouts" in Chinese cuisine. Very detoxifying, these beans are high in iron, vitamin C, potassium, and are a complete protein. They are, however, still awfully difficult to digest even when sprouted, and along with adzukis can have some "duds" that don't sprout and feel like a stone in the mouth. The best way to enjoy them, besides saying "mung" to people on the street, is sprouting them fully into thick and crunchy long white vegetables using the pressure method described on page 87 if you'd like to add these fresh, mild legumes to your diet and cuisine.

Method: Bean Sprouts (preferred), Bag or Jar

Oat

Oats are a source of gentle but potent fiber, nutritious, and one of my favorite grains. I was quite surprised when I first concocted a "living oatmeal", expecting to trade my usual light and vibrant feeling for the comforting flavor of a cold-weather breakfast, but found the opposite to be true. Throughout the digestive process my "sproutmeal" gave me a buoyant energy that was a far cry from how I used to feel after eating Quaker Oats. Now this treat is a frequent part of my diet in colder months. See "Kitchen Sink Farming Volume 4: Homegrown Living Recipes - What to Do with Your Sprouts and Krauts" for the recipe.

I may have been previously prejudiced against oats because the many variations of commercially available products remove much of their nutrition and life force. Hulled ground oatmeal is made the same way as white flour and is not much better; steel cut, or groats, are missing many of the key factors that work together with the germ to create complete nutrition and digestibility. Pre-cooked instant or microwaveable products are utterly devoid of benefits. Oats will only sprout in their complete, unshelled form, available as "unhulled" or "sprouting oats" which I've rarely seen in stores, and are very much worth the effort of ordering them online. They are rich in protein, phosphorus (which is essential for the development of the brain and nervous system), and silicon (necessary for the development and renewal of bones and connective tissue). Nutritionally-bankrupt cereal-and-milk or pastries do more harm than good, when "enriched" wheat products with their synthetic vitamins and minerals that are unusable by the body block the cells' recepetors to actual nutrients. Feeding our children living oatmeal for breakfast can help reverse this "overfed, undernourished" epidemic and help make a generation of vibrant young people with full access to their natural intelligence.

Oat is the third leading ceral crop in the US and it fares best in cool, moist climates. This is why oats are such a popular staple in the British Isles of Scotland, Ireland and Wales, and shows that they prefer a dry wit. Today, nearly half of the world's oat crop, more than 4 billion bushels a year, is grown in the United States and Canada. The outer shell of oats is often ground into bran and bottled as a fiber supplement, but it doesn't hold a candle to the effects of whole oat sprout, finely ground in milk, cookies, smoothies, or anything that will merge with its very light, nutty and mildly grassy taste. The first time you try it you may be pleased at the ease of digestion and (especially) elimination. That is to say, a handful of sprouted oats and you'll be B.M.ing like a rockstar. They're also high in vitamins B, E, iron and calcium. The quality and quantity of the protein in oats is far superior to that of wheat and most other grains - oats have twice the protein of wheat or corn flakes. They also contain GLA (the omega-6 essential fatty acid gamma linoleic acid), which helps the body make other EFAs.

Oats sprout very easily, their thick hulls keeping them from retaining water or building up heat, so sprouting them in the jar they soaked in is just fine. Because their hull is so thick, a nice long soak (10-16 hours) is best, weighed down or in a jar filled up and lidded to keep their floaty selves submerged.

Method: Jar

Pea

The crown jewel of the legume family, fresh peas are only available for a month or so in early summer, and I highly recommend taking advantage of them then. They're available frozen during the rest of the year, their nutrients and enzymes in various degrees of degradation. Eating sprouted dried peas is a great way to get their nutrient-rich deliciousness in an easily-digestible form year-round.

Peas have been enjoyed for at least 8000 years for their mild, sweet taste and complex carbohydrates, calcium, magnesium, folic acid, vitamins A, Bs, C, and E. They're also 25% protein. The green variety also have the added benefit of being green, which comes from their natural oxygenating and detoxifying chlorophyll content. A molecule that's only one atom away from our own hemoglobin, which serves our blood's main purpose of carrying oxygen to our cells, chlorophyll is a nutrient that develops in sunshine, and therefore, often a rare commodity for apartment-dwellers.

Easily sproutable with the bag or jar method in their whole form (split peas won't sprout), peas are one of the few sprouts that don't get bitter if they're allowed to grow their roots into long white Fu Manchu beards. They also have a fresh, vegetable-y flavor and I throw them in every salad sprout mixture I make. Peas can also be grown into microgreens in soil or hydroponically. Someone must like them, as they're always available at my local natural foods store in this form, but I find them slightly tough and fibrous, and would rather just make sunflower greens. I also love peas because they're very inexpensive, so it will cost next to nothing to sow a handful of sprouted peas at the base of a houseplant or in a tray, and if you don't like the taste, just leave them alone and soon you'll have a full pea pod factory and your houseplant will enjoy the nitrogen-fixation legumes provide to soil. They're commonly available in green and yellow hues, though a wide range of colors, sizes, and mottling exist. There's even a blue one called the Butterfly Pea that's ground and used as a natural blue food coloring in Thailand.

Peas grow in a uniquely segregated fashion — the root on one side, the shoot on the other, and the spherical pea ball in the middle. For this reason, it's fun to pull them apart while they're eaten, especially for kids.

Method: Jar or Bag

Peanut

More pea than nut, peanuts are actually legumes that, unlike nuts, will poke out a tail when sprouted. Peanuts, or groundnuts as they used to be called by folks dressed like Col. Sanders, originated in South America and are now grown throughout the tropical and warm temperate regions of the world. They were widely cultivated by the natives of the New World at the time of European expansion in the sixteenth century, and were subsequently taken to Europe,

Africa, Asia, and the Pacific Islands. Peanuts were unknown in the present southeastern United States until colonial times, where they stayed a specialty garden crop until the civil war, when soldiers on both sides began to grow peanuts for themselves and their livestock. When the war ended, they took their taste for peanuts home. They soon became available from street vendors and at baseball games and circuses.

In 1903, George Washington Carver, an American scientist, botanist, educator, inventor and former slave began researching peanuts at Tuskegee Institute in Alabama. Though peanut butter had been created by then, Carver developed more than 300 other uses for peanuts and improved their horticulture so much that he is considered by many to be the "father of the peanut industry." He recognized the value of peanuts as a cash crop (currently #2 in America) and proposed that peanuts be planted on a rotation basis in the cotton fields where the boll-weevil insect threatened the region's main crop and financial stability. At the time, many people still saw African Americans as intellectually inferior to whites, and the fame of Carver's achievements helped dispel this myth.

Peanuts grow underground, attached to the roots of the shrub. For this reason, they have more enzyme inhibitors than many other seeds, so soaking and sprouting them is non-negotiable to get even a modicum of their nutrition. Peanut butters sold in stores are obviously unsprouted and stale; any vitamins and delicate healthy oils have long since hit the road. To get the most out of them, meals must be at the peak of their freshness and nutrition and prepared right before we eat them. Though it's cheap and easy to do it this way, I haven't seen any products that come close to this integrity that aren't astronomically priced, and on the rare occasions I can find them in big city specialty stores. I'd rather just make them on my kitchen counter or spare bookcase shelf with a handful of humble seeds and couple of minutes' effort.

There are four common varieties of peanut: Virginia, Runner, Valencia, and Spanish; this list goes from largest to smallest. Harder to find, but well worth the search are "wild jungle" peanuts, beautiful heirloom nuts from the Amazon. These peanuts are rich, aromatic and earthy, with a familiar yet exotic flavor and a beautiful mottled red color. As with most wild or closer-to-the-source foods, these peanuts are lower in fat and higher in nutrients. And unlike the hybridized peanuts so many people are allergic to, heirloom peanuts are free of aflatoxin, peanut's allergy-causing component. They do cost 3-4 times more than the others, understandably.

Statistics show that about 1% of adults and 25% of children in the US report an allergy to the peanut, and 25% of these children will grow out of it. (The 1%-6% discrepancy between current and future adults' allergies is probably due to the fact that allergies are more likely to be recognized and reported now than when the adults surveyed were kids.) Recent research in the UK shows that 100% of allergic children were able to build up a tolerance to the allergen through "oral immunotherapy", or taking slightly increasing amounts of peanut flour daily for a 3 week period. It's unclear whether or not this treatment will make peanuts safe for everyone, but it has been shown to protect allergic children from the dangers of accidental consumption of up to ten peanuts, which is in fact the leading cause of food-related deaths.

A pound of peanuts is high in food energy and provides around the same caloric value as 2 pounds of beef, 1½ gallons of milk, or 36 eggs. Cultivated peanuts contain about 30% protein and 45% oil, and are very high in vitamin E (a dietary antioxidant that helps to protect cells from oxidative stress, an inevitable damaging physiological process sometimes referred to as aging), folate (needed for cell division, which means that adequate folate intake is especially important during pregnancy and childhood when tissues are growing rapidly), niacin (a B vitamin that helps to convert food to energy), riboflavin, magnesium, phosphorus, phytochemicals, and fiber.

Peanuts sprout easily in bags and jars, the already-present point growing into a root. They're best after just a day or two, while they retain most of their fat and nuttiness; they'll taste detectibly vegetable after that. Peanuts are dicots like sunflower seeds, meaning that the seed itself is the first leaves the plant will grow into. If you let them grow for a week or more, or plant one in the dirt of a houseplant, point down, they'll grow a few inches then split into a pair of spectacularly large leaves. A fun botanical drama for the young or curious.

Method: Jar or Bag

Quinoa

A staple of the ancient Central and South Americans, quinoa is currently enjoying a surge of popularity. The Incas, who called it the "mother grain", grew quinoa on terraced plots in the Andes Mountains in Peru, Chile, and

Bolivia, many of which are still in use today by the descendants of the original farmers. The indigenous people would grind the tiny seeds, which grow in clusters at the end of the stalk of an annual herb, for breads or use them in hearty stews, use the leaves as vegetables, burn the stalk for fuel and even use a sticky resin released from the soaking seeds as soap. But beginning with the Spanish attempt to destroy the Native South Americans culture by burning fields of quinoa and levying severe punishments against anyone caught growing it, and continuing with the mass marketing of refined wheat products, quinoa lost its illustrious status and even developed a negative association among locals, ignorant to their land's potential of being a nutritional mother lode.

Quinoa is 16 to 20% protein, more than any other grain. Even better, it's an unusually complete protein, supplying all the essential amino acids. Not only is quinoa's amino acid profile wonderfully well-balanced, which makes it a good choice for vegetarians and vegans concerned about adequate protein intake, but quinoa is especially well-endowed with the amino acid lysine, which is essential for tissue growth and repair. It has more calcium than milk (the "mother grain") and contains an abundance of the cofactor magnesium, which is necessary to assimilate calcium, as well as silicon, another invaluable nutrient for bone and joint health. It's also very high in iron, B vitamins, phosphorus, vitamin E, and contains no gluten and is therefore not allergy-producing. Its high levels of magnesium relax blood vessels, allowing for increased blood flow and nourishment of the cells and a lower risk of plaque build-up and heart disease. Quinoa can also help prevent type-2 diabetes, as magnesium is also a co-factor for more than 300 enzymes, including ones that regulate glucose and insulin secretion. Quinoa is also a very good source of manganese and copper, two minerals that assist anti-oxidants to combat free radicals that cause aging and cancer.

There are hundreds of varieties of quinoa, from yellow to red, purple to black. The yellow variety is the most common, though an heirloom red variety is starting to show up on supermarket shelves. I prefer this one, which has a more rich and nutty taste, because its ancestors' DNA have been messed with less by selective breeding and chemical influence. All quinoa are naturally coated in a bitter gel called saponin, foreshawdowed above. Before quinoa can be packaged and sold, it must be washed several times to remove this inedible coating, but much of it still remains on the seed. This can be seen in the soak water, which quickly becomes foamy and cloudy. As popular as quinoa is becoming, not many people realize that it must be soaked for 8 or more hours, the water changed at least a couple of times, to remove this digestive inhibitor before it's cooked or sprouted. It also has to be rinsed more thoroughly than the average sprout, because its enzymes inhibitors are more tenacious than most. For this reason, it's best sprouted in bags where a large volume of water can be passed through it easily, instead of filling and dumping a jar many times.

> "About one hundred and fifty years ago, bananas were unknown to the United States and peanuts were only eaten by slaves. So what's to say that an old South American grain called quinoa (pronounced keen-wa) won't become a popular American staple." Author Steve Meyerowitz,

Quinoa is a very quick sprouter, though (24 hours yields a ¼ inch tail, and in a day or two more your crop is at its nutritional apex), so the little bit of extra effort that goes into rinsing is made up in time, and is more than made up for in nutrition and flavor. Quinoa happens to be delicious, with no acquired taste to acquire, which makes it perfect for people transitioning to a less- or no-meat diet. It has a fluffy, creamy, slightly crunchy texture and a somewhat nutty flavor, is great warm or cold, and mixes well with other grains, vegetables, and flavorings, and is great ground or whole in breads, salads, dips, butters, or sauces.

Method: Bag

Radish and Daikon

A leafy green sprout with a zesty spice, common radish is a crucifer-like cabbage, mustard, and turnip. Its heat is stimulating to the digestive system, helping to remove mucous in the intestines and respiratory system, and fires up elimination. It's both anti-parasitic and antiseptic (good news for Candida sufferers) and supportive to beneficial bacteria. Radish sprouts have 4 times more vitamin A than milk, and more vitamin C than pineapple.

A little bit of radish sprouts go a long way, but they've no equal in meat sandwiches or with other rich foods. Grow them for a week with the basket method or, more efficiently, throw a little bit into a salad mix in a bag or jar.

Method: Basket (preferred) or Bag (for us lazy)

Rice

White rice, like white flour, is made so by removing the bran, or shell. Eliminating most of its nutrients, this process also renders the seed un-sproutable. The milling process that converts brown rice to white also removes about 10% of the product, resulting in an over 40-ton yearly loss of food worldwide. Brown rice will sprout like any other seed, though its sweet, starchy flavor makes it unappetizing raw. Cooked germinated brown rice is far superior to any other form of cooked rice nutritionally because 1) the removal of phytic acid and other enzyme inhibitors that bind nutrients and make them unusable to some degree by the human digestive system (see pg 23 for more on enzyme inhibitors), 2) increased nutrient content, and 3) activated enzymes, which will begin to predigest complex starches and proteins into a simpler and more readily-available form.

Germinated brown rice, or GBR, also tastes much better when cooked than un-germinated rice, and requires less cooking time and therefore retains even more nutrients. Increased 15 times is the amino acid gamma-aminobutyric acid, or GABA, a chief neurotransmitter that helps block anxiety- and stress-related impulses from reaching the motor centers of the brain. A deficiency in this amino acid has been linked to panic attacks and PMS symptoms, and it's used in massive doses as a non-toxic tranquilizer in epileptics. The small amounts available in food can induce calm and serenity, and in its role as a hormone regulator it can increase muscle tone and sexual vitality and promote weight loss. Other remarkable improvements are shown in the amounts of dietary fiber, magnesium, potassium, zinc, E and many B vitamins. It's included in this list of otherwise living foods because rice is so pervasive in so many of the world's cuisines and economies. Rice is the world's main food crop for humans, accounting for more than one-fifth of all calories consumed worldwide[9]. Rice is included in this book to inspire maximization of its potential both as a food and as a commodity.

Incidentally, according to Japanese food economist Ito Shoichi in his 2004 presentation for the Rice Conference held by the Food and Agriculture Organization of the United Nations, there's some evidence that the ancient Japanese germinated all of their brown rice. Another too-common example of modernization changing the inner value of food while keeping the outer form intact. I desperately hope that with the current rapid evolution of both modern science and the popular desire for real food, the best of both worlds will soon be commonplace.

GBR requires a much longer than normal soak time, 1 to 3 days depending on the temperature. The reason rice needs to be soaked so long is its relatively low quantity of phytase, the family of compounds that are activated during germination to neutralize EIs. At 85-100 degrees F, germination takes about 24 hours, at 80 degrees it's about 2 days, and at 60 degrees it's about 3 days (with the soak water changed daily). A low-temperature hot plate or aquarium heater can be used to keep the water the optimal 85-100 degrees. When germination has finished, the rice will change color and the end will begin to bulge. If

---

[9] Smith, Bruce D. *The Emergence of Agriculture*. Scientific American Library, A Division of HPHLP, New York, 1998

drained and rinsed for several days, a root system will emerge and the flavor will intensify. Sprouting rice past the germination phase isn't advised, except for specialty culinary applications like rice pudding and amasake, because it gets pretty sickeningly sweet.

Japanese researchers at the Shimsu University's Department of Bioscience and Biotechnology and the Fancl-Domer Company's Food Science Research Center concluded in 2000, "Continuous intake of GBR can lower blood pressure, improve brain function, and relieve some symptoms of menopause. It also may prevent headaches, relieve constipation, regulate blood sugar, and even prevent Alzheimer's disease and some cancers, including colon cancer and leukemia." As profound as that proclamation is, it's important to remember when reading comparative statements like this that we don't know exactly *what kind* of diet it is being compared to. If you're eating White Castle several times a day, all these benefits and more will most likely apply if you add some GBR. If you're already eating an organic diet rich in living veggies, fruits, and sprouted seeds, you're probably already in good shape. The quotation is included more to give the reader a sense of what the effects of such a simple action like soaking rice before its cooked can have on the undernourished, whether by lack of resources, knowledge, or self-discipline.

When cooking GBR, because the outer shell has been softened by germination, it cooks as quickly as white rice, in a little less than half the regular time.

Method: Long Germination - 1-3 Day Soak, depending on water temperature

Rye

Rye is a relatively young grain; its cultivation began in around 400 B.C, when farmers became interested in a wild grass that grew untamed in the wheat and barley fields in what would become Germany. A hardy plant, rye thrives in poor soil and cold climates, sometimes as far north as the Arctic Circle. In the dark ages, rye was relegated as a food for the poor, and as standards of living improved rye began to take a backseat to wheat. Though it is a "gluten grain", rye has less gluten than wheat, as well as several beneficial properties missing from that "strip-mall of grains". Since it's difficult to separate the germ and bran from the endosperm of rye, it's never been available as a "white" version so its flour retains a large quantity of nutrients, unlike refined wheat flour. Rye contains fluorine, a rare mineral that strengthens teeth and tooth enamel, and its photoestrogenic lignans can help normalize hormone activity. For women going through menopause, this subtle effect can be enough to reduce or prevent symptoms like hot flashes, which are thought to be the result of plummeting estrogen levels.

Because rye has less gluten than wheat, it yields a denser loaf of bread with a rich and hearty, sweet-sour flavor. I recommend a combination of kamut and rye sprouted anywhere you'd use wheat, but it's best grown into its slightly bitter grass form and juiced, which has powerful cleansing properties. You can also sow a little bit into a tray of wheat and barley grasses or use it to make a delicious probiotic water (see Kitchen Sink Farming Volume 2: Fermenting) for a sweet-sour flavor reminiscent of NY delis.

Method: Grass (preferred), Jar or Bag

Sesame

These small, flat seeds are the first recorded seasoning, and have stayed popular for more than 5000 years since. According to Assyrian legend, when the gods met to create the world, they drank wine made from sesame seeds. In ancient India, the seeds were a symbol of immortality, the God Vishnu's consort Maha Sri Devi was associated with sesame seeds, and it's still considered the most auspicious oil next to ghee (clarified butter) in Hindu rituals and prayers. They were used in Ayurvedic medicine to help people achieve a healthy weight, whether they needed to gain or lose. Available in light and dark brown and black, sesame seeds are ground into a nut butter called tahini, a main component in hummus, and are quietly popular in just about every type of cuisine. Especially high in calcium, containing almost 1000 times as much as milk, sesame seeds are also rich in phosphorus, potassium, magnesium, and vitamin A.

Sesame seeds must be in their commonly available shell-on version (which still contains all the healthy oils and fiber) to sprout, though of course soaking the soft, white hulled variety will improve their digestibility, flavor, and nutrition. An easy and quick sprout, soak them for 4-6 hours and sprout them for 2 days. They can be placed on a sunny windowsill for another few hours to develop their chlorophyll as they turn bright green. I love black sesame seeds in my salad mixes and nut butters for their rich and oily middle-eastern taste and gorgeously contrasting color.

Method: Bag or Jar

Soybeans

A complete protein in and of itself, soybeans can produce at least twice as much protein per acre than any other major vegetable or grain crop, ten times more protein per acre than land used for grazing milking cows, and fifteen times more protein per acre than land set aside for meat production. Even so, 98% of soybeans grown in America are used for livestock feed, which yields 20 times less food. Accordingly, Monsanto attacked the soybean first with their bioengineering and legislative muscle; now almost all the soybeans grown in America are from the company's patented "Terminator" seeds that are engineered to only grow once, and genetically-modified to resist the same company's herbicide, Round-Up. This way, farmers need to buy both the especially toxic pesticide as well as new seeds every year instead of using the time-honored tradition of saving their best seeds for the next planting, otherwise the farmer risks government-sanctioned bullying by the company's private police force. This disgusting greed and incredible waste while over 40 million Americans, including 17 million children (one in four) face a daily struggle against hunger.

During the Great Depression, it was discovered that soybeans had the ability to replenish nitrogen in the soil, and great tracts of drought-pummeled dust bowl land were regenerated by this little bean. Henry Ford, of "Built Ford Tough", originally designed the first automobiles and tractors to run on soy oil, with the idea that farmers could grow their own fuel. By 1935, soy was somehow involved in every step of the manufacturing process in his plants, from soy-based paints to plastic panels. He was said to have a suit made entirely of a silky soy fabric, and would give dinner parties with nothing but soybean items on the menu. And you thought I was into this stuff.

An integral part of Asian cooking, soybeans are fermented to make tasty and healthy miso, natto, tempeh, soy sauce, and tamari. The most common usages of soy are in milk and tofu, both of which are unfermented and made from the endosperm, or white part, of the bean and are therefore not much better than white bread. Whole soybeans also contain high levels of lecithin, necessary for the digestion of fat and breakdown of fat deposits in the body. They're also especially rich in iron, omega-3 fatty acids, tryptophan, molybdenum, manganese, fiber, vitamin K, magnesium, copper, B12 and potassium.

> "There's a crack in everything. That's how the light gets in."
> – Ayn Rand, *Anthem*

Raw soybeans contain "anti-nutrients" that affect humans and animals, and bind and prevent mineral absorption, binding to red blood cells and suppressing regeneration in adults and growth in children, and contain anti-coagulants which keep the blood from clotting. These attributes can be reduced by heat or broken down even more by sprouting, but the only way to enjoy all the benefits of soy with none of the drawbacks is by fermenting your sprouted beans. A few days of sprouting and a few days of fermenting will give you all of the goods and none of the bads. Soybeans can also be fermented into any of the appetizing items listed at the top of the previous paragraph with just a little more effort and patience.

Method: Jar or Bag, and Fermented

Spelt

Spelt is the ancestor of modern wheat, and one of the first known cultivated grains. Perhaps the first grain ever to be used to make bread, it originated in Southeast Asia and was brought to the Middle East more than 9000 years ago. As populations migrated throughout the continent, they brought this hearty and nutritious grain with them to their new lands. Spelt became especially popular in Germany, Switzerland and Austria, where it was called einkorn, or "one seed", for the single grain that grows in each of the plant's small flower spikes. The 13th Century Christian mystic and Benedictine Abbess St. Hildegard said of spelt: "Spelt is the best of grains, warming, lubricating and of high nutritional value. It is better tolerated by the body than any other grain. Spelt provides the consumer with good flesh and good blood and offers a cheerful disposition. It provides a happy mind and a joyful spirit. No matter how it is eaten, spelt is good and easy to digest." Spelt remained popular until the 19th century, and has been making a comeback in the last two decades, from 40 hectares in 1987 to over 3200 in the US just ten years later.

What brought the decline of spelt in the early 1900's is exactly the same reason it's growing in popularity now. Spelt has a tough hull, or husk, that makes it more difficult to process than modern wheat. The husk, separated just before milling not only protects the kernel, but helps retain nutrients and maintain freshness. Also, less pesticides are needed, so even spelt that's not organically grown (which is rare) is less toxic and more environmentally friendly. Wheat dominates the modern world's grains not because of its nutritional content or digestibility, but because of its commercial convenience. It's been bred for centuries to be easier to grow and process, so yields are higher and cheaper, and to have a high gluten content for the production of high-volume commercial baked goods. Spelt does have gluten, but it's water-soluble, making it much easier to digest than wheat, and is therefore an option for some people with wheat and/or gluten sensitivity. And unlike wheat, spelt has retained much of its ancient nutrition and flavor.

Spelt is naturally high in fiber and has up to 25% more protein than wheat. It's plentiful in B-vitamins, as well as mucopolysaccharides, special carbohydrates that are an important factor in blood clotting and stimulating the immune system. Spelt looks generally like wheat or oats, a small light brown cylinder with pinched ends and a deep crease running down the side. Its many health benefits are best enjoyed when it's grown into a highly nutritious grass and juiced, though it can be hit or miss because the necessary removal of the hard shell can sometimes be too much for the seed. It's always fine for sprouting if the inner shell has been broken or much of the germ has been removed, but since grass requires two weeks of growing it can be dicey. Kamut is a more reliable wheat grass; spelt is most useful in sprouted loaves that call for a lighter, sweeter flavor than Kamut's rich butteriness.

Method: Bag or Jar

Sunflower

As mentioned elsewhere, sunflowers are among my very favorite seeds to sprout. In their hulled form they sprout very quickly, less than a day from soak to spoon. They have as much protein as the same weight of chicken breast, and are a rich source of vitamins A, B complex, E, and even D, and minerals including calcium, copper, iron, magnesium, potassium, phosphorus, zinc, and linoleic acid (LA), an omega-6 essential fatty acid. Sunflower sprouts are also a good source of dietary fiber and contain phytosterols, which can help reduce cholesterol levels. They are also abundant in lecithin, necessary for the metabolization of fat and EFAs, both in the diet and stored in the body (lose the love handles).

Sunflower seeds contain the amino acid tryptophan that is responsible for processing serotonin, a neurotransmitter that creates a relaxed and content feeling – for this reason, sunflower seeds combat depression and stress. They blend up smoothly and make a nutty and delicious milk, and add a potent protein boost when used as a base for smoothies, soups, salad dressings, or desserts. And since they're so quickly at their best (8 hours of soaking and 8 hours of sprouting), they can be soaked along with non-sprouting seeds, which will drain as the sunflowers are sprouting. Throw in some pumpkin seeds, walnuts, millet, or hemp hearts, and soak them overnight. Drain them when you get up and let them sprout until you're ready for breakfast, then blend a handful of your mix in water with some vanilla and/or raw honey and/or cardamom, pour the fresh nut milk over the rest of them, add some dried fruit, and enjoy an outrageously easy and nutrient-rich living granola. Save a bit to combine with some honey, drop them on dehydrator sheets and enjoy amazing cookies after dinner.

Shell-on sunflower seeds can be grown into crunchy and succulent microgreens, delicate long white stalks with two thick green leaves on top. They're great added to sandwiches, veggie juices, wraps, dips and soups and can be the main lettuce in a salad. In fact, they may just be the top best-tasting, most nutritious sprouts in both the leafy green and nut-seed sprout categories. This makes them ideal for brand new sprouters and veteran kitchen sink famers alike.

Method: Hulled – Jar or Bag

With Shell: Grown into micro-lettuce

Triticale

A combination of wheat and rye first bred by French botanists as a possible solution to world hunger because it's very quick and easy to grow, and it's rich in simple and complex carbohydrates. It was hybridized in a laboratory setting, and though it's popular as a grass with some folks, I prefer to devote the space on my windowsill to time-tested ancestors of ancient, wild food. Triticale is still under development, though, and is listed here as an option for those working out large-scale solutions to pandemic hunger concerns.

Method: Grass (preferred), Jar or Bag

Wheat

What wheat has going for it is that it's widely available, though in its organic, sproutable form, it's not much more common than its superior cousins, spelt and kamut. It will grow into a nutritious grass and culture the right bacteria for a healthy probiotic water (see Kitchen Sink Farming Volume 2: Fermenting), but the small amount of extra effort to find wheat in its ancestral forms, which haven't been hybridized and genetically manipulated to yield an overly gluey, gummy texture, is well worth it.

For grass growing, it's available as a whole grain, called a berry, in several varieties; you'll want "hard red wheat berries", or one that's specifically labeled for grass.

Method: Grass (preferred), Jar or Bag

Wild Rice

Neither rice nor grain, wild rice is actually the fruit seed of a tall marsh grass native to the Great Lakes region of North America. Harvested by Native Americans for at least 10,000 years, wild rice was collected by canoe in shallow ponds and lakes. Look for organic "heirloom" varieties; descendants of these same plants that yield a shiny, black cylindrical pod with a nutty and satisfying flavor, because much of the wild rice sold today comes from hybridized seeds grown in man-made pools with no circulation for the toxic chemical fertilizers and pesticides that are liberally applied.

Wild rice is rich in calcium, iron, magnesium, phosphorus, vitamins C, E, and B-6, is 15% protein, and is a medium-length sprouter. Its sprouts are best after 4-8 days of rinsing when its hard shell bursts dramatically open to reveal a light-colored, creamy germ center. They're alive and more nutritious just a few hours after they're first drained, so if you're going to cook them, anytime after that is fine. But I recommend you wait and try them when they've opened – they're so soft and flavorful (and full of enzymatic life force) that I bet you'll want to eat them living after all. They are a little on the starchy side, so are best in a salad mix. Their flavor is rich and strong so can add a nice deep nutty taste to an otherwise mild mix. Their unusual color and shape adds a striking contrast to any dish.

Method: Jar or Bag

Herbs and Spices

These seeds will add interesting flavors and/or more subtle, medicinal benefits to sprout mixes; you wouldn't want to eat a handful of coriander or fennel seed sprouts, but throw some in with some pea and lentil sprouts and your pre-dressed mix will have built-in yum. Sprout some garlic seeds for a few days, then add garbanzo and sesame for another day for premixed hummus. I always have a jar of mustard sprouts in the fridge to add to salad dressings, and a tablespoon of cumin sprouts get ground up in anything remotely Latin.

Herbs have a rich history and mystical presence; I'm a fan of foods that are said to both increase vitality by stimulating the healing energy of the body as a whole, and more fancifully, purporting benefits like making one win in court cases (a surprising number of herbs advertise this advantage, actually), and can still be found under a grocery store chain's fluorescent light. Though many herbs are rich in nutrients, I haven't focused on their nutritional profiles here, because the small amount that most people use as a flavoring isn't really enough to nourish on a straight nutrient level. Instead, I'm expounding on their culinary use, fun histories and anecdotes, and their real or perceived effects on health, sometimes in a quite ensorcelled vein.

Herbs have been used since prehistoric times for all manner of denouements, so a good number of their agreed-upon values might just be passed-down superstition. Though there's medical evidence of garlic sprouts lowering cholesterol and fighting off infections and fenugreek seeds have been proven to lower inflammation and lessen dementia, I've always enjoyed herbs more for their culinary uses, leaving their more esoteric properties to my mom's friends that contribute to NPR. However, as a drop of poison in a million gallons of water can have an immediate and potent effect on human health, the subtle energetic qualities of food, the electrons of as-yet unknown chemical compounds vibrating just so, can have equally potent effects on well-being.

As with all seeds for sprouting, it is important to get organic, untreated seeds. Almost all non-organic herbs and spices are irradiated, which renders them biologically (and in all other ways) inactive and unsproutable.

Anise

Anise is a relative of dill, fennel, coriander, cumin and caraway. Many of these relations have been described as having a licorice flavor, but anise is the true taste of licorice - its oils are distilled into the flavoring for licorice candy, and ironically not from the herb licorice. Anise is native to the eastern Mediterranean region and Egypt. It is one of the oldest known plants that's been used for both culinary and medicinal purposes since ancient times; there is evidence that anise was used in Egypt as early as 1500 B.C. To aid digestion, the Romans enjoyed anise-spiced cakes after heavy meals and it was thusly spread throughout Europe by Roman legions. In the Bible, there is mention of paying tithes with anise, and in the 14th Century it was listed by King Edward I as a taxable drug, and merchants bringing it into London had to pay a heavy tax which went towards the repair of the London Bridge. Of the many qualities attributed to anise, I like what one writer puritanically warned: "it stirreth up bodily lust". It was also said to keep away nightmares if placed under one's pillow. Called "Tut-te See-Hau" by Native Americans, meaning "it expels the wind", anise's carminative (or anti-gas) properties have been known since antiquity. It helps with digestion and sweetens the breath, so it is chewed after meals in parts of Europe, the Middle East and India. Anise is a mild expectorant, often being used in cough mixtures and lozenges. It's also antispasmodic (suppresses muscle spasms), soporific (calming, or sleep-inducing in larger quantities) and a few seeds taken with water will often cure hiccups.

Anise is a long and tapered, light brown or greenish seed, about the size and shape of rice. It is a very strong seasoning, so it's best grown as a flavoring agent alongside grains for sprouted breads, and in desserts like fig pudding. Star anise, native to Asia, comes from an entirely different plant. It refers to the dried fruit which will not sprout.

Method: Jar or Bag

Caraway

Caraway seeds are native to North Africa and the Mediterranean, where they're sometimes called "Persian cumin". It's been used for at least 5000 years, making it one of the oldest known spices. Old herbal lore says that caraway can keep things from being stolen or lost, maybe because it was attractive to fowl and was used to keep chickens and pigeons from straying. It was also common for wives to flavor a straying husband's meal with the herb, possibly for the same reason.

It has a sweet warm aroma with a flavor similar to anise seed and fennel. It figures prominently in the cuisines of Germany, Austria, Eastern Europe and Scandinavia, and is traditionally paired with rye, resulting in that robust deli flavor. It's another rice-shaped seed, sometimes striped with lovely alternating bands of green-tinged brown and black.

Method: Jar or Bag

Cardamom

A wild plant native to Southern India, today cardamom is also cultivated in Sri Lanka, Guatemala, Indo-China and Tanzania. Cardamom is the fat seed-pod of a ginger-like plant, ranging in size and color from black and brown to light green, and is best just given a long soak. If you're set on germination, most likely for growing a cardamom plant, the pod's thick coating must be scarified to allow enough water in to the hidden seeds. Shake them in a container with some natural sand, then soak them for 24 hours, rinsing twice daily afterwards. The pod will open and the seeds will begin to sprout in three to six weeks. They can be planted anytime after the first soak, the soil kept warm and tropically moist.

Pungent and aromatic, with a eucalyptusy and lemony perfume, cardamom is said to be a digestive aid and aphrodisiac. It is indispensible in Indian cuisine; try the Mung-Cardamom Sundal in "Kitchen Sink Farming Volume 4: Homegrown Living Recipes - What to Do with Your Sprouts and Krauts".

Method: Long Soak, or scarify and germinate in a Jar

Celery Seed

Though it's relatively unknown in Western medicine, celery seed has been used medicinally for thousands of years in other parts of the world. From ancient times through today, India's Ayurvedic school of medicine uses celery seed to treat colds, flu, water retention, poor digestion, various types of arthritis, and diseases of the liver and spleen. Recent scientific studies have shown celery seed to be effective in the treatment of high blood pressure, cholesterol, and arthritis and can protect the liver from damaging substances such as acetaminophen (Tylenol). It helps reduce muscle spasms, calms the nerves, and reduces inflammation. Oils from the seed also act as a mosquito repellent.

Preliminary studies show that celery seed may help prevent the formation of cancerous tumors in mice[10]. In humans, researchers have found that people who eat a diet rich in lutein, which comes from spinach, broccoli, lettuce, tomatoes, oranges, carrots, and greens, and in which celery seeds are especially high, were significantly less likely to develop colo-rectal cancer.

Celery sprouts can be grown a little or a lot; thrown them into salad mixes or grow them into microgreens to add a beautiful elegance and mild celery flavor to sandwiches, soups, or tuna salad.

Method: Jar or Bag

---

[10] Banerjee S, Sharma R, Kale RK, Rao AR. Influence of certain essential oils on carcinogen-metabolizing enzymes and acid-soluble sulfhydryls in mouse liver. *Nutr Cancer*. 1994;21:263-269. Abstract.

Coriander

The small round seed from which the cilantro plant grows, coriander probably originated in the Middle East but has been used in Asia for millennium. It's the main ingredient in curry powders, and sprouted coriander makes an exceptional flavoring for salsa, especially for people who don't like cumin.

Coriander has been used to ease stomach upset for thousands of years; in India breastfeeding mothers drink coriander tea to ease their baby's colic. It can alleviate nausea and vomiting. Both the sprouted seeds and full-grown leaves have a cooling effect on the body so it's great for spicy Indian- or Mexican-themed summer meals. Buddhist monks grow coriander in monastery gardens to cool down their sexual urges and help maintain their celibacy.

Method: Jar or Bag, can be soil-grown into Micro-Cilantro

Cumin

Cumin is a medium-sized brownish seed, shaped like a thin tube tapering at each extremity with a tiny stalk attached. It's a stomachic (tones the stomach and stimulates appetite), diuretic (alleviates fluid retention and symptoms of PMS), carminative (anti-gas), stimulant, emmenagogic (promotes healthy menstruation), and antispasmodic (suppresses muscle spasms). Cumin is being researched as a natural way to increase breast size with positive results. In the ancient world cumin symbolized greed; thus the avaricious Roman Emperor, Marcus Aurelius, was given the offensive nickname "Cuminus".

Cumin has a spicy-sweet aroma and a pungent, powerful, sharp and slightly bitter flavor. It's very popular in spicy dishes all over the world: it features in Indian, Asian, Middle Eastern, Mexican, Portuguese and Spanish cookery. Cumin is an ingredient of most Indian curry powders, many Middle Eastern savory spice mixtures, and is the spice most people associate with Mexican salsa.

Method: Jar or Bag

Daikon

Daikon radish is an Asian cousin that's Japan's most common sprout with a thicker stem and slightly hotter flavor. It's otherwise just like a radish, and sprouts the same way.

Method: Basket (preferred) or Bag (not as leafy but way easier)

Dill

"Therewith her Veruayne and her Dill, That hindreth Witches of their will." (Michael Drayton's *Nymphidia*, 1627)

Dill is a light brown seed, winged oval in shape with one side flat and the other convex. Appearing in ancient Egyptian writings of 5,000 years ago, dill, from the Norse word "dilla", or "to lull," was once used in sleep tonics to aid insomnia and relieve colicky infants. In the Middle Ages it was used to dispel witchcraft, hence the above quote. Most North Americans associate its aromatic, fresh and slightly sweet flavor with pickles, and in Europe it's a common pastry flavoring. Dill sprouts easily and its pleasant, fresh taste gives a unique flavor to salad mixes, spreads for wraps, and nut cheese.

Method: Jar or Bag

Fennel

A native to Eurasia, this ancient and celebrated member of the carrot family was introduced to North America by Spanish priests, and it still grows wild around their old missions. It has been called the "meeting seed" by the Puritans who would chew it during their long church services. That may have been because of fennel seed's ability to freshen the breath, suppress the appetite (making it a powerful weight-loss agent), or its reputation as an anti-flatulent. The Puritans were a considerate bunch, as long as you weren't a witch. It could have also been for pure enjoyment; fennel seeds have a warm, sweet and aromatic flavor similar to a mild anise.

Fennel is one of my very favorite flavoring herb seeds to throw into a salad mix, as its refreshing licorice-y flavor, which goes with everything

> "Money is the most envied and least enjoyed. Health is the least envied and most enjoyed"
> - Charles Caleb Colton

always seems to be just the right amount.

Method: Jar or Bag

Fenugreek

Fenugreek, along with just about every other herb seed listed, is a digestive aid. Fenugreek contains natural expectorant properties ideal for treating sinus and lung congestion, reduces inflammation, and loosens and removes excess mucus and phlegm. Fenugreek is also an excellent source of selenium, an anti-radiant which helps the body utilize oxygen. But fenugreek's most exciting properties lie in its benefits to diabetics and those with blood sugar imbalances by slowing carbohydrate absorption and inhibiting glucose transport with several compounds, one of which, appropriately called fenugreekine, and is currently being researched for these effects. Fenugreek may also increase the number of insulin receptors in red blood cells and improve glucose utilization, thus demonstrating potential anti-diabetes effects in the pancreas and other organs. The amino acid 4-hydroxyisoleucine, contained in the seeds, may also directly stimulate insulin secretion. If your blood sugar drops and you get crabby when you don't eat, carry around some fresh or dried fenugreek sprouts and you may notice that everyone around you becomes less irritating.

Fenugreek has a powerful, aromatic and bittersweet flavor, likened by some to burnt sugar. It's used mainly in curries, especially vindaloo and the hot curries of Sri Lanka. It's also a classic component of mango chutney, a key ingredient in Yemenite Jews' unleavened Passover bread, and common in Ethiopian cooking. Fenugreek has mainly been used as a cattle fodder because of its tendency to quickly get bitter, making it a perfect young sprout. Its name actually comes from *foenum-graecum,* or "Greek

Hay" in Latin, illustrating this fact. Best for people after only a day or two of sprouting.

Method: Jar or Bag

Garlic Chives

Neither garlic nor chives, this unhurried sprout tastes like a mild cross between the two. Garlic doesn't produce seeds, only bulbs and shoots, so any reference to "garlic seeds" actually refers to this plant. Best sprouted by itself with the basket method, because garlic chives take a week and a half or two to grow into pungent and delicious microgreens, with most of the taste (but much easier on the stomach) than raw garlic bulbs. Garlic chive seeds are also extremely expensive; an actual garlic plant can be easily and cheaply grown by sticking a bulb into a bowlful of soil (see Kitchen Sink Farming Volume 3: Growing) and cutting its fast-growing tubular shoots as needed.

Method: Basket or Grown into Chives in a dish of soil

Milk Thistle

This one is purely for medicinal use – I doubt anyone would eat this hard-shelled, spicy-bitter sprout for its flavor, but everyone *should* for its wonderful liver-cleansing and -strengthening properties. The liver is our second largest organ, after the skin, the first focusing on removing toxins and the second on eliminating them and protecting against new ones. The liver pulls toxic substances from the bloodstream and digestive system, adds co-factors to make them inert, and sends them into the intestines to be eliminated. These toxins can be anything from environmental pollutants, cigarette smoke and smog, to pesticides, free-radicals from heated oils and fried or improperly digested foods, to drugs and alcohol, stress, food allergens, and negative emotions. The Chinese call the liver the "seat of emotions", and many massage therapists will tell you stories of sudden and major emotional releases while working on that area of their clients. But without proper support, the liver fills with poisons and is unable to neutralize them; essentially using the liver's working space for storage.

It's estimated that the average adult's liver is operating at around 20%; at just half-powered liver function it's possible to have radiant skin, limitless energy, ideal weight, and a consistently good mood. You may have noticed that young children in smoking households, who eat fast food for every meal and junk food in between still have glowing skin, boundless energy and enthusiasm. This is because their livers are not yet bulging with toxins and that incredibly powerful and efficient machine is still able to keep up with demand from its punishing bosses. These qualities can be regained at any age with liver cleansing and nutritional and herbal support.

Method: Jar or Bag; sprout for two days and chew them straight like gum if you can take the taste, otherwise toss them in the blender with sweet salad dressings or other blended goodness that will mask the flavor. Sweet cancels bitter and vice versa. They can also be dried, ground, and encapsulated.

Mustard

Though small, spherical mustard seeds are available in a hive of colors (from very light yellow to black); there are two types – normal ("dry") and mucilages. The mucilaginous form of the seed (forms a slippery encasement when wet) is generally of the darker brown varieties and the dry seeds are usually yellow, but there are exceptions to this rule. I prefer the ease with which mucilages sprout – just put them in a dish with some water and you're golden. Actually, different commercially-prepared mustards use different ratios of mucilages to dry, letting them sit for hours or days to achieve just the right dry-to-slime ratio before they're ground up and painted on brats and pretzels.

Mustard is classified in the brassica genus along with cabbage, broccoli, kale, and horseradish, all of which evolved from a common ancestor. This family of plants has a unique root system - after two or three days of sprouting, microscopic hair-like roots will begin to develop when the plant is dry, and will retreat back into the main root after watering. In a few more days, the tiny root-hairs will show up as a distinctive "fuzz" which some people will think is mold but now you know better. They are also quite tenacious and will cling together like puppies in a storm, and have to be separated after a week or so by vigorous rinsing or manual pulling apart. All sprouts produce heat, but mustard becomes especially toasty. For this reason, it's best grown when the weather is less than 80 degrees, and frequent cold-water rinsings can't hurt.

From a study done on the ability of sinigrin, a compound found in black mustard sprout juice, to protect against carcinogenic (cancer-causing) chemicals: "In conclusion, our findings indicate that i) mustard juice is highly protective against B(a)P-induced DNA damage in human derived cells and ii) that induction of detoxifying enzymes may account for its chemoprotective properties. iii) Furthermore, our findings show that the effects of crude juice cannot be explained by its allyl isothiocyanate contents." [11]

In simpler terms, i) black mustard protects the cell against free radical damage ii) if it's in its living state, but iii) they can't figure out why based on isolating its chemical components. I.e. - there's an as-yet unexplainable power in a living seed, a vitality beyond the scope of current scientific knowledge. Hey, they said it, not me.

Mustard sprouts are wonderful in sauces and soups, anything that begs for a bracing bite, and are indispensible in salad dressings not only for their distinctive sharp flavor but also for their role as an emulsifier – a stabilizer that keeps two unlike liquids, like oil and vinegar, from separating.

Methods: Mucilages: (usually brown) Long Soak or Clay

Dry seed: (usually yellow) Jar or Bag, or Soil-Grown into Micro-Mustard Greens

---

[11] *Teratogenesis Carcinog. Mutagen. Suppl. 1:273-282,* 2003 Wiley-Liss, Inc.

Onion

Like garlic, onion is an allium that takes 2 weeks to sprout, and is ridiculously expensive. Radish is cheaper, quicker, and also adds a bracing kick to dishes. If you love onion, try growing onions or scallions (green onions, the tops can be used in the same way as onions and will continue to grow like grass) in dirt-filled yogurt containers. Your choice: one seed = one continuous 6" plant or 50 seeds = one bite of onion sprouts.

Method: Basket

Poppy

Poppy seeds come in two varieties – "blue" or European, and "white" or Asian. I can't tell the difference in color or flavor, and as far as I can tell the names are based on region, not culinary differences. The opium poppy that's native to the Middle East and also grown in Southeast Asia is a different species. An inert variety grows wild and is also cultivated in Europe and North America. The Eastern variety yields opium and other narcotics, and it is grown solely for this lucrative purpose. Poppy seeds sold for food use (and therefore home sprouts) have none of theoids that comprise any drug. Sorry.

The good news is that store-bought poppy seeds, unlike hemp (which is unnecessarily sterilized, as they can't be grown into an inert relative of marijuana) will sprout beautifully. High in protein and healthy oils, poppy sprouts also make an exotic, metallic-blue colored garnish. Like nuts, they tend to lose a little of their nuttiness and crunch when sprouted, but make up for it with a sublimely subtle sweetness. Poppy seeds are the very smallest seeds in the kitchen sink farmer pantry, so make sure to use a tightly-woven bag or fine mesh screen over your jar. Try them in Strawberry-Poppy Seed Vinaigrette or Almond-Citrus Poppy Sprout Cookies (both in "Kitchen Sink Farming Volume 4: Homegrown Living Recipes - What to Do with Your Sprouts and Krauts").

Method: Bag or Jar with fine mesh

Nuts

For the purposes of this book, nuts are the protein and fat-rich inner section of a hard-shelled seed. Because the shell is removed, nuts don't sprout. They do, however, contain valuable nutrients and their sometimes difficult digestibility and access to their nutrients is greatly improved by soaking. With the exception of wild peanuts, which aren't actually nuts and therefore not in this section (see pg 127) and almonds, which are actually "drupes" (shelled tree-fruit) in heavy rotation in my kitchen and are slightly sproutable due to the protection of their unusually thick inner shell, I don't eat a lot of nuts. Our ancestors probably avoided them in large quantities because of their hard shells; smashing them between rocks to get at the (then) mutilated tiny bite was not a wise transaction of energy, so we never really developed the ability to digest them in quantity. They're not strictly living and are still not a good bargain of digestive effort, especially for those that are used to a 100% living food diet. They can be a great way to transition to less or no meat, satisfying a craving for dense, protein- and fat-rich foods.

Nuts have better than no cholesterol: they're very rich in phytosterols, which block the absorption of unhealthy fats by the cells. These compounds can lower cholesterol and arterial plaque, and reduce the potential of heart disease by up to 15%. [12] There is some evidence, however, that phytoserols can lead to artheriosclerosis, a hardening of the arteries, so again nuts are a good transition food but not something that should have a permanently major role in the

---

[12] "Consumption of a Functional Oil Rich in Phytosterols and Medium-Chain Triglyceride Oil Improves Plasma Lipid profiles in Men" *Journal of Nutrition* (133): 1815–1820.

diet. If they can keep other, worse things out of your mouth then great, and they can be fun to play with in the kitchen, especially for crusts and creamy milk. Of course, their digestibility, fat content, and nutrition is greatly improved by fermenting them into nut cheese and yogurt, as the tenacious chemical bonds that keep them indigestible will be shattered by the work of our little fermenting friends, as the fats and nutrients are the building blocks of healthier compounds in their little paws. See Kitchen Sink Farming Volume 2: Fermenting for more info.

The harder the shell, the more powerful the enzyme inhibitors, so nuts must be dealt with conscientiously if they're to do more good than harm. Soaking them changes their very nature, taking them from hard, dry, and brittle to soft and creamy morsels with complex layers of flavor. They will lose some of their nuttiness, and won't have any of the roasted flavor you might be used to. In fact, soaked green pistachios might be mistaken for fresh peas, and soaked macadamias could be marketed as exotic and delectable fresh fruits. Drained, they'll last a couple of weeks in the fridge, and some of their rich nutty flavor, now more easily assimilable by our digestion, can be returned by low-temp baking or dehydrating.

Because nuts won't sprout, soaking them in salt water will provide all the benefits of soaking as well as enhance the flavor in some cases. The Aztecs soaked their pumpkin and squash seeds in seawater (1 part sea salt to 8 parts water) before they roasted them in the sun, and the process makes quite the delicious snack. Unless they're going to be used for a dessert (and sometimes even then), salt water-soaking makes a tasty, IE-free, vitamin enhanced nut.

Almonds

Today, almonds are grown mostly in California, Italy, and Spain. A law was quietly passed in 2007 which required pasteurization of all California-grown almonds, which presumably kills a pathogen found once on almonds that weren't grown organically and had no immune system of their own, but this heating process also destroys the enzymatic life of the seed. Pasteurized almonds are dead almonds. The only way to buy almonds that are still replete with life is to buy European nuts, the shipping of which can be expensive, or buy unpasteurized almonds directly from the grower at a roadside stand, which a loophole in the law allows. Fortunately, some crafty farmers have set up "internet farmer's markets", where unpasteurized organic almonds and other products can be bought cheaply and with free shipping. Check out the "Resources" section of this book for my favorites.

Almonds are the only alkalizing nuts (see pg 122), and the most nutritious, depending on how you classify them. They are a very complete food, containing generous amounts of protein (12% RDA), healthy fats, and all the "macrominerals", the minerals needed daily in large quantity by the body (except for sodium, which most of us get plenty of already). They contain more than double the amount of calcium in milk, 6 times the magnesium and 40 times the phosphorus, along with a good supply of potassium. They are also rich in many "microminerals", like folic acid, copper and zinc along with 35% of the recommended daily allowance of vitamin E.

They also contain an impressive amount of phytochemicals, a large family of compounds that have been used medicinally for millennia for varied health benefits, and are in use today in modern Western medicine for their effects against heart disease and cancer. Dr. Gary Beecher, Lead Researcher for the in-house research arm of the US Department of Agriculture, analyzed the phytochemical content of almonds and stated: "I have never seen this diversity of phytochemicals in a single food source" in a symposium entitled "Nuts in a Healthful Diet", as a part of the 1998 Experimental Biology annual meeting. Almonds are helpful in fighting heart disease in another way as they contain resveritrol, the ingredient in red wine oft-acclaimed at cocktail parties to maintain a healthy cardio-vascular system as an excuse to have another glass. Of course, almonds don't have the drawbacks of alcohol but you will not be popular if you share this fact.

Like most commonly available nuts, almonds have been shelled, but the protective barrier between the hard shell and the soft white flesh of the nut is so thick and fibrous that it will remain intact during the shelling process. This brown skin completely wraps the inner flesh of the nut and is full of enzyme inhibitors, and when fresh, organic almonds are soaked, the water will become quite mucky. Almonds should be soaked for 8-10 hours, becoming deliciously plump in the process. It's best to drain and refill the soak water a few times during the soaking stage, as clean, clear water will bring out the best in the almonds and keep them fresh longer. Because of this relatively thick protective skin, almonds can be sprouted slightly for a day or two after they're drained. Your newly alive almonds should be rinsed once or twice every 8-12 hours, which will cause a small green sprout to form inside the nut, which can be seen if the two halves of the nut are pulled apart and you look closely. Not the dramatic explosion of root and leaf like other sprouting seeds, but we've nonetheless gotten every possible microgram of nutrition out of this special little seed. Because we've removed the almond's natural protection against the elements, they should be refrigerated or low-temperature dried sooner than later, or they will quickly be enjoyed by your local microbial community. As they start to ferment they will get a smell and taste akin to an old-fashioned perfume, which is somewhat delightful in subtle amount but can become overbearing after a few days (kind of like some people who wear old-fashioned perfume).

When sprouted, almonds make a deliciously fresh and nutty butter when ground, and a creamy, frothy white milk when blended with water and strained through a sprouting bag to remove the flecks of brown skin, a totally optional step. The ground skin is slightly bitter and can be used for a skin scrub or dried and used in cookies and breads. This skin is indigestible cellulose, aka insoluble fiber, so if you dry it for future uses don't worry about the temperature or protecting non-existent enzymes and nutrients.

Method: Soak 8-10 hours, sprout in Bag (preferred) or Jar

Brazil Nuts

The seeds of a massive Amazonian tree, Brazil nuts are the largest and oiliest nut in common use, maybe because they have the hardest shell of all time. When soaked, they become quite a bit lighter in flavor as they swell with water. Brazil nuts are great for food preparation as they blend completely and add a subtly exotic deliciousness to a drink or dish. Rich in selenium, a powerful antioxidant for cellular regeneration and protection, Brazil nuts also have sulfur, potassium, and phosphorus.

Soak time: 4-6 hours

Cashews

The seed of a small pear-like fruit that is indigenous to Central and South America, cashews are today primarily grown in India. A relative of poison ivy and sumac, toxins in the shell must be destroyed by cooking the fruit until the nut's outer shell bursts, revealing a light brown hook-shaped nut with a succulent flavor. They have several flaws, unfortunately, such as containing the irritant urushiol, the same toxic oil in poison ivy that causes rashes. Cashews are also extremely high in oleic and monounsaturated fats. These omega-6 and 9 oils are needed in small quantities, but an overabundance will leach the more illusive omega-3's from our system and resulting in a cadre of health problems. For these reasons, I don't recommend over-using them in your food preparation, as most raw food restaurants seem to, with every item on the menu including them. That being said, cashews are pretty much the bacon of the nut world. They make everything taste better, and like bacon bits in salads, foods with cashew pieces in them become a game of "hunt for the nuts". They blend smoothly into a delicious creamy base for soups, sauces, or a whipped dessert topping, which is probably why they're leaned on so heavily by natural food chefs. The heating process destroys any vestigial enzymes that might be present however, and many cashews are treated much worse with the help of radiation and toxic gasses. In any case, they're not a potently enzyme-rich alkalizer like, for example, almonds or sunflower sprouts. Because of the two strikes of an unbalanced ratio of fats and that their life force is cooked away, judicious use is recommended.

Soak for 2-4 hours

Hazelnuts (Filberts)

Grape-sized reddish nuts, hazelnuts have creamy white inner flesh that has an instantly recognizable flavor that's amazing in both sweet and savory dishes. Rich in calcium, potassium, phosphorus, and healthy fats, un-soaked hazelnuts have a slightly bitter flavor. If you already like them, you're in for a real treat when you try them sprouted.

Soak for 8-12 hours

Macadamia Nuts

Native to Australia, the macadamia nut tree was originally brought to Hawaii as an ornamental, with no knowledge of the incredibly delicious nut which would become one of the islands' main cash crops. The sweet and oily marble-sized nut is great in desserts and as a sweet component chopped up in a salad, and their elegant richness makes them a great candidate for cheese (see Kitchen Sink Farming Volume 2: Fermenting).

Soak for 2-4 hours

Peanut

See pg 127

Pecans

An exquisite nut from the hickory family, pecans look somewhat like a walnut (both of which remind me of a dual-lobed wrinkly brain, and traditional medicine draws connections between the nut and the organ) and have a rich, buttery flavor. High in potassium, phosphorus, and vitamin A, pecans are native to North America and grown in temperate southeastern climates. They're thusly marvelous in recipes with an earthy Native American vibe or comforting southern feel, and pecan-crusted or -filled pies are the quintessence of cach.

Soak 4-6 hours

Pine Nuts (Piñolas)

Labor-intensively hand-harvested from the inside of certain varieties of pine cones, pine nuts are a torpedo-shaped rich and flavorful addition to tapenade and stuffed vegetables, and are an essential ingredient in pesto (though they are expensive, which is why I make pesto out of walnuts and/or sunflower seeds and sprinkle some pine nuts on top of the finished dish). Extremely high in Vitamins K and E, manganese, copper, zinc and magnesium, pine nuts are also a good source of niacin, thiamine, iron, and potassium.

Soak 2-4 hours

Pistachios

Native to the Middle East, pistachios are a long and lumpy nut with a distinctive green hue. Organic is essential here, as all sorts of nefarious things are done to pistachios conventionally grown, from steaming open the shells before they're ready, to chemically dying the whole thing red to cover up the bruising that happens when they sit on the ground for too long. Natural pistachios are a wonderfully sweet, nutty treat, and should be purchased without the shell if they're to be used for any other reason than keeping my brother and I quiet on road trips in the 1980's. High in protein, copper, manganese, B6, thiamine, and phosphorus.

Soak 8-12 hours

Pumpkin Seeds (Pepitas)

Though not strictly nuts, pumpkin seeds are included in this section because they won't form a root system in the edible form, and will start to rot if they're left moist like sprouting seeds. These seeds of the pumpkin squash are naturally encased in a slippery white shell that's all fiber, both soluble (the natural slipperiness creating a lubricating gel in the digestive tract) and insoluble (the cellulose casing is indigestible and acts like a scouring pad, scrubbing away undigested matter in the intestines and colon). Unlike nuts, this shell doesn't have to be removed from the seed to make it edible, but it does have to be dried before water can soak through it to work its magic on the enzyme inhibitors beneath. That's only if you're harvesting your own pumpkin seeds post Jack-O-Lobotomy; commercial harvesters dry the seed until the shell cracks and is easily removable, leaving the unsproutable flat, dark green seed behind.

Pepitas are one of my favorite nuts for their abundance in healthy oils, vitamins and minerals that are rare in the nut world, high fiber and distinctive taste. They blend up into a creamy froth and contribute equally to all world cuisines, from North and South American to Mediterranean and Asian, maybe because varieties of squash are found all over the world.

More than a third protein, just one cup of pumpkin seeds provides 68% of the RDA, as well as 115% of iron, 185% of magnesium, 96% of copper, 89% of Vitamin K, 162% of phosphorus, and 208% manganese.

Soak 8-10 hours, this is a good one for salt water-soaking), 1 part sea salt to 8 parts agua

Walnuts

Like pecans, walnuts are the woody-shell encased fruit from a flowering tree in the hickory family, but are more rich and deliciously bitter than pecans. There are two varieties: the English walnut which is golden brown in color, lightly sweet, and has a higher percentage of the illusive omega-3s than any other nut, and the black walnut which is more intensely flavored and higher in protein, vitamins and minerals. Walnuts are also anti-microbial, especially effective against Candida, and have been shown to decrease inflammation and lower cholesterol, both beneficial to the blood vessels. The hull is used for many medicinal purposes, not least of which is getting rid of parasites in the digestive tract and blood. These benefits are available to lesser degree, but a much better tasting one, in the nut.

Soak 8 hours or so

Appendix B: Sprouting Table

This chart is meant to be a quick and easy reference for sprouting. It won't hurt to do it "right" the first time, so you get it, then do what you like; the general rule is: soak overnight, drain and rinse a couple of times a day until your sprouts are to your liking. Soon you'll be an expert in how to get your favorite seeds, in your climate, to be the best they can be for your particular likes and needs. The seed is the real teacher.

NAME	SPROUTING METHOD	SOAK TIME (HOURS)	SPROUT TIME/DAYS	NUTRIENTS/PROPERTIES	NOTES
Adzuki	Jar or Bag	Long, 8-10	2	Protein, Iron, phosphorous, K, A, C	Adds beautiful red color to mixes; watch out for "duds"
Alfalfa	Basket for Nano Greens; though Jar or Bag is fine if with Salad Mix	Medium, 6-8	2-3 in Salad Mix; 5-7 for Nano Greens	Abundance of enzymes and hard-to-find trace minerals and micronutrients, from its special root system	Very healthy, mild and a little boring. Will grow 16 times their size, so start 1 T seeds for every 1 C. of sprouts desired.
Amaranth	Bag	Zero	0	Protein (including the aminos lysine and methonine), calcium and its cofactors magnesium and silicon	Quick sprouts; will get bitter after 2 days. Though the seeds are small like alfalfa and clover, they'll yield only 30% more sprout than seed.
Black Beans	Jar or Bag	Long, 8-10	1-2	Molybdenum, folate, fiber, tryptophan, manganese, protein, starches	Difficult to digest – best as a garnish, or ground, rinsed, and fermented. Or, if you're going to cook them anyways, it's best to sprout them first.
Barley	Tray Method for Grass; Jar or Bag for Sprouts	Prolonged, 10-12	2-3 for Sprouts; 6-9 for Grass	Chlorophyll, enzymes including SOD, iron, folic acid, C and B-vitamins	Can lower cholesterol and regulate blood sugar. Fairly bitter flavor.
Broccoli	Basket for Nano Greens; though Jar or Bag is fine if with Salad Mix	Medium, 6-8	2-3 in Salad Mix; 5-7 for Nano Green Sprouts; 7-10 for Micro Greens	Cancer-fighting SGS, vitamins A C, and E, calcium, phosphorous and magnesium	Will grow 16 times their size, so soak 1 T seeds for every 1 C. of sprouts.
Buckwheat	Tray Method for Grass; Jar or Bag for Sprouts	Prolonged, 10-12	2-3 for Sprouts; 6-9 for Grass	Chlorophyll, Iron, Lecithin, Potassium, Vitamins A, and C and Calcium	Mild, very tender leaves are a great addition to a salad or way to ease into drinking grass juice; plant 50% buckwheat to start.
Cabbage	Jar or Bag, never a basket	Long, 8-10	4-8	Very high in vitamin C; glucosinates have anti-cancer and anti inflammatory properties	One of the most nutritious sprouts. 5 to 1 yield. mild cabbage flavor.

NAME	SPROUTING METHOD	SOAK TIME (HOURS)	SPROUT TIME/DAYS	NURIENTS/PROPERTIES	NOTES
Chia	Long Soak or Clay Method	Continuous Soak	2 days for Long Soak (a small tail may or may not be visible), then refrigerate. 5-6 days for Nano Greens	Very powerful food. The most Omega-3s of any plant source and without the toxic heavy metals of fish sources. Calcium, phosphorous, magnesium, iron, niacin, zinc, manganese, copper, molybdenum.	Like flax the world's easiest sprout/ micro green to grow.
Clover	Basket for Nano Greens; Jar or Bag is fine if with Salad Mix	Medium, 6-8	2-3 in Salad Mix; 5-7 for Nano Greens	Vitamins A, B, C, E and K, Calcium, Iron, Magnesium, Phosphorus, Potassium, Zinc, Carotene, Chlorophyll, Aminos, Trace Elements, Protien	Nutrient profile is excellent for women. Will grow 16 times their size, so soak 1 T seeds for every 1 C. of sprouts.
Flax	Long Soak or Clay Method	Continuous Soak	2 days for Long Soak, until the shell opens and a small tail pokes out, then refrigerate. 5-6 days for Nano Greens	Omega-3 EFAs, awesome fiber, complete protein. A recommended daily health boost.	The world's easiest sprout/ micro-green.
Garbanzo	Jar or Bag	Long, 8-10	2-3	Fiber, molybdenum, manganese, folate	Still starchy even after sprouting, a coarse grind and rinse is suggested. Essential in hummus and falafel.
Hemp	Jar or Bag	Prolonged, 8-12	2-3 – refrigerate when tail is as long as the seed; sterilized seeds will stop sprouting and begin to mold after a few days.	Best vegetable source of protein, better than animal by some points of view. EFAs galore, fiber, vitamin E, lecithin, potassium, magnesium, iron, zinc, sulphur, phytosterols, inositol, edestin	Hemp seeds are sterilized by law in the US; they will only grow a tiny tail no matter how long they're grown. Stop after 2-3 days, before they mold.

NAME	SPROUTING METHOD	SOAK TIME (HOURS)	SPROUT TIME/DAYS	NUTRIENTS/PROPERTIES	NOTES
Kamut	Tray Method for Grass; Jar or Bag for Sprouts	Prolonged, 10-12	2-3 for Sprouts; 6-9 for Grass	40% more protein than wheat, magnesium, niacin, thiamine, and zinc, healthy fats. May be untroublesome to people with wheat and gluten allergies.	Adds a rich buttery taste to sprouted loaves.
Lentil	Jar or Bag	Long, 8-10	2-3	26 % protein and high in calcium, magnesium, sulfur, potassium, phosphorous, and vitamins A, B, C, and E.	Best when the tail is as long as the bean.
Millet, Unhulled Only	Jar or Bag	Long, 8-10	2	Serotonin and tryptophan regulate mood, appetite, sleep, muscle contraction, memory and learning. Also rich in anti-oxidants, magnesium (can help reduce the affects of migraines and heart attacks), niacin (can help lower cholesterol), phosphorus (helps with fat metabolism, tissue repair and energy production) and nutrients that protect against diabetes, cancer and asthma	I've only ever been able to find unhulled online; see "resources" section.
Mung	Growing into bean sprouts is recommended, otherwise jar or bag	Long, 8-10	If sprouted by the rinse method, 2-4	Chlorophyll, iron, vitamin C, potassium, and are a complete protein	Watch out for duds if sprouting by the rinse method.

NAME	SPROUTING METHOD	SOAK TIME (HOURS)	SPROUT TIME/DAYS	NURIENTS/PROPERTIES	NOTES
Oats, Unhulled Only	Tray Method for Grass; Jar or Bag for Sprouts	Prolonged, 10-12 or more	2-3 for Sprouts; 6-9 for Grass	Amazing source of both kinds of fiber, a natural laxative, intestinal scrubber, and stool bulker. B vitamins, E, iron calcium, and GLA	The fibrousness of the husk varies a lot from company to company; less husk = less fiber but also less it has to be ground to break up the somewhat unpleasant tough fibers, which are like hard and sharp tiny strings in the mouth. See "Resources".
Pea	Jar or Bag for Sprouts; Tray Method for Pea Shoots	Prolonged, 10-12	1 day or more for Sprouts; for Pea Shoots 3-4 days covered or in the dark then 3-4 days in sun	Complex carbohydrates, calcium, magnesium, folic acid, vitamins A, Bs, C, and E. 25% protein. Green peas have chlorophyll.	Delicious and tender at any age. Will not get bitter so start a big batch and eat it for weeks. Huge variety of colors and sizes.
Peanut	Jar or Bag	Medium, 6-8	2, just after the point (the germ) has protruded	30% protein and 45% oil, very high in vitamin E, folate, niacin, riboflavin, magnesium, phosphorous, phytochemicals, and fiber.	A legume, not a nut, peanuts are an easy sprout and great way to bridge the mental gap between an inanimate everyday food and a growing seed.
Quinoa	Bag	Medium, 6-8	1-2	A complete protein, and higher in protein than any other grain. More calcium than milk and the cofactor magnesium, as well as silicon, iron, B vitamins, phosphorous and vitamin E, and magnesium, important in the fight against heart disease and diabetes. Manganese and copper fight the free radicals that cause cancer and aging.	A vital grain for a healthy population, fights heart disease, diabetes, and cancer, and could solve many of the world's biggest problems if it was the planet's primary protein source. Contains no gluten and is therefore not allergy-producing. High levels of enzyme inhibitors; change the soak water a couple of times. When rinsing, continue until there are no more foamy bubbles.
Rice, Brown	Germinated	Soaked 1 – 3 days		Fiber, GABA reduces anxiety and stress, magnesium, potassium, zinc, E and many B vitamins	Must be cooked. Improves health, digestibility and flavor, but is also a simple step that could lead to large-scale increase in food mass and amplified nutrition for much of the world.

NAME	SPROUTING METHOD	SOAK TIME (HOURS)	SPROUT TIME/DAYS	NURIENTS/PROPERTIES	NOTES
Rye	Tray Method for Grass; Jar or Bag for Sprouts	Prolonged – 10-12	2-3 for Sprouts; 6-9 for Grass	Fluorine strengthens teeth and tooth enamel, and its photoestrogenic lignans can help normalize hormone activity, helpful for all, especially the menopausal.	Less processed than whole wheat and retains more nutrients. Less gluten than wheat yield a dense, sweet-sour loaf. Grass juice is powerfully cleansing. Makes a sour-sweet probiotic water reminiscent of rye bread, pickles, and NY delis.
Sesame, Unhulled Only	Jar or Bag	Medium – 6-8	2	1000 times the calcium as milk, phosphorous, potassium, magnesium, and vitamin A.	Very easy to digest, rich oily flavor is great in both savory and sweet dishes, like hummus and halva, a sweet, dense confection popular in India, the Middle East, and North Africa.
Soybeans	Jar or Bag	2-12 depending on the seed; check every 2 hours for softness. Will fall apart if soaked too long.	2-5, depending on preference	A complete protein, also rich in iron, omega-3 fatty acids, tryptophan, molybdenum, manganese, fiber, vitamin K, magnesium, copper, B12 and potassium	Produces much more protein per acre than any other major vegetable crop, and much more than land used for meat or milk production. Can also rejuvenate nutrients in the soil. Sprouts are best ground, rinsed, and fermented.
Spelt	Tray Method for Grass; Jar or Bag for Sprouts	Prolonged – 10-12	2-3 for Sprouts; 6-9 for Grass	High in fiber, up to 25% more protein than wheat. Plentiful in B-vitamins, and special carbohydrates that assist in blood clotting and stimulating the immune system	Wheat's ancient ancestor. Not the best choice for grass juice, should be used in sprouted loaves that require a lighter, sweeter flavor than Kamut's butteriness.
Unhulled Sunflower, for Lettuce	Soil Method	Prolonged, 10-12	2-3 days covered with a wet towel, 5-7 days in the sun until the seeds mostly fall off, but before the second set of leaves come in.	Chlorophyll galore, all the vitamins and minerals below and more.	Will float insatiably in the soak water – submerge a filled sprout bag and weigh it down, or fill a jar until the seeds are high above the rim and screw on the lid, pushing all the seeds into the water.

NAME	SPROUTING METHOD	SOAK TIME (HOURS)	SPROUT TIME/DAYS	NURIENTS/PROPERTIES	NOTES
Sunflower Sprouts, Hulled	Jar or Bag	Medium, 6-8	1	33% protein, vitamins A, B complex, E, and D, and minerals including calcium, copper, iron, magnesium, potassium, phosphorus, and zinc. Omega-6 essential fatty acid. Phytosterols can help reduce cholesterol levels, lecithin is necessary to process EFAs and fats, both new and old. Tryptophan combats depression and stress.	Super easy sprout done before the first rinse. Can be therefore soaked with unsproutable nuts, like walnuts for an EFA balance, pumpkin seeds for a savory snack, or macadamias for a rich desserty treat. Won't sprout and will therefore lose a little nutrition if soaked in salt water, but won't trade their nutty flavor for a sprouty freshness – nice every once in a while.
Triticale	Tray Method for Grass; Jar or Bag for Sprouts	Prolonged, 10-12	2-3 for Sprouts; 6-9 for Grass		A combination of wheat and rye first bred by French botanists as a possible solution to world hunger as it's very quick and easy to grow, as well as rich in simple and complex carbohydrates.
Wheat	Tray Method for Grass; Jar or Bag for Sprouts	Prolonged, 10-12	2-3 for Sprouts; 6-9 for Grass		Use "hard red wheat berries" for grass juice. Good for grass and probiotic water (though not as good as Kamut, and not much cheaper or more available in an organic form.)
Wild Rice	Jar or Bag	Prolonged, 10-12	4-8	calcium, iron, magnesium, phosphorous, vitamins C, E, and B-6, is 15% protein.	Not rice nor grain, the fruit seed of a tall marsh grass enjoyed by Native Americans for the past 10 centuries. Will not grow a tail; is done which wild rice kernel split in two.
Herbs/Spices	Method	Soak, hours	Sprouting, Days	Flavor	Notes
Anise	Jar or Bag	Medium, 6-8	2	The true taste of licorice; digestive aid since Roman times.	

NAME	SPROUTING METHOD	SOAK TIME (HOURS)	SPROUT TIME/DAYS	NURIENTS/PROPERTIES	NOTES
Caraway	Jar or Bag	Medium, 6-8	2	Sweet, warming – pair with rye in probiotic water or sprouted bread for a robust deli flavor	
Cardamom	Jar or Bag	Prolonged, 24	3 – 6 weeks, if growing into a plant	Pungent and aromatic, with a eucalyptusy and lemony perfume, a digestive aid and aphrodisiac	A seed pod with a thick hull, must be soaked and ground (preferable) or germinated
Celery	Jar or Bag for Sprouts, Basket for Nano Green Sprouts or Soil for Micro Greens	Medium, 6-8	2-3 for Sprouts; 5-9 for Micro Greens	Mild celery flavor is wonderful in many dishes	Very medicinal; can help fight cancer and cholesterol
Coriander	Jar or Bag, or Soil for Micro Cilantro	Medium, 6-8	2-3 for Sprouts, 5-9 for Micro Cilantro	Cooling and delicious	
Cumin	Jar or Bag	Medium, 6-8	2	Featured in Indian, Middle Eastern, and Latin cookery in both Europe and N. America	Many wonderful digestive benefits
Dill	Jar or Bag for Young Sprouts; Basket for Nano Greens	Medium, 6-8	2-3 for Young Sprouts; 5-9 for Nano Greens	Aromatic, fresh and slightly sweet flavor; equally at home in micro-green salads, spreads, and seed cheese	
Fennel	Jar or Bag for Young Sprouts; Basket for Nano Greens	Medium, 6-8	2-3 for Young Sprouts; 5-9 for Nano Greens	Warm, sweet and aromatic flavor similar to a mild anise.	Freshens the breath, suppresses appetite, digestive benefits; a wonderful addition to a salad mix.
Fenugreek	Jar or Bag	Long, 8-10	2-6 days; great very young or just after the first leaves show	Powerful, aromatic and bittersweet flavor; use in curries and with to balance very sweet tropical fruit, both in flavor and nutritionally.	Preferably yellow and tender; a quick sprout that doesn't need sun. Expectorant, anti-inflammatory, regulates blood sugar.
Garlic	Basket	Medium, 6-8	4-8	Garlicky! Easier on the stomach than raw garlic, but prohibitively slow and expensive	Better to just plant some garlic in a yogurt container and cut its fast-growing tubular shoots as needed.

NAME	SPROUTING METHOD	SOAK TIME (HOURS)	SPROUT TIME/DAYS	NURIENTS/PROPERTIES	NOTES
Milk Thistle	Jar or Bag	Long, 8-10	1-2	Unparalleled liver cleanser and strengthener for better sleep, skin, and mood.	Hard-shelled; won't soften up much. Super bitter - best ground in juices in a high-speed blender, chewed up as a crunchy snack, or grond and put in capsules.
Mustard	Clay Planter Tray for Mucilages (Usually Brown); Jar or Bag for Dry (Usually Yellow)	Mucliage - Continous Soak. Dry Seed in Jar or Bag – Medium, 6-8	Long Soak – about 2, until a small tail protrudes, then refrigerate. Jar or Bag - 2-3	With a little apple cider vinegar, raw honey, and savory spices, makes a better mustard than you've ever had	Preferable yellow and tender, don't need sun. An emulsifier, go in almost all of my salad dressings and all soups and sauces inspired by Eastern European cuisines
Onion	Basket	Long, 8-10	4-8		Slow and expensive, better to use radish sprouts, or plant some green onion and cut its grass-like shoots
Poppy	Bag	Medium, 6-8	2 – will get bitter after	Not much flavor in small quantities so can be a versatile garnish; in larger quantities has a fresh and sweet taste, like candied bean sprouts.	Adds a beautiful metallic blue color to a dish when sprinkled on top.
Radish/Daikon	Basket for Micro Greens; Jar or Bag if with Salad Mix	Medium, 6-8	2-3 for Sprouts; 5-6 for Micro Greens	Spicy and zesty! Its heat is stimulating to the digestive system, removes mucous in the intestines and respiratory system, fires up elimination.	Will grow 16 times their size, so soak 1 T seeds for every 1 C. of sprouts. Move to a sunny spot after a couple day's growth. Antiseptic, anti-parasitic, and supportive to beneficial bacteria, so good for Candida sufferers (perhaps 85% of the population)

Fermenting - The "How?"

This chapter won't teach you how to make more food for less dough like the ones on sprouting and growing will, but you will learn how to make the food you have more nutritious, digestible, interesting, and last a whole lot longer. Fermented foods also have longer-lasting health benefits, as the beneficial bacteria you'll be cultivating will devotedly colonize your digestive system and, given the right conditions, can continue to enthusiastically propagate for the rest of your life.

> "Bacteria keep us from heaven and put us there." - Martin H. Fischer, 19th-century physician and writer

Fermentation is what happens when microorganisms 1) digest sugar, whether from cane, fruit, dairy, or starch, turning it into new and beneficial compounds, and 2) break the bonds of hardy molecules into their easier-to-digest, simpler components. This healthful process changes the nature of food and drink, giving us cheese, sauerkraut, yogurt, beer, soda, and countless other new and wonderful foods that come from all around the world. Home growing and sprouting is an significant way to take control of your health, but fermentation, though cheap and easy, is just as important.

A Brief History of Slime

For as long as humans have been on the planet, fermented foods have been appreciated for their distinctive flavors and nutritional benefits. They have sustained people through long winters and sea voyages, frequently and dramatically changed the course of human history, and their creation has been attributed to the gods. The real agents in the mystical transformation of honey into intoxicating nectar, cabbage into sauerkraut, grapejuice into wine, and cyanide-laden tubers into nutritious food that sustains the native peoples of Central America, are the oldest, wisest, and most mysterious life forms on the planet.

> "Bacteria have studied us more closely and more lovingly than any other creature. Even your dog can't give you the devotion that bacteria do." - Abigail Salyers, Ph. D, Professor of Microbiology at the University of Illinois.

Microorganisms, recognized for their health-giving benefits since the end of the 19th century, were thought to battle the disease-causing putrefaction of foods in the human digestive system. They are, of course, also responsible for said fermentation, but though ye olde scientists were wrong about the source of disease, they were onto something about the pro-biotic (good-for-life) potential of some of those unseen beings. In the two centuries since, beneficial single-celled organisms have been recognized not only as guards against pathogens but also as intelligent collaborators without whom life, and certainly vibrant health, would be absolutely impossible. Many people are surprised to hear that bacteria make up 10% of our body weight, and the percentages of those organisms that are helpful, neutral, or harmful is mainly the result of lifestyle choices. Even more surprising is that 90% of the cells in our body are bacterial cells, so only 10% of the cells in our bodies are actually human cells, "us" by the common mode of thinking. (The discrepancy in those two percentages, you clever rabbits, is due to the varying size of cells, microbes being very small and animal cells being very large.) In fact, it's a common expression in the bacteriological world that "we're just a colony of bacteria carrying around a little bit of person." A good reason to find out what microscopic organisms are all about.

> "Support bacteria - they're the only culture some people have." - Stephen Wright

DNA Sluts and Your Guts: *Genetic Promiscuity* and its effect on human evolution and happiness

An amazing behavior of microorganisms hints that the evolutionary enlightenment of the quadrillion (that a 1 with 15 zeros) little buddies we are hosting in and on our bodies ("we" and "hosting" have already been shown to be meaningless words, but we'll stay in the point of view of humans, for now) may have a lot more to do with the quality of our lives than whether or not we're constipated.

Bacteria have a strange and extremely effective way of learning. They share their experiences with any microbe who'll listen, and learn what their billions of neighbors know just by making a little cell-to-cell contact. They do this by something bacteriologists (and now you!) call "parallel gene transfer", or genetic promiscuity. This is the process whereby bacteria can exchange pieces of their DNA with neighboring organisms right through their cell membranes whenever they're in contact, just like plugging your ipod into a friend's computer. What's even more surprising is that they don't distinguish who they share with, even passing new traits, like how to resist new antibiotic drugs, between species, those naughty little critters. This is how they've been able to evolve so quickly into the incredibly efficient examples of evolution they are. When I say quickly, I'm talking about 4 billion years of evolution, each minute of which they're used with superlative efficiency.

Human DNA is a few tens of thousands of genes, compressed into the nucleus of our cells, which contain the codes for every part of our body, from the color of our eyes to the shape of the tiny connective tissues in our little toes, as well as many of our personality traits, as shown by studies of identical twins adopted by different families. Only 2%-3% of this information codes for proteins, so modern science calls the rest "junk DNA" (though some scientists feel that non-coding DNA might be more important than the rest.) Bacterial cells, on the other hand, are wall-to-wall DNA, containing 300 times more genes than humans. And they have only *one* cell to blueprint.

This fact alone (and there are many, many others) proves that they, not us whose laborious evolution happens not every few minutes like bacteria, but every 20 or so years, are the epitome of evolution. So when a bacterium develops a resistance to a certain antibiotic in Paris, for example, bacteria all over the world will have the same inside information in a matter of *hours*. This is only one way microbes communicate and probably not the most fantastical, considering new research which shows that some bacteria can also conduct electricity, sharing news by zapping their neighbors with charged electrons imprinted with data. Or that "magnetotactic" bacteria DNA create organs that contain magnetic crystals, which, sensitive to the Earth's magnetic field, tell a bacterium where it is on an unimaginably vast planet. We think of microbes living out their insentient lives in a square centimeter of soil or floating along aimlessly in a drop of water; why would a microscopic organism need a GPS? So when you consider the fact that "you" are 9/10ths bacteria, and that most of the other 1/10th of your cells are very recently *evolved* from bacterial cells, the nature of those organisms seems a matter too important to leave to chance or superstition.

Public Enemy #1: The War on Bugs

In ancient times, the Egyptians, Chinese, and Natives of Central America, and other primitive cultures used molds to combat infections, presumably without understanding the antibacterial property of mold and its connection to the treatment of disease. It wasn't until the turn of the 19th century that the surgeon Joseph Lister noticed that urine contaminated with mold wouldn't allow bacteria to grow freely.

In 1928, the world of disease-causing bacteria was checkmated when Alexander Fleming, a bacteriologist working at St. Mary's Hospital in London, observed that a petri dish of staphylococcus had been contaminated with a blue-green mold and that cultures of the bacteria adjacent to the mold were dissolving. Studies confirmed that this "penicillin" would be humanity's first and final weapon against sickness, Nobel prizes were awarded, and large-scale production was begun. Antibiotics, from the Greek "against-life", would ease suffering, save countless lives, and make the Earth more sanitary for all.

Then, only a year later, there was a problem. Strains of bacteria began popping up in hospitals that wouldn't bat a microscopic eye at penicillin. They had developed "resistance" to that weapon, and stronger tools became necessary. So steady-handed early-1940's biologists began coming up with more powerful antibiotics that would take final care of these misfit microorganisms, and attempted to strike the delicate balance between strong enough to kill the bacteria but not so strong that they would kill the patient. They sometimes succeeded. And so began the war *with* drugs that rages on to this day.

As discussed above, while humans like to think that they're highly evolved compared to microorganisms and therefore the "pages" making up the book of our DNA are also more advanced, but in fact the opposite is true.

> "This body ain't big enough for the both of us". - Bacterium Bill

There are no wasted letters or no wasted space in their genes, which are essentially wall-to-wall efficient data. Bacteria have become perfect machines of function and evolution. These are the unseen "cultures" we've decided to do battle upon, so that now, in our weakened state, debilitated by the slightest contact with a pathogen, we have no choice but to soldier on in the fight.

And this is a war that science is losing. "'In several member states between 25 per cent and more than 60 per cent of bloodstream infections caused by one type of pneumonia bug were found to have combined resistance to multiple antibiotics', the ECDC [European Centre for Disease Control] said.

'For the patients who are infected with these bacteria, few last-line antibiotics ... remain available,' said Marc Sprenger, the ECDC's director."[13] He's referring mainly to thanklemesien, the nuclear bomb antibiotic – physician's last-ditch effort against the super-bugs popping up everywhere from Berlin to New Delhi.

> "The sheer tonnage of antibiotics that [are] used in the world ever year... contributes to the problem of resistant bacteria in the community, which then becomes a problem in the hospital... I can't think of a microbiologist that would say that the wide application of antibiotics will do anything but select for antibiotic-resistant organisms. That's a consequence of... strains that won't be resistant to that antibiotic in the future." Michael Scheld. M.D., Professor of Surgery, University of Virginia Health Sciences Center

Even so, over 18 million antibiotic prescriptions were written last year for colds, which are caused by viruses, and *not* bacteria. It seems obvious, based on this track record, that we'll soon be out of options. In fact, a Tokyo patient recently died due to a thanklemesien-resistant strain of staphylococcus. A microorganism that, with all my sympathies and condolences to the families of people that have lost the battle with this infection, is easily overcome by a strong immune system.

13
  "EU doctors turn to last-ditch antibiotics as resistance to superbugs grows" Reuters London, Kate Kelland, Nov. 15 2012

It was in fact, Louis Pasteur himself, who first discovered how to kill microorganisms with heat by a technique named after him, who said: "It's the microbes that will have the last word."

Bacteria, microorganisms, probiotics, microflora – whether scary or sought after, these little critters make our existence possible. They're intimately involved with our birth, death, first meal and our last one, and pretty much everything that happens in between.

> "Science is the first word on everything, and the last word on nothing" – Victor Hugo

Your First Fermentation: Probiotic Water

The easiest and cheapest way to supplement with beneficial organisms is "probiotic water". This recipe makes use of fresh grain or seed sprouts to invite advantageous microflora to gently ferment water, which we can (and should) drink every day. It can also be a potent starter for other fermentations, like seed cheese.

Probiotic water (called "rejuvelac" by the old-timers) is very simple to make. It's a two-step process, the first is something you already know how to do from Volume 1 of Kitchen Sink Farming: Sprouting. First, seeds are sprouted (grains from the wheat family make the most popular flavor, though it can be made with any sprouted seed), then they're thrown into water and left to brew for a day or two. Some o' them old timers also talk about what grains make the "most nutritious rejuvelac", but this is an unnecessary occupation. Because the seeds don't have to be eaten, only the liquid used, taste is the only consideration, so experiment. Wheat is the most popular because of its yeasty-lemony flavor, and spelt, with its buttery quality, makes a slightly effervescent, cloudy tonic like I imagine Harry Potter's butterbeer to be. Rye's flavor translates nicely as a probiotic water, and the addition of some sprouted fennel or caraway seeds will take the imbiber back to their childhood among New York's Jewish delis, whether or not they had one. These are all great on their own as delicious health tonics and digestive aids, but the culinary possibilities are quite limitless, such as a base for tomato soup with a hint of pickle and pumpernickel, or a red-lentil marinara with the divine sparkle of life.

Probiotic water is rife with lactobacillius bacteria like acidophilus and bifidus and is a great alternative to store-bought probiotics. Homemade probiotics take just minutes of effort to brew over the course of a week, from seed to sprout to sip, are more potent and, as I once found while looking at an opened capsule of acidophilus next to a drop of probiotic water under my microscope, are about 40,000 times cheaper. Additionally, I've tried a few times to make "designer" probiotics, that is, to use those expensive, name-brand flora to start a little culture of home flora, and wouldn't you know it, those ridiculously expense little pills of bacteria would always go bad in the relatively gentle environment of my home-made probiotic water. Either the bacteria in my kitchen are a super-strength strain, or a fresh, living, lovingly-cultivated culture is unrivaled in vitality and potency to lab-grown, cryogenically frozen bacteria stagnating in bottles on supermarket shelves.

The recipe is as follows:

1 cup dry Seed or Grain

Sprout in a jar with a screen on top in the normal fashion (See Kitchen Sink Farming Vol. 1: Sprouting, or google it)

When the seeds have been growing tails for a day or two (not just poked out, but not longer than the seed itself), either rinse them one last time or don't. The reason FOR rinsing them would be to remove the last bit of enzyme inhibitors that are clinging to them; the reason for NOT rinsing is to leave be the probiotics that have slipped in and settled. The first depends on what seed you're using: soy beans and quinoa could use an extra rinse, and the second is determined by strength of the flora in your local environment. Have you been culturing for months or years? Then cleaner is probably better. Is this your first ferment in a Manhattan high-rise? Then you should probably treat your microbes with kid gloves. It's a fairly unimportant difference and I'm sure you'll be fine either way, but if you're nerdy by nature like me, now you know.

Fill the jar with pure water (now you know why we used a jar. You don't even need to take off the screen) and set it somewhere warm, clean and dark, with good air circulation. If you have small bugs around you can replace the screen with a cloth. The top of a refrigerator or in a warm cabinet with the door ajar work nicely - it will ferment more quickly in a warmer, moist environment. Leave it for 24 hours, then taste it. If it tastes like water, leave it for another day. We're looking for a lightly sour, pleasant taste; if the taste is too much, toss it and start over. One of the benefits of that 1:40,000 dollar ratio.

Probiotic water is a delicate, largely unprotected brew and there will be a point where unhelpful "bad" bacteria will move in and take over. This will be characterized by an increasingly foul smell and flavor; and we obviously want to stop the fermentation before that, while still cultivating the most numerous beneficial bacteria.

When the brew is at its peak, screw a lid on the jar and put the whole thing in the fridge, or you may want to strain just the liquid into a bottle for two reasons: 1) to take up less room in the fridge, or 2) to immediately start another batch of brew using new water and the same sprouts. The sprouted grains or seeds are generally good for two batches; after that they tend to start floating to the surface and attracting unfriendly bacteria. Putting an active fermentation in the refrigerator is called *cold stabilization* by wine geeks and thick-bearded home brewers, and refers to the fact that bacteria slow way down in the cold and stabilize their metabolic processes – fermentation pretty much stops. A half day in the warmth of the world equals a week or two in the refrigerator. Your probiotic water is ready to be drunk straight, used in food preparation, or used to start other fermentations, and the sprouted seeds can be tossed, or (preferably) used as more flavorful versions of their unfermented selves.

Recap:

Sprout 1 cup of any seed or grain with the jar method

When the tail is as long as the seed, fill the jar with water, leaving the screen on, and place in a dark, temperate place.

In 2-3 days, put it in the fridge, or strain out the probiotic water (putting that in the fridge) and cover the sprouts with new water, fermenting once more.

Local Flora - Sauerkrauts and Other Fermented Veggies

As we've discussed, bacteria are everywhere on Earth, from the cold and lifeless ocean depths to the upper stratosphere, where powerful ultra-violet light that would instantly vaporize a less adaptive organism. Thriving in the boiling geysers of Yosemite, active volcanoes, and nuclear reactors, bacteria effortlessly colonize every surface of your kitchen. On your skin, in your digestive tract, and within your very blood they flourish, and no amount of scrubbing with anti-bacterial soap is going to change that. And why would we want it to? Bacteria have been here long before us, preparing the world for our presence in a myriad of ways, and will be here long after us, whatever the reason for our demise.

Enough time has passed, I suppose, from the sanitation craze of the 50's that extended past countertops into relationships and politics, though never as thoroughly as we were led to believe. Now many people accept the benefits of probiotics in neat little capsules or yogurt, much of which has been ungratefully re-pasteurized; once the lactobaccilli have served their intended purpose they're warily cooked up under watchful, darkly circled eyes. There's even a growing market for raw milk products, whose microbial populations remain intact along with the natural compounds, usually boiled away or uselessly caramelized, that allow the benefits of milk, so noisily marketed, to be actually used.

Importing specifics types of microflora, like in the cases of kombucha and kefir, allows us to predict and benefit from their actions. Utilizing wild bacteria, however, yields a universe of flavors and health benefits that we can suppose and experience but to a full extent only imagine. Fermented vegetables in Ecuador will have a different community of probiotics than ones from Alaska, and so a different taste and effect on our health. And so much the better, if the people consuming them are in Ecuador and Alaska. By eating local fermentations by wild bacteria you'll connect on the deepest level with your community and build immunity to pathogens and allergens that the local bacteria have already overcome. You'll invite the untamed life force of the natural world to your table and body, especially important in the urban jungle where the only wilderness hides on this microscopic level.

Fermenting vegetables is a simple process (from a human point of view) though a very rewarding one, and no special equipment is needed. Just a vessel to hold the vegetables, some salt to keep out unwanted organisms, and a way to keep the veggies down. I started with gallon olive jars, gotten for free from bars, and rocks. Not rocket science. The salt can be either sea salt (preferred) or pickling salt, which is table salt without the added iodine, an anti-microbial agent. Kosher salt can also be used, but as the grains are much bigger and have less surface area for the mass, about 50% is needed.

Any fruit or vegetable can be fermented, but let's start with sauerkraut made from cabbage. Enjoyed the world over and a welcome addition to many foods you probably already eat; cabbage is inexpensive and already rich in the lacto-bacillus that will team up with your local wild flora. In my opinion, cabbage is by far the world's #1 fermented veggie because its glucosamines (see "what to sprout" in "Kitchen Sink Farming Volume 1: Sprouting"), act as a natural pesticide, deterring larger bugs from populating and leaving room for the probiotics to flourish. Others believe that cabbage, being an autumn and early-winter vegetable, was a better candidate for long-term storage by pre-fridge cultures, and the world has developed a taste for it. Though the reason why sauerkraut, and it's incarnations in various cultures, is so good may be as matter of debate, the fact that it *is* so good is just common knowledge.

Basic Sauerkraut Recipe

You'll need:

One head of cabbage per 1 quart of container, 4 heads for a gallon jar

1 ½ Tbl Sea Salt per head of cabbage

Chop or grate the cabbage. Thick or thin, with the heart or without; whatever you prefer. The light green and dark purple varieties are interchangeable, and can be mixed to make a light pink kraut. Other chopped or grated veggies, fruits, or sprouted seeds can be thrown in now as well; garlic, beets, carrots, greens (mustard and others), apples, seaweeds, or herbs like dill or sprouted celery seed are common options.

> Why Salt?
>
> For the biochemistry–minded, salt is added to fermenting veggies and fruits for two reasons. One is to induce osmosis; the fluid inside of the plant material will be sucked out in nature's desire to balance salt content on both sides of the cell wall, and the resulting liquid is a wonderfully full of sugars and growth-promoting factors. The other reason is that salt will inhibit the growth of spoilage microorganisms and pathogens. The lacto bacteria
>
> that fermented fruits and veggies into delicious sauerkraut or pickled tangerines, for examples, are already present on the skin and leaves of all produce.
>
> But again, as humanity, and un-aided nature actually, has been fermenting for longer than the word osmosis existed, it's not necessary to understand the principals behind the

> process, it's just important to do it. As the old yoga aphorism says: "99% practice, 1% theory".

Toss the cabbage with the salt. Pack it tightly into your container and find something to hold it down like a plate that fits inside your container with a rock on top. The combination of pressure and salt will draw out the liquid; eventually we want everything submerged under the anaerobic protection of salt water.

The easiest, and cleanest method (besides a fermenting crock) is to fill a sprouting or produce bag (see "Resources") with the chopped veggies and weigh it down with a heavy rock that's been sterilized. The best rocks I've found are the smooth round rocks businesses use in their landscaping, about the size of a fist. I'm positive that they'll give you a couple if you ask nicely. To sterilize your rock, scrub it with dish soap and hot water, then put it in a pot of boiling water for 10 minutes, covering the rock completely. You can also put the rock in an oven set to 350° F for 15 minutes. BE VERY CAREFUL as the rock could have air bubbles inside which will heat, expand, and explode. Wrap the rock in a dish towel, which won't burn until it reaches 450, and will possibly contain an explosion.

> Other Methods:
>
> As the veggies are acted upon by the breathing bacteria, bubbles will attach to individual shreds of leaf which will want to float to the surface of the water. At this point, the guides say to put a plate on top of the cabbage that just fits inside of the container and weigh it down with a rock. I've never been able to find so perfect a match. Even grated
>
> vegetables held down by a well-fitting plate will often find an opening, and like weeds growing up through the crack in a sidewalk will find their way to the surface and out of the safety of the brine. Veggies in a sprouting bag won't have

this problem. Another option is to fill a plastic freezer bag with brine (in case it leaks) and use this to hold down the veggies; the benefit (besides being cheap and already in your possession) is a complete seal. The drawback is a messy surface; often a harmless white mold will form where the water meets air. This bloom should be scooped out as soon as it forms to allow the bacteria under the water free access to oxygen, which is why I like to keep the surface of the water free from obstructions. If you let the mold overgrow, it can smell quite bad and cleaning is more difficult. I use my plastic strainer (the same one I use from my kefir) to skim the surface. The plastic makes it easy to squeeze it into the vessel, if the mouth is not as wide as the body. Rinse it upside down with hot water in between scoops. You can also use a very clean cloth for each pass. The plastic bag technique makes cleaning virtually impossible, and if it's in and out of the water as handfuls of kraut are scooped out every once in a while, it'll turn messy fast.

The last option I've tried is a bottle that fits inside the mouth of the fermenting vessel, filled with water, holding everything down. This has the same problems as the plastic bag but to a lesser degree, as it can be easily and cleanly pulled out and replaced after the mold has been cleaned from it and the water. I've found that Voss water bottles fit pretty well into wide mouthed canning jars (which have the same sized mouth in both the quart and half gallon size), but the most perfectly-fitted bottles are Corralejo tequila, with beautiful bubbly, colored glass. Keep out bugs by covering the whole thing with a clean piece of cloth, clean old t-shirt, or a coffee filter is nothing sticks out over the rim, and rubber-band it down. Put the vessel on a plate or shallow bowl, in case of spills or

overflow. Or, if the vessel has a lid, screw it on. The fermentation that's going to happen in this case is anaerobic, so it doesn't need oxygen.

Through osmosis and pressure, the liquid will slowly draw out of the vegetables. Push down on the weight every couple of hours to squeeze out the water, either with a clean hand or kitchen tool; the tamper from a high-speed blender works well. This is the main benefit from using a bottle; very easy to grab it like a dry handle and press down. Be careful not to raise the level of the water so much that it spills out! If after 24-48 hours the vegetables aren't entirely submerged in their own juice, add more brine, 1 cup of fresh water to ¾ tablespoons of salt. Wine can be substituted for the extra brine; it will give the kraut a more delicate taste that some who haven't yet acquired a taste for strong fermented flavors may appreciate.

Cover the whole thing with a towel or t-shirt to prevent bugs from getting in and leave your veggies to ferment. A dark corner of a kitchen counter works well; a cool cupboard is also good. Probiotics like darkness and 60-75° Fahrenheit. The colder the temperature the slower the fermentation process, which can make a mellower flavored kraut. Above 75 or 80° and a new type of bacteria will feel at home, which could be a problem.

Your kraut or other fermented veggies will start to be ready in just a few days, and will continue to mature for months. If you're going to let them go that long, you will want to look for a cool place to let them work, after the initial few days of getting started in the kitchen. I like to start eating my kraut in about a week, and keep dipping in until it's gone. I start a batch of something when I'm nearing the end of the last, so that I always have something working (usually several somethings). Whenever a friend has an over-abundance of a fruit of vegetable, or when I get a great deal at a farmer's market at the end of the day, it gets fermented.

The original reason people started fermenting, a way to store produce for when times were lean, is still a great reason to do it. Delicate greens will last a few days in the fridge, or months in the fermenter. Wherever you live, fruits and vegetables are only available certain times of the year, and are shipped in from across the globe during the others. An expensive process, both to the wallet and the environment. While the health benefits of fermented veggies are many, the environmental benefits may be even greater.

Sterilization

When a home fermenter wants only beneficial organisms in their brew, they need to work with clean tools. This way, they can make sure that no soil-based organisms, for example, are going to be competing with the lacto-bacteria in a vegetable culture, or that the delicate yeasts and bacteria in a young kombucha cuture won't have to fight with free-floating mold spores as they establish themselves. Obviously, sterilization is a new process, and judging from the millennia of successful fermentation that happened before its discovery, not a totally necessary one. But it does make the process simpler and more consistent. There are four ways to sterilize your equipment, boiling, baking, chemicals, or UV light. Bacteria can't survive past 250° F (120° C) for any length of time, at least the ones we're generally exposed to, so boiling your jars, bags, rocks, etc, for 10 minutes will do the trick. Tools can also be sterilized in an oven, which takes longer because any cooling water in or on the object must evaporate before the desired temperature can be reached, about 2 hours at 300° F. I also have a UV sterilizer wand that is fast and handy; about a minute per jar does the trick, and it's convenient to use on kitchen sponges, hotel pillows, or other places unwanted bacteria might develop. Simply washing equipment with hot water will almost always be enough, but an ounce of prevention is worth it in the case of weeks or months-long ferments.

Hydrogren peroxide (see "Kitchen Sink Farming Vlume 3: Growing"), iodine, colloidal silver, or a citrus-based commercial sanitizer can also be used.

Now that you're an expert in fermenting veggies at home, try these:

Kimchi – cabbage, carrot, ginger, garlic, onion, chili

Cabbage with apple, cranberries (halved), and a bit of shallot

Tangerines with cinnamon, clove, and honey

Cabbage, shredded carrot, onion, radish, and ginger

Carrots, beets, and raisins

> **Cultural diversity is as important in our guts as it is in our communities!**

Fermented veggies and wonderful on their own, on a slice of sprouted bread or dried cracker, or in many recipes but fermented condiments might be the apex of the art. A perfect blend of sweet and sour that enliven any food, the following condiment ideas will hopefully inspire you to include a dollop of a fermented goodness on the side of every meal. Even cereal and desserts will benefit from "Almond Cream Cheese" (see "Kitchen Sink Farming Volume 4: Homegrown Living Recipes - What to Do with Your Sprouts and Krauts").

Try these:

Raisins, garlic chives, cilantro, sprouted anise and cumin, ginger, whey (see Kitchen Sink Farming Volume 3: Fermenting)

Plum and Apple Chutney with carrot, cinnamon, allspice, ginger, and blackberries

Apricot and Rosemary

Green Tomato and Basil

Celery-Pear

Seed Cheese and Yogurt

Fermenting sprouted seeds and nuts into a creamy vegan cheese takes them to the next level in nutrition, digestibility, and epicure. Macadamia nuts can transform into a delicious crumbly feta, and quinoa, hemp and corn can become a full-flavored and velvety cheese spread in just a day or two of fermenting. Using the air-born beneficial organisms that occur naturally in your home, fermented seed cheeses are full of active enzymes, predigested protein, easy-to-assimilate starches, new health-giving nutrients only available through the microbial action, and of course, live probiotic cultures. The "soy cheese" or "cashew cream cheese" in natural food stores or on raw restaurant menus are almost always just blended nuts with dead yeast and flavorings; this is the real deal. Remember – in seeds "raw" means nothing, "alive" means everything.

Simple Seed Cheese

To make cheese, we need to first make probiotic water (recipe above), a simple elixir that develops the existing friendly bacteria on seeds and grains and lures in additional helpers that will go to work for us. Probiotic water is also an easy and effective way to supplant varied bacterial cultures in our digestive systems. It has a light, mild flavor reminiscent of lemon and bread, and can be used instead of plain old water in every juice, soup, or recipe that's not going to be heated past 115° F (as this would kill most of our guests, which is not very polite), or just drunk straight.

The Next Step

Put your sprouted seeds or nuts in a food processor or blender with just enough probiotic water to cover them. Pulse grind them until they're pulverized but not smooth. The right texture is important – the ground mixture needs enough consistency to end be homogenousenough to end up a solid mass when the liquid is removed; pureed too thin and it will all drain away. You want a fairly smooth consistency, while still having some texture. If it is over-smooth, throw in some herbs and veggies to thicken it up, and you've got a delicious dip.

Wash the soaking/sprouting jar thoroughly with hot water and return the blended mixture to it. Leave it at least a third empty, as the fermenting cheese will bubble and expand. Re-cover it with the screen, coffee filter, sprout bag or fabric, screw on the ring, and put it in a room temperature place, 65-75° F. If your room is colder than that, the top of your fridge will probably keep it the right temp. If your room is hotter, try a dark closet or clean ground-floor or below-ground corner.

Start checking it at 6 hours. Don't shake, swirl, or otherwise molest your project. The microbes are working hard to make your cheese, and if you disturb them it sets them back. I could image slowing down a fermentation in this way, and I imagine this would make a more sour or pungent finished product. The cheese will be done around 12-24 hours. There will be a thick, light colored mass floating on top of a clearish liquid; the solid is curds, and the liquid is whey.

Now, carefully scoop the cheese out of the jar with a spoon and place it in a sprouting bag or piece of cheesecloth. The top layer of the cheese may be darker from reacting to the oxygen; this is completely fine to eat. If it's dry and crusty you may want to scoop it off first and discard it for aesthetic reaons. Squeeze the rest of the whey out of the cheese into the jar or a separate bowl. Whey will last a really long time in a sealed jar in the fridge, and is great for many recipes, including lacto-ferments and sodas, as well as many household things. (See page 139 for uses of whey.) The resulting lump of cheese should be dry and have a creamy or crumbly texture, depending on the seed, grain, or nuts used and the original consistency of the mixture. It's ready to be used immediately, can be mixed with flavoring agents like salt, soy sauce, lemon juice, peppers or herbs and spices, and stored for up to a week.

Crumble seed cheese on salads and soups or use it in wraps or as a spread on veggies or crackers – anytime you'd use dairy cheese but still want to feel non-mucousy and deeply nourished. Actually, seed cheese is so high in available protein that's easy to digest thatmany people that have trouble keeping on weight and body builders alike find that seed cheese is the best source for lean muscles, especially when made from hemp (see Kitchen Sink Farming Volume 1: Sprouting).

As we've discussed, the cheese is highly reactive with air, so put it in a sealed container in the fridge; I don't recommend wrapping the lump of cheese with plastic which may leach harmful chemicals into the food, but the less air there is in the container, the less drying out there will be.

Seed Cheese Recap

You'll need:

A cup of sprouted seeds, nuts, or grains

About 1/3 cup of probiotic water (see pg 72)

Do:

In a blender or food processor, cover the sprouts with the probiotic water. Gently pulse the blades until the mixture is a fairly smooth consistency, while still having some texture.

> Clean the sprouting jar and return the mixture to it. Recover with a breathable material and place in a temperate spot, 65-75° F.
>
> Your ferment is done when the mixture separates, curds floating on top of whey. Saving the liquid whey, scoop out the curds and squeeze dry in a sprouting bag.

"Advanced" Cheese Making: A 2-Day Degree

While simple seed cheese makes a quick and creamy result, colander cheese will produce a more intensely cheesy concoction, as the flavors develop slowly over the course of a few days, "pre-digesting" and breaking down the complex elements all the while. Still a very straightforward and easy recipe, colander cheese is the gourmet's choice.

What you'll need:

Sprouted grains and/or nuts and probiotic water, as mentioned above

A colander with legs, or some sort of strainer and a way to keep it lifted, like crossed chopsticks or rocks. Or just go buy a colander with legs, they're like a buck.

A bowl that fits nicely inside the colander

A heavy weight: a clean rock, jar or bottle filled with water, etc.

A plate or shallow bowl to go underneath the colander

Blend your soaked and/or sprouted seeds or nuts with the probiotic water into a smooth mixture that still has some texture (see simple seed cheese recipe above), and put the resulting half creamy, half chunky, and all wet paste back into a sprout bag, twisting or tying off the opening so nothing comes out. Put it into the colander. The plate or shallow bowl goes underneath to catch the whey, and the bowl goes inside the colander, on top of the bag. The weight goes in the bowl, which presses down on the cheese to squeeze out the whey.

Over the next 2 – 3 days, all of the whey created by the fermentative action of the bacteria will drain out of the cheese. It's a good idea to stir or knead the cheese once a day so it will ferment evenly. After the whey stops dripping into the vessel beneath, the cheese is done and can be scooped out and put into a non-plastic container in the fridge, or formed into logs and rolled in herbs, crushed black pepper, the same type of seed or nut, coarsely ground and dried, or whatever flavoring you choose.

Coconut Cream Cheese

This is a different process that slowly produces an incredible sweet cheese from coconut pudding. I discovered this cheese by accident, when some pudding was starting to go south after a week or so, and I went out of town, resolving to throw it away when I got back about a week later. When I returned home I found a jar full of coconut puree in my refrigerator with a fuzzy growth on top, varying in color from white to dark brown. As I started scooping the stuff into the garbage disposal, I fortuitously caught a whiff of it as it went by. It smelled sweet and delicious, and I decided to try it. I scraped all the fuzz off the top and tasted a small spoonful. It was amazing, and as much as I wanted more, I waited to see how I felt. The next day I felt great, so I ate a bunch. Still fine, so now coconut cheese is a staple in my repertoire.

Make coconut pudding by blending young coconut meat with its water (see "Kitchen Sink Farming Volume 4: Homegrown Living Recipes – What to Do with Your Sprouts and Krauts") A fairly thick consistency works best, as it gives the microbes something to adhere to. Scoop it into a jar and cover it with a screen, cheesecloth, sprout bag, or coffee filter so that your local flora will appear. If you're doing this in a sterile environment like outer space and don't have access to helpful organisms, or as an experiment, you can also use *koji*, a mold used to make sake and amasake, fermented rice beverages from Japan, available online or from some home brewing stores. Leave the pudding on a counter for 12-24 hours, cover the jar with a lid, and put in the fridge. You'll start to see growth in about 2 weeks, and the flavor will continue to develop as the microorganisms turn the complex carbohydrates into sugars, and in turn digests the sugars. When you're ready to use it, scrape the top layer off, cleaning off the spoon or spatula between scrapings. Still not as gross as bleu cheese or moldy green-veined ones..

The coconut cream cheese is ready to be used in desserts or to sweeten up and add a hint of champagne sparkle to spreads for fruits or vegetables. It's really so delicious that it can be served plain in a digestion-boosting scoop, as a side for anything from appetizer to dessert. It's also amazing blended with fresh orange juice, which turns into a tropical creamsicle, and (fortunately or unfortunately) covers up the fermented flavor.

Vinegar

For thousands of years, vinegar held a prime place on the healer's shelves for its many health benefits, and at some point found its way into the chef's tool kit as well. Its low pH (high acidity) stimulated digestion by giving a boost to the stomach acids, and it's been used over the centuries to treat everything from skin conditions like warts and eczema to internal issues like arthritis, infections, headaches, high cholesterol, and ulcers. Apple cider vinegar especially is a popular and effective elixir, especially as a weight loss aid because of its bowel stimulating and appetite suppressing qualities. It's been studied less, but I find kombucha vinegar equal to apple cider in benefits and taste. Many pet owners have noticed increased energy and shinier coats in their dogs, cats, horses, birds, and rodents when apple cider vinegar is added to their pet food, and the ancient Samurai, sadly unmentioned in the rest of this book, believed a daily shot of vinegar would increase their vitality and power in battle (tamago-su or egg vinegar, was made by dissolving a whole raw egg in rice vinegar for a week).

Vinegar is any acidic, or low pH, liquid that contains acetic acid, and along with lemons is the only very acid food. For this reason, it's irreplaceable for adding zip to many dishes, soups, sauces, and of course vinaigrettes. And luckily, it's so easy to make that juice and wine makers have to take precautions to make sure their products *don't* turn into it. It could be said that the sugars in many liquid foods will turn into acetic acid by accident, but consistently making a nice, mellow vinegar with just the right about of bite takes just a little bit of knowledge.

Any liquid with some sugar (or carbohydrates, aka starch, which is sugar molecules bound in groups, so another step is required to make the sugars available) can become vinegar, from all kinds of fruit and vegetable juices (common ones are apple and grape), grains like wheat or rice, or sweeteners like honey, molasses, agave, or sugarcane. Even vinegars made from roots, bark, and wood were once very popular. The two-step process of turning the sugar into alcohol, and the alcohol into acetic acid yields the most consistent outcome (like grape juice into wine into red wine veinegar), but just combining an active vinegar starter with any of the above liquids and letting them brew will usually give fine results.

We'll start with the more complicated version so you'll understand the process, maybe keeping it in the back of your mind until you'd like to try your hand at an exceptional vinegar for a special occasion. Also, this process doesn't need a starter culture to get going; it makes the most of the natural yeasts and bacteria that are present in the air. The super-easy classic Kitchen-Sink Farmer follows.

First, you'll need a sweet liquid: a sweetener like honey, molasses, maple syrup or sugar and water, or fruit or vegetable juice. Apple juice has a good balance of sugars and acids that make it an ideal choice for a first vinegar. Put the liquid in a clean bottle or jug, filling it all the way up to the top. Next, you'll need an airlock which lets carbon dioxide out but doesn't let oxygen in. These are available from homebrew stores, and are a curved tube with water inside. The water lets the CO2 bubble away but air (particularly oxygen) can't pass through in the other direction. You can also make your own airlock, of course, by drilling a hole in a rubber stopper , a wine bottle cork, or a corn husk or piece of soft wood, carved to fit the bottle neck. Put a piece of flexible plastic tubing (available from hardware, medical supply or aquarium stores) into the hole and put the other end into a glass of water. Air can get out but not in. DIY airlock - check!

As the fermentation begins, you'll notice bubbling in the water. This, as mentioned, is CO2, a waste product being emitted by the microorganisms. The other waste product is alcohol, and when the bubbling stops (2-4 weeks, depending on how much sugar is in your original liquid) you have made alcohol. Hard cider if you've used apple juice, mead if you've used honey water, etc. You have probably already realized, but your newfound tools and knowledge of yeast fermentation can be applied to all kinds of home-made wines. Wine or champagne can also be used make vinegar by simply starting with the next step.

The next phase is to turn the alcohol into acetic acid, the classic flavor that's consistent throughout all vinegars. This process uses a new set of microorganisms that thrive in the presence of oxygen, or aerobically. The more oxygen these organisms can use, the faster the fermentation will happen, so you'll want to maximize the surface area of the brew. Pour the liquid into a wide-mouth jar or bucket, or divide it into a few bottles. Cover the opening with a light cloth or coffee filter secured by a rubber band and leave it for as long as you like. If you have some vinegar starter, or "mother" it can be added to speed up the process. It will, after a couple of weeks, continue to get stronger and more acidic, and will quickly surpass the potency of store-bought vinegars. It can even be looked at as a "vinegar concentrate", with water or juice added to achieve the desired zip. Bottle and cap it when it's reached the strength you like, and because it won't have access to oxygen it won't get any stronger but will continue to deepen in flavor as its bottle-aged. After you're an adept at this process, you may like to flavor your vinegar between steps 2 and 3, "acetic acid fermentation" and bottling, by putting herbs, fruit, sprouted grains, chilies, horseradish, onions, garlic, flowers, or other flavorings in the vinegar for a day to a week. These will add another layer of sophistication and potentially a lovely color to your homemade brew. The finished product can be so beautiful that you're tempted to put it in clear glass and display it, but remember that sunlight can break down living vinegar.

The yeast and acetic acid fermentation can also be done at the same time, but this process is just a little more fickle. If you're a gamblin' man (or lady), you can just put juice in a wide-mouthed jar, cover it with an air-permeable light cloth, and leave it for a few weeks, letting the different stages of microbia come and go. If the surface gets covered by a very fuzzy layer that breaks up when you swirl it, this is a somewhat volatile wild yeast and it's best to abandon the project. If a SCOBY forms in the juice (symbiotic colony or bacteria and yeast, like a rubbery white pancake) you've created a thriving metropolis of beneficial organisms, and you'll soon have delicious vinegar. A bit of this living condiment can be saved and added to the next brew as a starter. If possible, I recommend adding an unpasteurized, unfiltered vinegar at the outset of a vinegar brew to solidify the bacteria's foothold in its new colony. Unpasteurized apple cider vinegar is the most commonly available in stores, with "Bragg Organic Raw Apple Cider Vinegar" being the most widely available. Whether you used a store-bought or homemade starter, the easiest way to stay in vinegar is to do a continuous fermentation: when you take some vinegar out of your jar, add some new juice, as mentioned in the sections on kombucha and kefir. You will be missing the mellowing effect of bottling with this method, but once you've established your culture, continuous fermentation makes it a snap to keep it going forever.

Vinegar can also be made with kitchen scraps and peels, already full of beneficial bacteria because of their exposure to the air while growing. If you've washed your fruit and veggies in hydrogen peroxide (see "Kitchen Sink Farming Volume 3: Growing") you're guaranteed the lack of uncooperative anaerobic bacteria (oxygen-hating) while maintaining the aerobic ones (oxygen-loving). Put the peels and scraps in a wide mouthed jar and cover with filtered water and a light cloth or coffee filter. Continue to throw in kitchen scraps now and then to give the bacteria new sugars to feed off of. Start tasting the brew after a few weeks (dip a straw into the liquid then cover the end with your finger. You'll be able to lift the full straw out without losing any liquid, uncovering it when the bottom end is in your mouth. This testing method is called "thieving" in wine-making.) In 4-6 weeks it should be done. Apple cores and peels work especially well for this method, as well as peaches, pears, apricots, crushed grapes, and berries. If you don't like the taste of your kitchen-scrap vinegar, it's also an excellent plant nutrient.

> **Vinegar Flies**
>
> Wherever there's vinegar brewing, these pesky little friends (sometimes called fruit flies) show up. They love fermentation almost as much as I do, which is why they're often found around overripe bananas and oranges, or getting funky on an old batch of collard greens. I used to try to catch them in my fist and put them outside, until I learned that these are the critters most commonly used in labs to study genetics because of their short life cycle and hardiness. Then I thought: if I remove all the slow ones,
>
> leaving just the fast ones to reproduce, I'm inadvertently breeding a super-strain of ninja gnats. I've found that the best way to deal with them without direct violence is to put some vinegar in a glass or bowl and cover it with plastic wrap. Then poke a bunch of holes in the top with a fork (a piece of paper rolled into an downward-pointing cone with a small hole in the tip, above the level of the liquid, also works). The flies can get in but they can't get out. Kind of mean, but they are vinegar flies, after all, so I bet they die happy.

> **Super-Easy Apple Cider Vinegar**
>
> Get a bottle of raw apple cider vinegar
>
> Add it to a bottle of apple juice (no preservatives)
>
> Cover with a cloth and let ferment.
>
> Easy!

To make wild fermented apple cider vinegar and enjoy all the immunity-boosting and evolutionary benefits of aligning with your local flora, juice apples, which have probiotics and yeasts on their peels. You may also buy apple juice (with no preservatives, refrigerated means fresh). Wash and cut up an apple and put it in a bowl or wide-mouth jar, and fill with apple juice. Cover with a clean cloth and let it sit for a week or more, swirling the liquid a couple of times a day to inhibit mold (if a layer of white mold does grow on the surface, it can be scooped off.) Continue to ferment until it gets the acidity you like, then cover and stick in the fridge. Will stay "good" forever.

Specialty Vinegars

White wine vinegar is made by pouring double the amount of water over mashed raisins and leaving it for about 2 months. Strain the pulp out and use it again and again. Make raspberry vinegar by using fresh raspberries. Everyday for three days, add the same amount of fresh berries and enough water to cover. On day four, strain the liquid out and add one pound of sugar or honey, stirring until dissolved. Cover with a light cloth or coffee filter until it turns to vinegar - this takes about three months.

Make a lovely flower vinegar by dissolving (preferably raw) honey in twice the amount of warm pure water, less than 110° F so as not to kill the living organisms. Of course, any natural sweetener will do; raw honey isn't necessary for the process but it's just so much better for you and since it's made from pollen, goes wonderfully with the floral taste of this brew. Add several handfuls of edible flowers like marigold, clover, dandelions, nasturtium, citrus blossoms, jasmine, or herb flowers or leaves. Cover with a coffee filter or cloth and stir or swirl every day until it's done, usually 10 to 20 days. Strain the liquid and bottle it, though you may want to leave a particularly beautiful stem in the bottle, especially if the vinegar is a gift.

If you're curious about the actual acidity of your vinegar, which is a great way to determine if it's ready, there are three methods of finding out. One is a pH test kit, where a litmus paper will change color and tell you the acidity. There's also titration, a process using baking soda that determines the strength of the acid in the solution by finding out the smallest amount that's required to react with the baking soda (remember vinegar or lemon juice and baking soda volcanoes from middle school?) Instructions are available online and the benefit is that you only need household items: jars, water, baking soda, and a colored liquid of some kind. The other method is a laboratory pH tester, which starts at about $20, and I find extremely handy in all sorts of projects. I use my pH tester to determine when my brews are done, from kombucha to kefir to kraut, and I highly recommend picking one up. The pH tester won't tell you how much of *which kind* of acid is present, but that you can easily figure out by taste if you're interested.

Mead and Ginger Beer

Mead, or honey wine, is the simplest process described in this book, and by far the easiest thing you'll ever do that results in something to sip or chew (and that includes microwaving a tv dinner). And though it's so easy to do, perhaps *because* of it, brewing your own mead, like enjoying a sunset or howling at the moon, is participating in the most original amusement of our species. Some anthropologists believe that mead altered the course of humanity more than any other factor.

Raw honey is full of both probiotic bacteria and natural antibiotics that protect it from invasion by other microbial species. In fact, several-thousand year old honey was found in Egyptian tombs, quite fresh. But when wild honey mixes with water by nature or human design, it dilutes honey's natural protections so that wild yeasts and bacteria are able to get in to the candy store and enjoy the sweet nectar, converting it in their special way into a bubblingly living ferment. In just a few days to a few weeks, the honey-water will be mead, its sugars having been converted to alcohol and CO_2 by the action of the microorganisms.

> "I in my grandeur have surpassed the heavens and all this spacious earth.
>
> Have I not drunk of Soma juice?
>
> ...O Soma flowing on thy way, win thou and conquer high renown; And make us better than we are.
>
> Win thou the light, win heavenly light, and, Soma, all felicities; And make us better than we are.
>
> ...When purified within the jars, Soma,... golden-hued... flow on to us and make us rich. Drive all our enemies away.
>
> ... Send down the rain from heaven, a stream of opulence from earth."
>
> *Soma Pavamana, HYMN IV.*

The theory is that a caveperson happened upon a bubbling, golden liquid in the crook of a tree: honey that had been rained on, and was now being transformed by invisible forces. The caveperson carefully tried it, liked it, tried some more. Maybe the caveperson called some cave friends over and a cave party ensued, complete with, as is the case with many neophytic drinkers, much rowdiness, finding formerly uninteresting things fascinating, and animated declarations of love. The intoxicating elixir was seen as a mysterious gift from the gods. Songs were sung, offerings made. Actually, it's interesting to note that the *Vedas*, the large body of poems from ancient India (called apauruṣeya or "not of human agency") that kicked off the Hindu religion and influenced all the other ones, were unabashedly written under the influence of a mysterious drug called "soma", literally "juice" or "nectar" in Sanskrit, which historians believe was either mead or the juice of the ephedra plant, pounded out of the stalks, filtered, fermented and mixed with milk.

By some accounts, it was not the cultivation of crops or livestock but the desire for the altered state that fermentation provides that inspired primitive nomadic man to decide to stay put. Mead, which predates the cultivation of fire, influenced our hunter-gatherer ancestors to convert from a wandering lifestyle to a sedentary one, a way of life that had been working for at least 2 million years. It was this shift that cultural theorist Claude Levi-Strauss says marks the transition from nature to culture in prehistoric man. Describing a hollow tree he writes, "…which, as a receptacle for honey, is part of nature if the honey is fresh and enclosed within it, and part of culture if the honey, instead of being in a naturally hollow tree, has been put to ferment in an artificially hollowed-out trunk" (*From Honey to Ashes*, 1973).

Mead was also my first attempt at fermentation, as a teenaged way to get an alcoholic buzz and, I like to think, the buzz that a curious soul gets from cultivating mysterious forces. A friend of the family described to me the process in a few sentences, my curiosity was peeked, and I gathered my materials: a gallon water jug and a plastic bear container of honey that had been collecting dust and crystallizing in our kitchen pantry for as long as I could remember. The honey went into the jug which was then filled with water, and I put it under my bed, checking it every day when I got home from school. I noticed it start to bubble after a few days, and though I didn't understand why (wild yeasts, which had floated on the air towards the sweet vapors like the steam from a cartoon pie, were releasing carbon dioxide) I knew that *something* was happening, much like my ancient ancestors probably did. I watched the bubbling decrease over the course of a couple of weeks, both hesitant and fascinated. When I finally worked up the nerve to take a sip, I was surprised to find that it wasn't sweet at all, for the same reason that it had stopped bubbling: the yeasts had eaten all the sugars. I wasn't ready for the exotic taste exposed by the removal of the sugar, nor the layer of bugs that had sunk to the bottom of the jug. I tossed the mixture (probably a good thing, or I'd still have the toxic PCBs in my fat cells that had been leached out of the soft plastic) and didn't come back to the memory for about ten years, when I had learned enough to use a glass jug and cover the mouth. Now it's ten years after that and I'm playing with herb and fruit flavorings, homemade airlocks, and different kinds of honey. And the evolution of our species continues.

Mead recipe not in story form:

Ingredients:

A 1 gallon glass juice jug or jar, or a 5 gallon glass water jug (harder to find, a hard plastic one will also work, but don't let the ferment get too acidic or it will begin to leach the plastic)

3 cups or 750 mL of honey, preferably raw

A breathable piece of cloth, coffee filter, or sprouting bag

A rubber band and the jug's lid (you can also cover the opening with your palm during shaking, if you don't have the lid)

Directions:

Put the honey in the jug, fill with water, cap it. Shake it vigorously until the honey is dissolved. Remove the lid and secure the breathable material over the opening with the rubber band.

Put it in a warm place, out of the sun, and swirl it a couple of times a day to keep it mixed and aerated. The more oxygen and honey the yeasts can get at, the faster the fermentation. You can also stir it with a clean, long spoon.

In a few days you'll notice gentle bubbling; it will slow down and eventually stop over the course of 2 or 3 weeks. The brew will become less sweet the longer it ferments. Start tasting it after 2 weeks, and you'll notice it becoming drier, higher in alcohol, and more viscous. There's no rule about when it's best enjoyed, and it's nice to have a little bit of simple, plain mead every few days and experiencing the arc of its life cycle.

Flavoring Your Mead

Other ingredients can be added at various points in the process; adding fresh foods to mead or vinegar was once necessary to preserve them; it's likely that appreciation for the new flavors came second. It's easiest to add berries, herbs, fruits, roses, etc along with the water at the beginning of the brewing process, though much of the flavor will go out of them as their sugars are used as a food source by the yeasts along with the honey. Adding flavoring agents at or towards the end will generally yield a more flavorful brew, though you may want to play with partially or fully fermenting extra ingredients for added flavor, kick, and medicinal benefits. Be careful though, because many delicious herbal and medicinal flavorings are actually anti-microbial, and will prevent the fermentation process altogether. Cloves, eucalyptus, chilis, garlic, lemon, burdock, marigold, and grapefruit seed are anti-microbial, so add them only after the initial fermentation.

When fruit is being used as an ingredient, it has the habit of floating on top of the mead, creating what is called a "cap". This can cause a couple of issues with the fermentation, the most crucial of which is the potential for contamination. When the cap sits for an extended period of time on top of the mead, it can begin to dry out, creating a crust on which mold can grow. This mold will then contaminate the mead, creating off flavors and potential health risks. The cap can also restrict the bubbling off of the carbon dioxide, which will build up in the mead and slow down the fermentation. To prevent the cap from drying out and to aid in the release of the CO_2, the cap needs to be punched down a couple of times a day. This requires nothing more than to gently stir the fruit back down into the mead using a clean spoon.

Adding pureed ingredients anytime before the very end will make them ferment too quickly, the bacteriological equivalent of putting a bunch of toddlers in a pool filled with cotton candy. Freezing pieces of fruits or whole berries will burst their cell walls and make the juices more available to the fermentation, while decelerating the process by giving their cellular innards a little privacy. Traditional flavors include apple and cinnamon, the lemon herbs (-grass, -thyme, -basil, -balm, and -verbena), and mulling spices. I've tried lemon/ginger, raspberry/tangerine/goat milk kefir (citrus is best sliced into disks, peel on), clove/cinnamon, and cacao/mint, and like them all. Some people even throw in multi-vitamins, why the heck not? The following is a recipe from Edward Spencer's "The Flowing Bowl", 1903:

"Take of spring water what quantity you please, and make it more than blood-warm, and dissolve honey in it til 'tis strong enough to bear an egg, the breadth of a shilling; then boil it gently near an hour, taking off the scum as it rises; then put to about nine or ten gallons seven or eight large blades of mace, three nutmegs quartered, twenty cloves, three or four sticks of cinnamon, two or three roots of ginger, and a quarter of an ounce of Jamaica pepper; put these spices into the kettle to the honey and water, a whole lemon, with a sprig of sweet-briar and a sprig of rosemary; tie the briar and rosemary together, and when they have boiled a little while take them out and throw them away; but let your liquor stand on the spice in a clean earthen pot till the next day; then strain it into a vessel that is fit for it; put the spice in a bag, and hang it in the vessel, stop it, and at three months draw it into bottles. Be sure that 'tis fine when 'tis bottled; after 'tis bottled six weeks 'tis fit to drink."

> "Wine is constant proof that God loves us and loves to see us happy. -Benjamin Franklin

Works for me. Note – most mead recipes recommend boiling honey, which kills all the bacteria and yeasts already present. This allows for an easier foothold for the wild yeasts that come in to ferment the mead. This may be true but I dislike removing any benefits, and as mentioned in the section about raw honey (see "Kitchen SinkFarming Volume 4: Homegrown Living Recipes – What to Do with Your Sprouts and Krauts") heating honey can release toxin compounds the bees picked up from the flowers they visited. I prefer honey raw, unadulterated and alive.

Alcohol

The alcohol content of your mead is determined by a couple of different things. First, the kinds of yeasts that are in your brew have different tolerances to alcohol, which is their waste product (along with CO_2), and poisonous to them. Once the level of alcohol goes higher than their ability to live in it, they will die and their contribution to the ferment will end. These tolerances are well-documented in commercial yeast, but in wild fermentations every batch can be excitingly unpredictable.

The second factor is how much honey is in the brew. A starting ratio of more water to less honey will give the yeasts less food to convert to alcohol, and therefore lower alcohol in the finished product. More honey will yield the opposite result. More honey can also be added a few times during the fermentation, which will make the mead both sweeter and higher in alcohol. It's important to note that the higher the alcohol content, the less susceptible your mead will be unwanted secondary fermentation, that is, new wild microorganisms coming into your mature brew and producing less-than-desirable flavors.

Once the fermentation has slowed, the bubbles being few, you can enjoy your mead right away or bottle it, or just remove the permeable top from the mouth of the container and screw on a lid, another reason I use canning jars

> "It has been my experience that folks who have no vices have very few virtues." - Abraham Lincoln

for everything. Since the CO2 has nowhere to go, it will build pressure and create a slightly sparkling beverage. It can also be strained to remove the cloudy sediment and yeasty flavor common in high-end champagne but that some people don't love. Other flavors can be added at this time, or more honey or other sweetner to start an anaerobic secondary fermentation. Fruit juice fills both categories.

The exact alcohol content can be measured with a handy tool called a hydrometer, which measures the specific gravity, or thickness, of a liquid. Since alcohol is thicker and stickier than water, it's as easy as measuring before and after.

I'm not going to mention the numerous negative effects of alcohol here, but for our purposes it's worth noting that it can kill the probiotics you've so carefully cultivated in the digestive system. It can also adversely affect every system in the body. But of all libations, home-brewed mead might have the least detriment, and its benefits might possibly tip the scales.

I highly recommend the sections on mead and yeast in "Sacred and Herbal Healing Beers: The Secrets of Ancient Fermentation" by Stephen Harrod Buhner

Ginger Beer

Ginger beer is a refreshing sparkling soda made with the help of wild yeasts. As far as I've seen, even the best bottled ginger ales sold today uses cultivated yeasts and cream of tartar, and so lack the olde-timey flavor that makes authentic, wild ginger beer so special. Once again, the best foods and drinks are only available to the DIY-er and their friends, and for a fraction of the price of the counterfeit.

The first batch of ginger brew requires a "starter" (called a "bug" in Jamaica) which can then be stored for subsequent batches. A starter is a recipe of some sugar and ginger in water that lures the right kind of wild yeasts in. It's handy to have a grater or zester for the ginger (about $10), though it can also be finely chopped or grated with a very clean wood rasp, if you're the type that uses woodworking tools in everyday life. You'll also need some glass bottles that seal, like ones with screw-on lids or bail-wire tops, like old Grolsch beer bottles. The water you use is important; it must be totally free of chlorine so that the yeasts can live and thrive, so if you don't have access to filtered water then get some from the tap and leave it out for 24 hours to let the chlorine evaporate away. A much easier but less traditional and crisp ginger brew can be found in "Kitchen SinkFarming Volume 4: Homegrown Living Recipes – What to Do with Your Sprouts and Krauts".

A slightly more advanced version – worth trying if you're sensitive to sugar is using a combination of raw sugar (also called "turbinado") to feed the yeast, and palm sugar to sweeten the soda; microscopic organisms prefer the simplest form of sugar, which shocks our more complex system.

Ginger Beer Recipe (makes a gallon):

Ingredients

Ginger, skin and all

2 Cups raw sugar (or ½ Cup raw and 1 ½ Cups palm)

2 Lemons

1 Cup Warm Water

Cheesecloth or similar

A small bowl

Bottles

For the "Bug":

Combine 1 cup of pure water, 1 teaspoon grated ginger, and 1 teaspoon raw sugar in a small bowl. Put in a warm place with access to fresh air, like a window sill, and cover with something that will keeps bugs out and let yeasts in, like

cheesecloth. Feed the bug every other day by adding another teaspoon each of ginger and sugar and stir, until the

liquid starts to bubble, should be between 4 and 8 days. It's most efficient to grate 6 tablespoons ginger all at once on day one and keep it in the fridge.

The brew can be made anytime the bug is active – keep feeding it until you use it. If you plan on multiple batches, save a few teaspoons of the living starter for future batches in the fridge, where it will stay viable for a couple of weeks.

For the Ginger Brew:

In a pot, combine 2 quarts of water, 2-4 teaspoons grated ginger (depending on how strong you want the ginger flavor) and 1-1 ½ cup sugar (I prefer palm sugar at this point but more raw sugar is fine). Boil the mixture for 15 minutes, then let it cool for about an hour. If you're in a rush, you can use less water then add ice to make up the difference. Make sure the sugar water cools down to less than 110° F, so as not to kill your carefully cultivated bug. It should be a comfortable temperature to your finger. Add the juice of the lemons, a few tablespoons of the strained ginger bug and stir.

Pour the soon-to-be soda into bottles, seal, and leave them to ferment in a warm dark place for 2 weeks or more. There's very little chance of an explosion, but as you're probably using used bottles it's not a bad idea to store them somewhere with detonation in mind, like an unused shower stall or a plastic tote container. Start testing the brew in about a week; the longer it ferments the less sugar and more carbonation it'll have, as the yeasts eat the sugar and produce CO_2. Refrigerate when done to "cold stabilize" the fermentation, and make sure it's cold when opened to avoid a frothy mess.

Fermented Bread

Picture cakey, soft slices of living bread with a hint of sour, slathered with savory vegetable tapenade, rich nut butter, light and velvety clarified butter, or creamy avocado sprinkled with sea salt. As easy as grinding up some sprouted grains and spreading them onto dehydrator trays, the next day pulling off warm, spongy pieces and eating them straight away. Or painting a thinner layer on the sheet to get crispy crackers. As with everything else in this book, enzyme and nutrient-rich sprouted grain loaves require little time and even less effort, and as we'll see in a moment, the very forces as work might be so misunderstood that they're attributed to gods or angels (though it may be me that doesn't understand). Though we'll cover the history, techniques, and benefits as thoroughly as I know how, this delicious nourishment is mostly the result of experimentation by fairly primitive people. I encourage you to prepare food with as much curiosity and abandon.

Grinding sprouted grains and baking them in the sun is commonly credited to the Essenes, a religious sect that lived near the Dead Sea from 200 BC to 100 AD, though I'm certain that these nutritious living loaves have been around for much longer. Whether or not you stick to raw foods, it might be an unusual experience to eat a couple of slices of moist and flavorful bread and feel light and vibrant afterwards. Sprouting the grain, as discussed in previous chapters, unlocks its full spectrum of nutrition and low temperature baking keeps its living enzymes intact, allowing for complete and effortless digestion and assimilation of all that goodness. We know that enzymes, the chemical components of food that account for its freshness and life begin to degrade at 110° F. However, the same characteristic that allows seeds to go dormant, retaining their potential vitality when sitting for years in the hot sun, can be used for culinary benefit as well.

We first sprout the seeds and grains we'll be using for our breads. Then we slowly turn up the heat, putting the already activated seed *back* into hibernation, allowing for higher-temperature baking that's safe for enzymes. It works like this: if living foods are heated just under 110° F for a half day or so, the enzymes are triggered to go into a dormant state, protecting themselves and their "host" seeds from harm, seeds which we've already made as nutritious and digestible as possible. The heat can be gradually turned up to about 160° F, and the enzymes will stay biologically active. It's a fun experiment: sprout some seeds (I've tried sunflowers, quinoa, and wheat) and separate them into two piles. Put one pile in the dehydrator at 108, or the oven on the "warm" setting, with the door slightly open, and carefully monitor the temperature. After 12 hours, turn up the heat to 150 and put the other group of sprouts in, remembering which group is which. After another day or so, take them out and re-soak them separately for a few hours, then start sprouting them again. You'll notice that the sprouts that were given a low-temp chance to go dormant will continue to sprout, while the other group has passed over to the other side. The group that does sprout will probably do so in a somewhat sluggish and stunted fashion; this can be fixed by slowly turning up the temperature more slowly. It could be quite important to know at what temperature each seed goes dormant and how high its enzymes can survive – please send me the results of your experiments at jp@KitchenSinkFarming.com (and why not subscribe to the blog while you're at it?) and I'll compile a chart so we can know (before we eat them and feel the effects) how to maintain the life-force of our breads. This info might have benefits for storing and distributing high-quality foods in emergency situations as well.

> From the Essene Gospels:
>
> *"Let the angels of God prepare your bread. Moisten your wheat, that the angels of water may enter it. Then set it in the air, that the angel of air may embrace it. And leave it from morning to evening beneath the sun, that the angel of sunshine may descend upon it. And the blessings of the three angels will soon make the germ of life to sprout in your wheat. Then crush your grain, and make thin wafers, as did your forefathers when they departed out of Egypt, the house of bondage. Put them back again beneath the sun from its appearing, and when it is risen to its highest in the heavens, turn them over on the other side that they may be embraced there also by the angel of sunshine, and leave them there until the sun sets. For the angels of water, and air and of sunshine fed and ripened the wheat in the field, and they likewise must prepare also your bread. And the same sun which, with the fire of life, made the wheat to grow and ripen, must cook your bread with the same fire. For the fire of the sun gives life to the wheat, to the bread, and to the body. But the fire of death kills the wheat, the bread, and the body. And the living angels of the living God serve only living men. For God is the God of the living, and not the God of the dead."*

Pretty much the same as what we're saying here, but descriptive in their own way. I wonder why those ancient cookbook writers weren't more specific about what to put the loaf on, how to keep animals away, etc. Maybe it was common knowledge at the time, and in 2000 years people reading this are going to wonder why I didn't explain how to open the refrigerator door. The things we think.

My basic recipe for modern Essene bread calls for 2 cups unsprouted wheat, ¾ cups raisins, and a pinch of sea salt. The wheat is sprouted a little until the root starts to protrude (see "Kitchen Sink Farming Volume 1: Sprouting"), coarsely ground in a food processor or high-speed blender with the raisins, hand-shaped into a loaf, and baked at a low temperature. I find that wheat, with its high gluten content, makes a hearty and dense loaf which some people prefer, but low-temperature air has trouble penetrating to the center. This can be fixed, as in the passage above, by making "thin wafers". I prefer a loafy loaf of bread, with a crisp outer crust and a chewy, slightly moister center, so I go easy on the wheat, instead substituting sprouted grains like quinoa, millet, and amaranth, which have a light texture that allows for low-temperature baking, and a mild nutty flavor that's great in bread.

Naturally Yeasted

The *"it is risen to its highest in the heavens"* part can only refer to fermentation by wild yeast, and one of the best flavorings you can add (or more accurately, "let come in") to your bread. Sprouted breads don't have to be fermented to be nutritious and delicious, but the natural addition of beneficial bacteria will add a layer of health and a natural sourdough flavor so heavenly that you may never want to go a day without it.

If you're going the more traditional route of dehydrator or oven, the exposed fermentation can be duplicated or assisted by first making probiotic water out of the grains and seeds for a few days before grinding them. Bacteria and yeast will cling to the seeds, and they'll be blended into dough that's already biologically active. Obviously, it's better to get into the habit of making each thing for its own benefit and using the leftover "waste" for another project, as opposed to carrying out the several-step process of sprouting grains, then using them to make probiotic water, then making bread out of them, with bread being the purpose of the whole process. Each step has its benefits, and if you have some recently finished grains from probiotic water continuing to gently ferment in the fridge when you run out of bread, you'll be that much more supported by the whole Kitchen Sink Farming process. I prefer using pre-fermented grains than naturally-yeasted bread dough – I'd rather not cruelly tempt those beaks and talons. If I was a bird and found a luminous paste of freshly ground sprouted organic grains and raisins, warmed by the sun, lying out on some dude's balcony, I'd work pretty hard to get at it. If and when we have to find a way to feed ourselves without gas or electricity, (or camping, or a fun challenge) I suppose a clear plastic box or large glass vase would do, turned on its side so that the sun can shine through the top and the opening securely covered with a cloth would be a simple solution. A glass-block wall with broken sides could be an effective cookie machine, maybe the easy-bake oven of the future. A bird cage with a shelf inside… Lots of choices abound for enterprising apartment farmers.

See the "Bread, Crusts and Crackers" Section in "Kitchen SinkFarming Volume 4: Homegrown Living Recipes – What to Do with Your Sprouts and Krauts"

Cultivated Flora

As opposed to wild cultures as discussed above, cultivated floras are in their own section because, though they're fermented foods like the rest of this chapter, Kombucha, jun, apple cider vinegar, and kefir are the names given to distinct cultures, colonies of specific bacteria and yeasts that are often thousands of years old, and require a little more initial effort than putting out a bowl of candy and a welcome mat like the rest of our ferments. You'll first have to get a bit of this culture, then give it the opportunity to thrive. This will usually be the traditional method, but there are countless ways to use the culture to ferment other things, like in the case of "Coffee-boocha", or kefir-fermented apple butter.

In this section, you'll learn how to find the culture cheaply or freely from locally store-bought products or from folks willing to give the stuff away. The following sections will go over these cultures' many health benefits, safe and simple techniques for home-brewing, ways to procure the culture for cheap or free, and other, secondary products you can make at home with the cultures, like cheese and yogurt in the case of kefir, and vinegar, beer, and champagne ('booch hooch) for the kombucha.

Kombucha

Enjoyed for at least 2,000 years in Asia and Russia, kombucha is rapidly growing in popularity in the rest of the world, where it's sold in natural foods stores for $3-$4 a bottle, though it's really easy to make at home. Many people drink it every day for increased energy, nutrition, immune system and liver function, better digestion, and a plethora of other benefits. Its fermentation is caused by colonies of bacteria and yeasts, all working together and getting along in a way that'd make Rodney King proud, that modern science doesn't fully understand. Though the active organisms are microscopic, the evidence of their cooperation can be easily seen with your own eyes in a quite dramatic way.

The microorganisms in question build a Mother of Kombucha, or "SCOBY", an acronym that stands for "Symbiotic Colony Of Bacteria and Yeats". More accurately called a "zoogleal mat", this structure resembles a rubbery pancake and isn't the actual culture, but a *polysaccharide* matrix the organisms build to support themselves, and a really cool indication that something's happening. Even cooler – this germ home will reproduce itself in a week or two so you can start another batch, more quickly ferment in the container you're using, or trade it to someone for something else. The very definition of sustainable, all started from a few ounces of a store-bought drink.

To get your very own SCOBY, you'll need to do one of two things. Find someone willing to give or send one to you (try the craig's list barter section or the worldwide kombucha exchange at www.kombu.de). The SCOBY is rich in the organisms that will be brewing your tea, but all that's needed are the organisms, the SCOBY is just a hangout they've built. The easiest method of getting the kombucha creatures is from a bottle of unflavored, unpasteurized kombucha tea, available at most natural food stores, and when conditions are right they'll build a SCOBY on their own. When you buy a bottle of the drink, you're also buying the culture or "seed" which, just like an avocado pit, banana peel, or apple seed, can feed hundreds by cultivating what to most people is something between litter and compost. Be aware that many kombucha companies use a engineered culture designed to be more consistent in terms of fermentation and low alcohol content, but will die off after a couple of brews.

Kombucha Tea Recipe

What you'll need:

5-6 bags of caffeine tea or 10-12 grams of loose tea in a tea ball or sprouting bag.

1 ¼ - 1 ½ cups of sugar (400 grams or so)

¾ Gallon of filtered water

(more info on water, tea, and sugar follow this recipe)

A gallon jar (I get mine from bars; just ask the bartender or barback for an empty olive jar. A busy bar will throw away or recycle a few of these a week, so if you time it right they'll be happy to share. And if you're slowly sipping a dirty martini with extra olives and tip well, you might increase your chances.)

Something to keep out bugs but let in air, like a sprouting bag, coffee filter or piece of clean cloth and rubber band

A bottle of kombucha (unpasteurized, unflavored)

What you'll do:

Clean your gallon jar with soap and hot water. You can sterilize it with UV light, H202, or an oven if you're nerdy by nature like me (see pg 71).

Heat about half of the water to almost boiling; remove from heat and stir in tea. If you heat 2 quarts jars full of water in a microwave for 10 minutes then pour it into the gallon jug and brew right there, there's one less thing to wash. The hot, empty jars will quickly dry and be sparklingly clean.

After the tea has brewed sufficiently (some people go 5 minutes, others overnight) pour in the sugar and stir to dissolve it. Don't add the sugar to the boiling water because it will caramelize, though semi-hot water will help the sugar dissolve. Next add the rest of the water and let it cool to room temperature; there should be enough room at the top to allow for the kombucha starter and bubbles. Stick a clean finger in the tea to make sure it's comfortable to touch. If it's too hot for your skin, it's too hot for your new microscopic pets.

Pour in the bottle of kombucha tea, cover it with a coffee filter, clean cloth, or sprouting bag and let it sit in a warm place (60° F minimum, 75-80° F is optimal) for about 1 ½ - 2 weeks. Take a peek every so often and witness the awe-inducing formation of the SCOBY. If you haven't taken any creative license with these very lenient directions, you should have the beginnings of your own light-colored rubbery circle in a few days, and it should be fully formed in 1 ½ weeks or so. It looks like mold or curd as it's forming, don't fear, just wait and see that it forms a nice smooth disk. Taste the ferment. If it's sugar-sweet, that means that your little friends haven't eaten all the sugar and have some more work to do. The yeasts will actually produce fructose, or fruit sugar, which will be pleasantly sweet in a different way. If left to ferment further, they'll convert the fructose into gluconic and acetic acids, the flavors that give vinegar its kick. I like a good balance between the three, not too sweet with a nice acidic bite. The brew is done when it's refreshingly sparkling, pleasant-tasting (as long as you like the taste of the tea you started with) and slightly acidic (a ph of around 3.5 for you sciencey types). Five minutes of work and a couple of weeks of waiting and you have a gallon of this probiotic and enzyme-rich elixir.

There are two different ways to continue your kombucha fun: when you get to the end of your gallon, save a little bit of the liquid, clean the jar, and start over from the beginning. The other way is to do a continuous ferment: adding the amount of tea that you remove every other day or so, an uninterrupted process. I prefer the second method for several reasons. There's no waiting involved – after you've taken out your tea for the day, add enough sweet tea to fill the jar back up and your already-existing SCOBY will immediately go to work on breaking it down, so it will be ready the next day. It's easier – very simple to make a few cups of tea and pour them into your jar, and there's no weekly cleaning necessary. It's more consistent - since you're just maintaining a powerfully established ferment, your brew is much less likely to be influenced by wild bacteria and yeasts. It's healthier – gluconic acid, the factor most responsible for kombucha's wonderful cleansing properties, doesn't appear until about a week and a half. Many other esoteric benefits don't develop until 2 or 3 weeks or more.

When I was first fermenting kombucha, I used two 3-gallon glass jars with spigots that were sold as lemonade or vodka infusion jars on ebay. They were $18 each. I let one of them get about half empty, re-fill it with sweet tea, and then switched to drinking from the other one until it gots half empty, going back and forth like this indefinitely. If you go out of town, bottle almost all the 'booch, cutting off the air and stopping the fermentation, and stick it in the fridge or take it with you. Use beer bottles with snap-on lids or old kombucha bottles with heavy-duty screw-on caps – both are made to withstand some pressure. You can also use wine bottles and pound the cork back in with a rubber mallet (synthetic corks work best). If you use a container with a metal cap, keep it stored upright so the acidic tea won't come in contact with it and eat away at the metal. When you're gone the tea still in the jars will become quite acidic, so when you get home and start 2 new batches of brew, it will be ready to drink quickly. This technique also works well if you have a surplus of finished brew. Stick your bottled tea in the fridge when it's at its peak, in your opinion, adding whole or pureed citrus, ginger, berries, herbs, or other flavorings for your personal peek at the sublime.

Secondary fermentation is what happens in the bottle with the cap on at room temperature. Without new oxygen, the yeasts become more active (as opposed to the bacteria, who were the star during open-air fermentation). The yeasts will continue to ferment any sugar left in your brew. Their waste product is carbon dioxide (the same thing that gives beer, champagne, and soda its bubbles), so as fermentation continues the pressure will increase. Most people like to flavor their 'booch with 10-20% juice and leave their closed bottled out for a few days before sticking them in the fridge. Bottles can be "aged" for months or years, flavors developing and bubbles getting smaller and softer in the process, just like a fine champagne.

On Water, Tea, and Sugar

Water

Purified water is best for all the recipes in this book. Tap water contains many additives meant to kill off unwanted microorganisms in the water supply. These chemicals will also kill your kombucha culture, as well as the probiotics in your own system. Buying water or getting it delivered can be expensive, time-consuming, and environmentally unfriendly, and almost all bottled water is just filtered tap water in pretty bottles. If they're plastic bottles, they've been leaching chemicals into the water. The best route is to filter water yourself at home. A filtration system that removes chlorine, fluorine, chloramine, pesticide residue, heavy metals, and other contaminants can be had for a couple of hundred dollars; reverse osmosis is unnecessary unless you're using untreated water from a private well or spring. Distillation removes everything.. For city-dwellers, carbon block or another simple filtration system that pulls water through a .5 – 1 micron screen is fine.

Though some municipalities use other sanitizers, chlorine is the most common and easy to get rid of. If tap water is your only option, pour a gallon into a pot and let it sit for a day; the chlorine, which is lighter than air, will evaporate out.

Tea

Black teas, such as Sencha or Darjeeling, are the standard for kombucha brewing, and they're what most commercial brewers use. They don't have to put this, or what kind of sugar they use, on the labels, as the kombucha is considered to convert them, which it does but not completely. Black tea is the fermented leaves of the tea plant, and has the highest caffeine content of any tea; about half of the caffeine in the original tea gets converted into the many acids listed above, and the other half remains in the brew. If you're sensitive to caffeine, green tea works just as well and has about a third the caffeine of black (as well as a host of anti-oxidant properties). Green tea is the unfermented, dried and steamed leaves of the tea plant. Black tea will produce a fruity, apple-y amber brew, while green will have a light and grassy flavor. Oolong tea is halfway between green tea and black tea, both in flavor and caffeine content. It's gently rolled after picking and allowed to partially ferment until the edges of the leaves start to turn brown.

Earl grey has bergamot oil which is damaging to the culture. Herbal teas will not work either, at least in the long run, because they have oils that could damage the culture, and are missing the nutrients and purines found in the tea plant that are necessary to produce the brew. There are two exceptions. Rooibos is a South Africa plant that is caffeine-free and is respected for its health benefits; it's anti-aging and anti-allergy, has oligosaccharides (compounds found to fight viral infections), combats high blood pressure, diabetes, and atherosclerosis, and is good for the skin. Honeybush is a different family of plants, though also from South Africa, and is slightly sweeter than rooibos. Neither rooibos nor honeybush contain tannins, so are fine for people with tannic allergies, and can be steeped much longer than true tea without becoming bitter.

Caffeine stimulates the reproduction of micro-organisms, so if you're using a caffeine-free tea and find your fermentation slowing down, you may want to do a cycle of caffeine tea to re-invigorate your brew. It can be given away if you're sensitive or allergic to caffeine.

It's much cheaper to buy tea "loose", that is, not in bags, and measure the appropriate amount into a sprout bag or tea ball. A kitchen scale is invaluable for this, as well as measuring the sugar, herbs and spices, and mail (if you print your postage out from home on usps.com you get free tracking). They start at $15 with free shipping on ebay, and my cheap Chinese scale has lasted me 4 years thus far.

Sugar

White sugar, also called "evaporated cane juice" or other creatively green-washed derivatives, is the best for kombucha. It's sugar in its simplest form, which the simple digestive systems of single-celled organisms appreciate. Other sweeteners might be better for us, like honey, palm sugar, or molasses, but these are more difficult for the culture to utilize and leave residual substances in the brew, which can ferment on their own by attracting unwanted organisms. There will be some sugar leftover in the brew that you drink (though some of the sweetness comes from sugar recombined into the fruit sugar fructose), but it's a small price to pay for the innumerable benefits. Use organic, free-trade if possible, unbleached sugar (though not brown or muscovado).

Health Benefits of Kombucha

First off, kombucha is a living beverage, complete with all the enzymatic and probiotic benefits discussed elsewhere in this book. But that's not all – ferment now and we'll also throw in these powerful compounds…

LACTIC ACID is found in kombucha in its most potent form L-lactic(+). Lactic acid is essential for the digestive system in breaking down foods, improving digestibility, stimulate peristaltic movement of the intestines to improve regularity, assisting blood circulation, normalizing acidity of gastric juices, which in turn helps maintain proper body pH (see section on Alkalinity in "Kitchen Sink Farming Volume 1: Sprouting" pg 122), and helps restore the level of healthy bacteria in the digestive system. It's also highly detoxifying. Eli Metchnikoff won a Nobel Prize in 1908 for his research on the benefits of lactic acid to our health and immune system.

GLUCORONIC ACID is responsible for "xenobiotic metabolism" (from the Greek xeno, stranger) that remove toxic foreign substances from the liver like drugs, pollutants, androgens, estrogens, corticoids, and retinoids.

ACETIC ACID inhibits harmful bacteria in both you and your brew. It is also gives the tea a nice kick. This is where the vinegar flavor comes from that will increase as the brew is fermented further.

MALIC ACID also assists in detoxification.

OXALIC ACID encourages the mitochondria, the cell's energy producer, and is a natural preservative.

GLUCONIC ACID is effective against many yeast infections such as candidiasis and thrush, and dissolves mineral deposits, those crunchy things that develop in chronically tight muscles.

BUTYRIC ACID is produced by the yeasts and when working with gluconic acid. Also helps combat yeast infections such as candida.

NUCLEIC ACIDS work with the body aiding healthy cell

regeneration.

AMINO ACIDS are the building blocks of protein.

GLUCOSAMINES **prevent or treat all forms of arthritis** by increasing synovial hyaluronic acid production. This joint lubricant functions physiologically to aid in the preservation of cartilage structure and help the joints glide, preventing arthritic pain. Hyaluronic acid and synovial fluid are the major difference between young joints and old ones, as this emollient decreases as we age. It enables connective tissue to bind moisture thousands of times its weight and maintain tissue structure, moisture, lubrication and flexibility, and elsewhere in the body lessens free radical damage while associated collagen retards and reduces wrinkles.

PROBIOTICS improve digestion, fight candida and other harmful yeasts, and remove carcinogens in the intestines and colon, fighting cancer in yet another way. These biologically active aspects of kombucha are being studied for their far-reaching effects, relieving **everything from symptoms of fibromyalgia to depression and anxiety.**

It's extraordinarily **ANTIOXIDANT RICH, boosting the immune system in both the short and long terms, and increasing energy levels.**

An in-depth study of several individual ferments found analgesic compounds, anti-arthritics, anti-spasmodics, hematinics (increase hemoglobin content of the blood so used to treat anemia, iron deficiency) and counteractions for hepatotoxins, anti-fungal compounds, and several anti-microbial/anti-bacterial compounds. They also contained beneficial enzyme inhibitors of glucuronidase, heparinase, hyaluronidase, and monoamine oxidase. But because kombucha is a living product resulting from the actions of dozens of organisms, what is in a ferment is not 100%

universal, except for gluconic, acetic and glucuronic acids, and fructose.

Kombucha hasn't yet been extensively studied by medical science because of its relatively recent debut on the Western stage. But based on the Russian discovery that entire regions of their vast country were seemingly immune to cancer, researchers at the Hokkaido University in Japan have isolated either glucuronic or glucaric acids, substances which help the liver in detoxification. Without the presence of these compounds, the liver will re-absorb whatever toxin it has just laboriously removed from the blood and bowels. It's also rich in many of the enzymes and bacterial acids our bodies use for detoxification, thereby easing the workload on the liver, pancreas, blood, and digestive system. This family of substances is being looked into for its anti-cancer properties and seeming ability to render some chemotherapy-related toxins completely inert. There is, however, overwhelming anecdotal evidence about kombucha's anti-cancer properties; Alexander Solzhenitsyn, the recently deceased Russian author and Nobel prize winner, claimed in his autobiography that kombucha tea cured his stomach cancer during his internment in Soviet labor camps. Because of this testimony, President Ronald Reagan used kombucha to halt the spread of his cancer in 1987. He didn't die until 2004, and that was from age-related disease, not cancer.

Billions of microorganisms of different species working together to feed, nourish, cleanse, and sustain. I'll drink to that.

Vinegar Flies

Wherever there's vinegar brewing, these pesky little friends (sometimes called fruit flies) show up. They love fermentation almost as much as I do, which is why they're often found around overripe bananas and oranges, or getting funky on an old batch of collard greens. I used to try to catch them in my fist and put them outside, until I learned that these are the critters most commonly used in labs to study genetics because of their short life cycle and hardiness. Then I thought: if I remove all the slow ones, leaving just the fast ones to reproduce, I'm inadvertently

breeding a super-strain of ninja gnats. I've found that the best way to deal with them without direct violence is to put some vinegar in a glass or bowl and cover it with plastic wrap. Then poke a bunch of holes in the top with a fork (a piece of paper rolled into an downward-pointing cone with a small hole in the tip, above the level of the liquid, also works). The flies can get in but they can't get out. Kind of mean, but they are vinegar flies, after all, so I bet they die happy.

Kombucha can also be used to ferment other things in the same way that vegetables are "pickled" with raw apple cider vinegar. Fill a jar with sliced cucmbers and kombucha with onions, garlic, dill, and a grape leaf (for crunchiness) and enjoy fresh zingy pickles in a few days to a few weeks. Put a SCOBY and some starter tea in coffee for "Coffee-Boocha®", one of my probiotic drink company's most popular products(SOMA evolutionary refreshment in Porltand, Oregon).

Jun

Very little is known about this very special culture, said to be from Tibet. It's hard to find, my company is the only I know of that producing it commercially, and I've never found any studies about it. Hard-core kombucha fans often try jun once and switch their allegiance, as jun gives a calm and grounded energy that's at the same time mellow and ecstatic.

While kombucha is a symbiotic colony of 30-40 different bacteria and yeasts, jun is just one of each. Jun lives on honey and green tea as as opposed to kombucha's sugar and black tea craving, and their difference is evidenced by their nearly identical fermentation time – but brew kombucha with honey and you'll likely triple or quadruple your wait. Honey has powerful anti-bacterial properties, some of which are enzymatic and therefore destroyed by heating, but even cooked honey has a compound that's antibacterial. More on honey in the "Desserts" section of "Kitchen Sink Farming Volume 4: Living Homegraown Recipes – What to Do with Your Sprouts and Krauts".

Jun loves raw honey and takes on an appley-pear flavor as it brings out honey's malic and citric acids with a fructose boost - the combination that gives pears and apples their distinctive crisp sweetness - a process that also takes place in nice wines though jun does it without making alcohol. It's interesting to note that kombucha doesn't like raw honey, and using it instead of sugar will slow kombucha's fermentation time to a month or longer (or kill the culture). Many jun cultures are actually kombucha, and fermenting speed is one way to test this. Jun SCOBYs also look darker, thinner, and less rubbery than kombucha's.

If you're lucky enough to find a jun mother, ferment it in the following manner:

Bring 3 liters of water to 200°F and remove from heat

Steep 12 Green Teabags (or 1 oz tea – twice as much as for kombucha) for 5-10 minutes

Add 2 Cups Honey (raw preferred, wait until water is under 110°F before adding)

When liquid is cooled to room temperature add jun mother

Pour all into a gallon jar and cover with a clean cloth

Drink after a week or two, depending on temperature and strength of your culture. Jun is very sensitive and goes dormant or dead much more easily than any other culture, and may require some coaxing or another starter. When you have a strong culture going, put a mother in the freezer as a backup.

Kefir (Dairy)

Kefir is another "imported" culture; here it refers to dairy kefir. There's a culture called "tibicos" that ferments juice anaerobically (as opposed to dairy kefir, which uses oxygen) and is also refered to as "juice kefir" – more on this in the next section. Dairy kefir is a group of specific bacteria and yeasts that the inhabitants of the Caucus Mountains in Russia have asserted for centuries or more are responsible for their longevity. Like kombucha, the organisms responsible for making kefir form a polysaccharide mass, in this case fluffy cloud-like chunks that can grow to the size of garbanzo beans, called *kefir grains*, which give the probiotics something to attach to. The various cooperating microorganisms that make kefir occur naturally in the Caucuses; the story goes that the inhabitants of the region used to hang large leather sacs filled with milk in their doorways, organically inviting in the benevolent microscopic visitors; guests would give the bag a friendly slap or sharp poke on their way in and out and thereby keep the brew mixed and fermentation even. Those of us with Russian grandparents aren't surprised at the harshness sometimes shown to objects of love and affection.

Kefir has been much more thoroughly studied by medical science than kombucha (maybe because its effects were more localized and therefore more obvious), and the amount of hard data is encouraging. Dr. Orla-Jenson, a noted Danish bacteriologist specializing in dairy research states that "Kefir digests yeast cells and has a beneficial effect on the intestinal flora". It's high in calcium, amino acids, B-vitamins and folic acid, can repair a damaged digestive system or help build a healthy one in babies, and has even been shown to protect against the negative effects of nuclear radiation. If it can combat radiation imagine how powerful it can be against the effects of environmental damage, pollution, stress, harmful bacteria, viruses, fungi, and yeasts such as Candida, a harmful parasite that grows in the bloodstream of over 80% of people. Kefir's friendly cultures also produce specific antibiotic substances which can control undesirable microorganisms and act as anti-carcinogens. It's also been proven to combat acne in more than three-quarters of teenaged sufferers tested.

For people who drink milk, the benefits of kefir are mainly due to the breakdown of the aspects of milk that make it difficult to digest, thereby allowing all the benefits to be fully enjoyed. Lactose is converted into the immensely beneficial lactic acid, so people with lactose intolerance (an estimated 75% of the world's population) can enjoy kefir without digestive anxiety. It also pre-digests the many proteins, which no longer stay hard and largely unusable by humans.

Eli Metchnikoff, an international Nobel Prize-winning researcher, found in 1908 that kefir activates the flow of saliva, most likely due to its lactic acid content and its slight amount of carbonation, and that it stimulates peristalsis (the wave-like motion of the bowels that push food along) and digestive juices in the intestinal tract. For these reasons, it is recommended as a post-operative food since most abdominal operations cause peristalsis (the waving motion of the bowels that pushes food through) to freak out and stop. It's also great to use whenever digestion has slowed, due to travel, stress, sleep deprivation, or pregnancy.

Dr. Johannes Kuhl conducted one of the foremost European studies of lactic acid, which he found in high amounts in kefir. Among many other benefits, he found that a well-balanced diet with liberal amounts of lactic acid fermented foods was a good protection against cancer.

For folks concerned about the safety of drinking milk that's been sitting out for days or weeks, it should be noted that lactic acid bacteria actually fight pathogenic organisms, killing e. coli and salmonella, while s. paratyphi and c. diphtheriae lose their pathogenic properties. Kefir cultures have also been reported to help treat achylia gastrica, peptic ulcers, cholecystitis, gastroenteritis, colitis, diarrhea, and dysentery.

Dairy Kefir: History and Mystery

The origins of kefir are shrouded in mystery and adventure. It was said to be given to the people of the northern slopes of the Caucasian Mountains by Mohammed, who told them to closely guard their secret, as the strength of this powerful health tonic would dissipate as more people learned about it. "The Grains of the Prophet" were seen as part of a family's wealth and were passed on from generation to generation like an heirloom, so for centuries the people of the northern Caucasus enjoyed this fizzy tonic and its benefits in secret.

Tales began to spread about kefir's existence, and Marco Polo mentioned a "magical" elixir of fermented milk in his writings. Most of the world remained largely ignorant of kefir, however, until the end of the 19th Century, when Russian doctors began studying the health of the people from the Caucus Mountains and deciding that kefir was worth looking into. Not being able to find a source for the grains, however, the All Russian Physician's Society enlisted the help of the Blandov Brothers, who not only ran the Moscow Dairy, but also had ties to the Caucus region. With the agreement that they would be the only commercial producers, the brothers became determined to procure some of the probiotic beverage.

In the summer of 1908 they sent a beautiful young employee, Irina Sakharova, to the court of a local prince, Bek-Mirza Barchorov. Her mission: charm the prince into giving away some kefir grains, and whisk them back to Moscow. The jealousy with which this mystical culture was guarded was underestimated, however, and when the prince discovered her plan he imprisoned her with a mind to keep her there forever as his bride. A daring rescue by agents of the Blandovs followed, the forced marriage was stopped and the foiled prince dragged before the Czar. It was decided that Irina Sakharova was to be given ten pounds of the grains as recompense for her insults, and the Blandovs began the cultivation and production of kefir which is immensely popular in Moscow to this day.

In the 1970's and early 80's microbiologists attempted to create kefir grains from the isolated organisms that make up the colony. They were unsuccessful, and it's still unknown how the bio-matrix that is a kefir grain is created. The researchers eventually gave up, capitulating to the fact that an unknown factor made the first propagation of kefir possible in the Caucus Mountains, for reasons that are unable to be duplicated in the lab.

Just as it was for the All Russian Physician's Society in the early 1900's, the hardest part for modern kefir culturers is finding the grains, but a quick internet search will yield lots of people willing to sell or share (check out the "Resources" section and the end of the book). Try to find grains that have been used in raw milk, which will be the strongest and most viable, with goat's milk preferred over cow's. I've never seen any that weren't grown in organic milk, but make sure to double check that. Gently put your grains in a glass jar, pour in some milk, (again organic raw goat milk is best, but your kefir will improve any kind of milk) and cover the jar in a way that lets in air and keeps out bugs; the old sprout bag or coffee filter and rubber band or screw-on ring method works fine. The grains can also be used to make kefir out of nut and seed milks, coconut water or milk, fruit and vegetable juice, or even water with sugar, maple syrup, honey or other sweetner. I heard about some people who kefir-ed Gatorade, dyeing their grains a neon blue. This didn't change the culture's effectiveness but I wouldn't recommend that for obvious reasons. Kefir cultures thrive in mammal milk, however, and I recommend a cycle in raw animal milk for every couple of weeks in other liquids, though I've had a stable group of grains fermenting in coconut water for several months.

To make kefir, put a couple of tablespoons into milk (raw is best, and though it will ferment any mammal milk, goat is recommended over cow because of many reasons, such as its easier digestibility and better nutrition. For humans). Cover the container with a clean cloth, sprout or produce bag, or coffee filter and secure it. Kefir stays un-refrigerated while it's brewing, and in a few hours to a day the whey will separate from the milk proteins, which rise to the top of the liquid, and a quick swirl or stir with a spoon or chopstick will blend them back together. I employ a continuous fermentation method like the one with kombucha.

Your kefir will be ready in a day or two – taste and smell your milk to determine readiness. When to enjoy your kefir is a matter of taste; the healthful lactic acid will produce a kind of sourness so the kefir is done when it's the sourest you can enjoy. Then, just like with kombucha, you have the choice to do an interrupted or continuous fermentation – cover and put the finished kefir in the fridge and start a new batch, or every time you strain some kefir out, pour some fresh milk back in. About a half day later, the whey will separate out of the fresh milk; a swirl or stir will mix it back in. Just like with kombucha, I recommend the continuous process; it's easier, gentler on the culture, and I have to imagine that (again, just like kombucha) new benefits are continually created over the weeks and months. I've been using this method for years and my potent culture is consistent and dependable.

When you're ready to enjoy your kefir, strain some through a screen strainer into a glass, and gently drop the grains back into the fermenting cuture. Or get a tea straw, like ones made for yerba mate or loose-leaf tea that has a little strainer at the bottom (glass is easy to keep clean), and just drink straight from your culture. Never rinse the grains, as you're washing away valuable probiotics, or press them to squeeze out the kefir. The grains will increase in size and quantity; soon you'll notice your fermentations speeding up, and you'll have enough grains to separate for other fermenting projects, give away, or eat, as they happen to taste sweet and delicious. The kefir produces carbon dioxide, and putting an air-tight lid on the finished product in the fridge will produce an effervescent potation.

I went through a phase of tossing kefir into most anything liquid I made: salad dressings, smoothies, dips and soups, slightly souring and adding a new dimension of flavor and health to each (check out the recipe for "Pepita Sour Crema" in "Kitchen Sink Farming Volume 4: Homegrown Living Recipes – What to Do with Your Sprouts and Krauts"). The kefir grains want to be able to get at all of the liquid; if it's so thick that there's no circulation, you'll just have a pocket of healthy fermentation happening in what's otherwise a jar of stuff sitting out on the counter. You want to avoid that so other bacteria don't come in and colonize the rest while the forces of good are trapped elsewhere. If the substance doesn't move freely you'll want to stir it a few times a day with a spoon or chopstick, and in a few days it'll taste like you added goat cheese, sour cream, or yogurt to whatever you were using. The health benefits of this are obvious, but the culinary aspects can be quite pleasantly surprising: kefir'ed cream of mushroom soup and tomato-basil bisque (just to mention a couple) are so good you'll never want to go back to the ordinary versions. If you can't find the grains to remove them, don't worry about it; they're delicious and also very healthy.

Kefir grains are acidic, and for this reason many people recommend not using metal utensils thinking that the kefir will leach metals from the substance. This is true only in the case of reactive metals such as brass, aluminum, copper, silver, zinc, and iron. Stainless steel is fine. When kefir was catching on in the early 20th century, these reactive metals were commonly used to make kitchen implements, so that's maybe where the thought came from. I only say this as a warning not to bring the above metals in contact with your culture, and also in case someone tells you that all metal is a no-no, a common misconception.

Kefir Recap:

Add kefir grains to milk (1 tablespoon to a quart minimum, there's no maximum. More grains = faster fermentation)

When separation occurs, swirl or stir the brew to keep curds (floating proteins) and whey (clear liquid) togetherIn 1-3 days, strain out some kefir with a mesh strainer and

> dump the grains back in, or drink straight out of the jar with a straining straw, and refill with fresh milk.

Kefir as Starter

Your living ferment is a delicious and probiotic beverage on its own, but it's also a versatile starter culture for anything from apple butter to sauerkraut.

Living kefir seperates into two parts: whey and laban. Whey, the clearish liquid that rises to the top of fermenting kefir, can be poured off and added to pretty much anything: chopped vegetables, like cabbage for kefir-kraut, and fruit butters are among my favorites - look for "Ginger-Kefir Apple Butter" in "Kitchen Sink Farming Volume 4: Homegrown Living Recipes – What to Do with Your Sprouts and Krauts". Sulfur-containing amino acid-rich kefir whey can also be used in place of buttermilk in any recipe, or subbed for water in bread for an easy sourdough (or even cake (see "Whey-Dough Bread" and "Sour Chocolate Cake" in "Kitchen Sink Farming Volume 4 – Homegrown Living Recipes – What to Do with Your Sprouts and Krauts). Whey-Good Ginger Cream Soda (pg 125) is much easier than capturing your own wild "ginger bug" and, as the name implies, the whey gives a delicious creaminess to the soda. Whey can also be used as a facewash, anti-dandruff shampoo, or mixed with aloe vera gel to make an emollient, anti-psoriasis lotion or shave cream. It can also be added to any drink or food for humans or animals for a nutritive probiotic boost.

Whey can be added to cream to make sour cream, which can then be shaken or churned to make real olde-timey butter (next section).

What's left after the whey and grains are removed is called "laban", or Basic Kefir Cheese, and is the other starter in kefir. The best way to remove all the whey is to pour the strained kefir into a sprout bag or pre-moistened cheese cloth, and hang it over a bowl for 12-24 hours. It can also be done in smaller quantities in a coffee-maker – spoon some kefir onto a coffee filter and put the coffee pot underneath to catch the whey.

The resulting laban is a flavorful cross between cream and cottage cheese, and is awesome right away, spread on sprouted loaves, with fruit (a traditional dessert from the Caucuses), or any other way you'd use the previously mentioned condiments. Blend 3 tablespoons oil per cup of Basic Kefir Cheese, along with herbs or vegetables for a delicious dip. Plain Basic Kefir Cheese can also be used to make hard cheeses.

Add a teaspoon of salt to each quart of Basic Kefir Cheese, and put it back in the sprout bag, cheese cloth, or coffee filter. Osmosis will pull even more liquid out, and another day of draining will yield a nice block of cheese that can be pressed into a wheel or brick and left to air dry for a week or two. To give it just a little air, put it into a sprout bag in a jar, hang the string over the lip of the jar, and screw the lid on. It can also be left on a counter with an upturned container over it, flipped daily. If a white mold covers the cheese, consider yourself lucky, as you have not one but two kingdoms of organism working for your dinner: bacteria and mold. The white fuzz is harmless and will add a magnificent depth of flavor to your fromage. If the mold starts to get colorful though, these could be pathogens (probably not, but it's hard to test outside of a lab) so it's best to toss it and start over.

When the Basic Kefir Cheese is dry to the touch, it can be waxed to ripen without drying further (in two months you'll have sharp cheddar, in 6 months to a year you'll get a robust parmesan). For kefir feta, drop your fresh cheese in a 7% salt water solution for two months (make sure it's dry and well-pressed prior to plunking it in the brine so it doesn't fall apart). A little blue cheese can be mixed into the Basic Kefir Cheese and it will propagate into the whole thing. Most hard cheeses are best after at least two months of aging.

Storing your kefir grains

If you'll be away for a week or less, your kefir grains will hibernate nicely sealed in the fridge in some fresh milk. The fermentation will slow greatly, so to them it'll feel like a day on the counter. If you're leaving for 2 months or less, the grains can be frozen in a sealed container – a little dry milk powder will help prevent freezer burn. Frozen kefir has been known to last a year or more, but the best way to suspend your culture for the long-term is to dehydrate the grains. They can be dried at under 110° F for a couple of days until they look like little yellow lava rocks. I find that drying them in a batch of kefir laban, spread out on a dehydrator sheet, helps them re-animate the fastest and most consistently.

Whey-Good Ginger Cream Soda

Ingredients:

1 ½ cups kefir whey
1 cup water
2 inches juiced or blended and strained ginger
4 Tbl sweetner – raw honey, sugar, etc
1/2 tsp salt

> **Do:**
>
> Combine all ingredients in a quart or larger mason jar. Cover with clean cloth, sprout or produce bag, or coffee filter, and allow to ferment at room temperature for 2-3 days. Optional: add juice of 5 oranges for a creamsicle treat.

Tibicos (Juice Kefir)

There exists another culture called water kefir or tibicos, and is from Japan. Like dairy kefir and kombucha, it makes a SCOBY, a symbiotic collection of bacteria and yeast, held together by a polysaccharide matrix. Water kefir SCOBY looks more like small clear crystals than rubbery rice-like dairy kefir grains, so for the sake of clarity I call it water kefir, crystal kefir, or tibicos, while dairy kefir retains the generic label "kefir".

Water kefir can live in any sugary liquid, producing readily available lactic acid bacteria and carbonation, and are the best choice for fermenting non-dairy beverages. These drinks will have less health benefits than kombucha and milk kefir, but coconut water "champagne", fermented juices and teas are a wonderful way to enjoy cultured thirst-quenchers. Water kefir is also a great way to remove sugars from sweet liquids. I always crystal kefir maple syrup for the master cleanse (a ten-day diet of maple syrup, lemon juice, and cayenne in water to purify the digestive system and detoxify the body). My probiotic drink company SOMA Evolutionary Refreshment® makes "Maharaj Cleanse®", crystal kefired and kombuchaed master cleanse with the addition of crystal kefired coconut water, and it's very popular as both a cleanse and beverage.

To make a sparklingly alive water kefir drink, gently drop a tablespoon or more of the grains into a juice, tea, or other liquid. Unless your liquid is naturally sweet, add a little sugar, raw honey, maple syrup or other sweetner, and seal. In 12-24 hours the juice or sweetened tea will be slightly everfescent and alive. Strain the crystals out with a strainer. Your finished crystal kefir can be put in the fridge to slow the fermentation.

The above process will slowly make more kefir crsytals as time goes by; if you'd like to make a lot fast there's another process: put your kefir crystals in a quart jar, add a cup of maple syrup, fill with filtered water and screw the lid on. This can be left indefinitely (open the top periodically to release pressure) and the grains will quickly multiply, making a thick crystally mud which will grow into crystals by the day.

Kefiring maple syrup with an airlock from a surgical glove

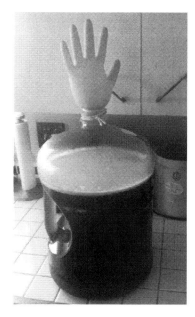

Crystal kefiring maple syrup, 1 part syrup (organic grade B) to 2 or 3 parts filtered water or coconut water. This polycarbonate container can't take much pressure so will explode after a certain point. To keep the fermentation anaerobic, use an airlock or a ballon. I like to use a surgical glove so I'll be greeted by various gestures as the pressure increases. I've since found a source for glass 5-gallon containers and switched to using those.

Fermenting Fats – Butter and Oil

Butter has been enjoyed for as long as milk-producing animals have been domesticated – it's a natural by-product of raw milk and an effective way to store milk fat without refrigeration. If you let un-homogenized milk (milk that hasn't been crushed, turning the components into a undifferentiated liquid of deteriorating nutrition) sit out for a few hours you'll notice the fat globules, which are lighter than the protein and water that constitute the rest of milk, rise to the top.

In our kefir-making, we stir or swirl to keep all parts together, but the milk fat can also be skimmed off of the surface, becoming cream. This is just what prehistoric man did, right before they beat it with sticks (how they started doing this I'll never know), until the fat globules stuck together and the protein-rich liquid, the buttermilk, was released. Their cream was already fermented by the wild lactic-acid bacteria in the environment, and in fact *all* butter was fermented for flavor and stability until the 1940's and the advent of butter-making machines. While cream needs a day or so to ferment and release its wonderfully rich flavor, the machines weren't going run only half the time. Unfermented "sweet cream" butter was continuously "churned out" (sorry), and people got used to the flavor, soon forgetting the ancient heirloom goodness of traditional butter.

In the 1915 *Principles and Practise of Butter Making* by McKay and Larson, there's no mention of sweet cream butter.

"To Produce Flavor and Aroma: The chief object of cream-ripening is to secure the desirable and delicate flavor and aroma which are so characteristic of good butter. These flavoring substances, so far as known, can only be produced by a process of fermentation. It is a well-known fact that the best flavor in butter is obtained when the cream assumes a clean, pure, acid taste during the ripening. For this reason, it is essential to have the acid-producing germs predominate during the cream ripening; all other germs should, if possible, be excluded or suppressed. . . . When cream has been properly ripened, it is practically a pure culture of lactic-acid-producing germs, while sweet unpasteurized cream contains a bacterial flora, consisting of a great many types of desirable and undesirable germs."

Good news: your kefir culture is the perfect starter for making fermented butter, a fun and delicious process.

Making Butter

Obtain raw cream, the higher the fat content the better the butter, and even though goat's milk is more nutritious than cow's, easier to digest and lighter in flavor, it's actually slightly higher in fat as well.

Put a few tablespoons of kefir whey into each cup of cream and stir well. Leave it to ferment for a day or two, or longer. I've gone up to two weeks (on a roadtrip) and the butter was amazing. Stir a few times a day - the cream is thick and the kefir has a harder time swimming around. You want every corner of the cream to be fermented.

Next, spoon the fermented cream into a jar or bottle with a tight fitting lid. It may seem counterintuitive in the next step, but the fuller the container, the faster the butter will come.

Now – shake shake shake. Just like our thick-browed ancestors did with their sticks, we're smacking the fat globules together, smashing their protein sheaths apart and letting the pieces get carried away in the water. In about ten or twenty minutes of hard shaking you'll have whipped cream, which (sorry) is even harder to shake. But keep at it - perseverance will soon yield small yellow lumps. Keep shaking and soon all of the milk fat will be separated from the buttermilk, which will look like floating yellow tapioca. Scoop it out, squish it into a ball and squeeze out the remaining liquid, and pat yourself on the back, if your arms can still move.

The paddle of a kitchen mixer can also do the job, as can a bunch of friends at a party or a kindergarten classroom passing the jar around. I've heard that butter was discovered by camel-riding traders in North Africa – when they reached their destination they opened their pouches of raw milk and by the many steps of their beasts, butter happened. A jar of milk in the pocket of a long-distance hiker will meet a similar fate if their gait is bouncy enough.

Ghee

Natuve to the Himalayans, ghee is "clarified butter", or butter that's had the protein and water have been removed, leaving only the fat. Ghee contains all the nutritive benefits of butter and none of the casein and lactose, so it's easier to digest for many people. Because it's 100% fat ghee will last a long time at room temperature, even unfermented. In Ayurvedic medicine, India's ancient "science of life", ghee is said to coat the nadis, the channels by which life force flow through the body, strengthening the energy field around the body, or aura. Because ghee is a simpler and therefore more easily digestible form of butter, its benefits to both the cardiovascular system and mental functioning are obvious to even more linear logic..

Traditionally, ghee is made by heating butter (made from yogurt) until the water evaporates out and the protein rises to the top and can be skimmed off. But we Kitchen Sink Farmers know better. Put butter in a dehydrator for a couple of days, and as the water vanishes, a white foam will form. Scoop it out as it grows (the liquid also can be strained at the very end to remove all traces of milk proteins), and you'll soon have unpasteurized, fermented, raw clarified butter. It's the best fat for cooking, if you do that, because ghee has one of the highest smoke points of all fats - 485° F. Scrumptious brushed on sprouted loaves or lightly dehydrated veggies; ghee's concentrated flavor from lack of water means that you need much less of it than butter in any food prep.

And Now The Crown Jewel of Fat… (and I don't mean Miss Piggy's Tiara)

The two healthiest fats together at last: kefir ghee and coconut oil. Coconut oil's succulent velvet added to ghee's nutty smoothness is, IMO, the quintessence of oils.

Coconut oil is the most processed food that comes into my kitchen. By this point, you know that I always start with whole foods, which I then attempt to use in a way that maximizes their nutrition, life force, and flavor. Coconut oil is something I don't often do at home[14], and I won't be without its many incredible health benefits and unbelievable flavor. Coconut oil fuses seamlessly into everything from dressings, smoothies, soups, and nut butters. It egolessly improves the flavor without trumpeting its presence.

---

[14] Make coconut oil by dehydrating freshly shredded coconut meat (store-bought coconut flakes have been de-fatted). Blend the dried shreds in a high-speed blender and sit the paste ontop of a dehydrator or other warm place for a day or 2. The oil will rise to the surface, ready to be scooped off and enjoyed.

Coconut oil helps normalize blood lipids, protecting against damage to the liver by alcohol and other toxins, and in small amounts prevents kidney and gall bladder diseases. It's associated with the prevention and management of diabetes through its ability to stabilize blood sugar and regulate insulin production. Coconut oil has anti-viral, anti-bacterial and anti-fungal properties, improves mineral absorption (which is important for all body processes including healthy teeth and bones), and is also the world's best skin and face lotion.

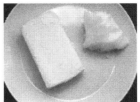

Homemade butter and coconut oil

It's important to use organic coconut oil, as conventionally-produced products use all sorts of nasty chemicals and can be exposed to pathogens. Raw is even better, assuring the quickest and most gentle processing. My favorite brands are Nutiva, sold on amazon, and Hummingbird (www.hummingbirdwholesale.com), only available in stores . Nutiva has a raw, in glass, coconut oil but their basic oil is so well-prepared that I don't think the considerable extra expense is worth it. Look for the amazing price on two 54 oz. tubs. Hummingbird's raw, organic extra virgin oil is incredible, packed in glass instead of plastic, and among the cheapest coconut oils I've seen. If you can find it near you, do.

As a saturated fat, coconut oil is solid at room temperature[15] so in colder seasons I leave mine on top of

---

[15] (<76ºF, actually). Saturated fats have only single bonds in their carbon chains which allows them to be neatly "packed". Unsaturated fats have a double bond along their row of carbon, causing it to have a kink. Because of this bend these molecules can't stack so easily, and remain liquid at room temperature. Saturated fats, because of their ability to stack so easily, build up more quickly in the body than unsaturated fats. That's why in large quantities (especially with

my dehydrator or fridge so it's always liquid. Pour it into liquid ghee, in whatever ratio you like, stirring every so often as the mixture solidifies to keep them from separating.

Raw Fats and Unrefined Oils for Weight-Loss and Well-Being

Lipase, the enzymes that breaks down fats and is missing from refined oils and pastuerized dairy products, is vital for health. Its not only a major player in fat diseases like obesity, heart disease, diabetes, stoke, Parkinson's and degenerative muscle disease, but is also a factor in skin problems, autoimmune diseases, cancer, degenerative diseases of the brain and nervous system, and general rejuvenation and regeneration.

Fats and oils are not only essential for our energy metabolism, but they also play an important role the structural integrity of our body. Most of our brain, nerves and cell membranes consist of fats, or "lipids". Lipase is important in maintaining optimal cell membrane permeability, allowing adequate nutrient supply into the cells and wastes to flow out. P.G. Seeger, the the world's

leading researcher on the relationship between nutrition and cancer, has clearly shown that the first biochemical step towards cancer is a deterioration of the cell membrane.

As we age the functioning of our pancreas, the body's lipase factory, naturally declines. Decreasing lipase production leads to reduced bile flow and less surface area in the intestines for nutrient absorption. The resulting

---

saturated fats derived from animals) this can be harmful to the body - these fatty acids can build up on the heart and blood vessels and affect their function.

deficiencies of fat-soluble vitamins such as A, D, and E, phospholipids and essential omega-3-fatty acids in turn

contribute to the common symptoms of aging and the development of degenerative diseases, such as aging skin, Alzheimer's disease, arteriosclerosis and atherosclerosis, auto-immune disease, cancer, cardiovascular disease, chronic fatigue syndrome, cystic fibrosis, dementia, depression, diabetes, eye diseases, fibromyalgia, lateral sclerosis (A.L.S.), liver diseases, malabsorption of nutrients, multiple sclerosis, muscular dystrophy, obesity, pancreatitis, Parkinson's disease, psoriasis, Raynaud's disease, stroke, and vertigo.

Fat vs. Weight

With a strong metabolism, we can easily gain or lose weight. Two-thirds of US adults and one-third of children are now classified as overweight. Research shows that lipase deficiency is a huge factor in this alarming state of affairs.

The problem is this: the less fat there is in a meal, the more quickly it is released from the stomach into the small intestine. The plentiful carbohydrates that might be present in the same meal rush past the scanty and slow-moving fats and are rapidly absorbed into the bloodstream, which can lead to damaging high blood-sugar levels. In an effort to prevent this, the pancreas releases large amounts of insulin. This helps glucose enter cells more quickly but if you are

not doing hard work or exercise at the time, the excess glucose is either converted to lactic acid (some of which is used by the brain, intestines, and red blood cells), thereby causing overacidity and mineral deficiency, or the glucose is converted to fat.

Fat is then stored in fat cells. When the blood sugar level drops, this stored fat can now be used to generate energy – but only if there is sufficient internal lipase. If lipase is deficient, fat remains in the fat cells and you need more readily-available energy, and so feel hungry again, having

another carbohydrate meal with a replay of the same story. After several years of repeating this cycle with habitually elevated blood sugar levels, diabetes is often the result.

This finely-tuned system was designed under two assumptions: 1) humans lead an acive lifestyle, especially when eating large amounts of starches, and 2) we eat unrefined, living fats - with lipase intact. These factors could be counted on in our ancestors' lives, but as the speed of changing culture has outrun the rate of genetic evolution, for the first time in

our planet's history a species has outsmarted it's own genetic mandate, with disastrous consequences.

Lipase-rich raw butter, for instance, is effective in the fights against psoriasis and tuberulosis but (lipase-deficient) pasteurized butter can cause or aggravates them. The same is true for heart and liver problems, which are created or aggravated by processed cheese and butterfat. These health problems were less common in the centuries before pastuerization, and in the modern-day inhabitants of the Caucasus region with their high intake of raw milk products. Cholesterol was a non-issue in the old days when mainly unheated milk products were used, and cardiovascular disease was almost unknown. This was not

because of lack of medical knowledge. Carnivorous wild animals have diets high in fat and cholesterol but show no signs of atherosclerosis and heart disease. In contrast, domesticated dogs and cats that live on canned food, pasteurized milk or cooked meat develop the same diseases as their caretakers.

There are two ways to solve this problem, and it's best to use both. First, get plenty of lipase, preferably from raw fats and oils, or though there are also lipase supplements. Second, slow down the absorption of carbohydrates. There are 2 ways to do this: either eat less carbohydrates, or

slowing down the emptying of the stomach by mixing carbohydrates with sufficient oil or fat. For example, eat fruit mixed with raw coconut or kefir, or grains mixed with raw oils or ghee.

Alternatively, one can eat mainly slow-digesting carbohydrates, such as sprouted legumes like garbonzos, mung beans or lentils, with vegetables and a raw oil-rich dressing. Another option that's very effective in bodies used to holding onto fat is snacking – small amounts of food at a time to space out the starch intake and absorption. Ingest only as much carbohydrate as you need to produce energy during the next 30 to 60 minutes so that

nothing is converted into fat. Then have another snack. Finally, be aware that if you do have a high calorie-meal in the evening your body may have no choice but to store in fat cells. Fat burning can also be accelerated by drinking enzyme- and probiotic-rich apple cider vinegar before meals.

All raw lipid-rich foods are high in lipase. However lipase is water-soluble so breaks down quickly without the protection offered by whole foods. There's not much lipase in pure oils; unless extremely fresh, the lipase in even

unrefined oils breaks down quickly. This includes avocado oil and coconut oil.

In order to obtain a high lipase intake from vegetable sources, we need to consume the whole food. This means eating the avocado instead of using just the oil, or pressing, juicing or blending the coconut flesh to make and use coconut milk or cream. This needs then to be refrigerated or frozen because the high enzyme content causes it to deteriorate rapidly at room temperature.

This is not a problem with fresh olives, avocado, coconut flesh or raw dairy as they usually retain enough water and

therefore most of their lipase. Cream, for instance, has about 60% water, butter 16% and egg yolk about 50%. Besides a diet high in refined and salty carbohydrates, the government ban on raw dairy products has done the most towards creating the epidemic of obesity in the country. The lawmakers can't be blamed, however, as they represent (usually) what their constituents want, or will accept. It started with the use of non-organic farming methods, leading to the breakdown of the immune systems in plants which were then not able to support a healthy immune system in dairy cows, and pathogens began to flourish. Chemical fertilizers and pesticides became commonplace because their use was accepted by the public and our "magic bullet" mentality, but long-term observation proves that quick-fixes rarely last.

Raw milk is illegal in many places, so dairy farmers that still understand the benefits of unadulterated milk has found creative solutions for getting real dairy to people. A popular method is "herd sharing", in which consumers will buy a "share" of a dairy animal, whether cow or goat, and have access to milk for a feed or packaging fee. Look at www.realmilk.com for herd shares in your area.

Oil-rich nuts and seeds are another great source of lipase, but need to be sprouted to receive the full benefit (see Kitchen Sink Farming Volume 1: Sprouting) Lipase is also available in supplement form, but is of course not as effective as a whole food source.

Fats and oils, or fatty foods such as egg yolk, ingested without thoroughly chewing together with other food (and thereby emulsifying it with the natural co-factor lecithin) are not absorbed effeciently and may cause indigestion and deficiencies. If, for example, you just swallow capsules of fish oil or vitamin E, or a spoonful of cod liver oil, the oil may just remain in a puddle and not be absorbed because lipase cannot penetrate. Always try to emulsify oils and

fats by shaking them with lecithin, or the natural way, by thoroughly chewing them in their whole food forms.

The "How?" - **Growing**

Sprouts and Greens

Sprouts are seeds that have formed a tail, and we eat the entire thing. Greens are sprouts that have taken a further step; their roots have burrowed into something that keeps them upright, and contains moisture and nutrients. Soil is one such thing and once the sprouts' roots have become one with the dirt, we eat just what has grown above. All leafy green sprouts can be grown in this manner: alfalfa, clover, watercress, broccoli, etc. and will become micro-lettuce, micro-greens, or nano-greens if they're really small. All of these are smaller than baby lettuces or greens, usually chopped at a couple of inches after 1-3 weeks. Grains such as wheat, rye, barley, and oats can be grown into grasses which aren't great eaten straight but make ridiculously nutritious and cleansing juice. This section covers the next step of planting your sprout seeds in a shallow growing medium to take them to their next level, and the couple of things you'll need to have and know to do it.

Grass and Micro-Greens

Growing grasses and micro lettuces is somewhere in between sprouting and gardening. After seeds are sprouted in the normal way, they're transferred onto a tray filled with growing medium, which is either soil or man-made (though I'll show you how to skip one or both of those steps in some cases). Then they're rinsed and drained twice a day, aka "watered", just like sprouts, for a week or more. Lighting must be taken into consideration, because these more mature plants need chlorophyll to grow up strong, and their oxygenating greenness is a major health benefit of your developing crops. The little bit of effort that goes into planning the space, getting the materials and taking an extra

step or two in growing will yield you diminutive fields of delicious salad greens and an unlimited supply of juice which is "literally condensed sunlight energy. It is one of the most potent healing agents on the planet" (author Steve Meyerowitz,
Wheatgrass: Nature's Finest Medicine), for pennies.

Why Grow Grass?

In the early 1900's, Edmond Bordeaux Szekely, a linguist and philosopher who held several Ph.D's and professorships was studying ancient texts at the Vatican. His laborious research uncovered four Aramaic and Hebrew volumes that would become the "Essene Gospels of Peace", manuscripts written by a sect of religious mystics that lived between 200 BC and 100 AD near the Dead Sea between present-day Jordan and Israel, and who were also responsible for the famous "Dead Sea Scrolls". A good chunk of these writings deal with the Essene's health practices, which were supposedly later taught to the abstinent ascetics by Jesus. In the books, the distribution of which became Szekely's life purpose, Jesus prescribes vegetarianism, eating living foods, and the benefits of grasses.

Though information about the use of grasses for human and animal health was available, it remained a fringe and esoteric knowledge until the 1940's, when future health pioneer Ann Wigmore cured her cancer with the wild grasses and weeds that grew in vacant lots near her home in Boston. After studying thousands of types of grasses, she and a physician colleague decided that a) all grasses are good for human and animal consumption, and b) wheatgrass was the best. Then in the mid-seventies, the Japanese owner of a pharmaceutical company, Dr. Yoshihide Hagiwara, became very sick from working with the drugs his company produced, many of which were his formulations. After several years of trying and failing to improve his health through medicine, he began looking into traditional Chinese medicine. There, he discovered the philosophy behind the writings of Shin Huang-ti, the father of Chinese medicine, who said: "It is the diet which maintains true health and becomes the best drug". Similarly, Hippocrates, the father of Western medicine advised: "Let your food be your medicine." After exhaustively studying over 150 plants during the course of 13 years, Dr. Hagiwara decided that barley grass was nature's most healing food and began to cure himself immediately.

"Green(s) should not be recognized by discussing the amount of their vitamins and minerals. The era of focusing on a single vitamin or mineral is gone... much more attention is being focused on biological phenomenon." - Dr. Yoshihide Hagiwara

"In a recent John Hopkins study, 95 percent of 200 arthritis patients found almost complete relief after taking two ounces of wheatgrass juice a day for three weeks. I can attest to this fact when witnessing a crippled lady unable to climb stairs do so after three weeks on wheatgrass juice and living food. In my own healing, my body has cleansed from toxins, I became emotionally sound, drug-free, had more energy, felt more self-worth, lost weight and returned home to live a more fulfilling life." - Loretta Harmony Kohn, former employee at Ann Wigmore's Hippocrates Institute

The Benefits of Wheatgrass Grass Juice

Wheatgrass juice is one of the most mineral-rich foods on the planet, and one ounce of juice contains about as many nutrients as 2.5 pounds of green vegetables. It's a complete food and excellent source of vitamins, including B12, which is very hard to find in a vegan diet. It contains 17 amino acids and about 80 known enzymes.

Wheatgrass juice is also the highest food source of a nutrient called chlorophyll, which is the green pigment in plants that let them turn sunshine into energy.

The chlorophyll molecule is remarkably similar to hemoglobin in human blood, the substance that carries oxygen in our body. The only difference is that hemoglobin has an iron element in the center of the structure, which is red, and chlorophyll has a magnesium element, which is green.

Dr. Yoshihide Hagiwara, president of the Hagiwara Institute of Health in Japan, is a leading advocate for the use of grass as food and medicine. He reasons that since chlorophyll is soluble in fat particles, and fat particles are absorbed directly into the blood via the lymphatic system, that chlorophyll can also be absorbed in this way. In other words, when the "blood" of plants is absorbed in humans it is transformed into human blood, which transports nutrients to every cell of the body. Wheatgrass juice is like a liquid oxygen transfusion. Oxygen is vital to many body processes: it stimulates digestion (the oxidation of food), promotes clearer thinking (the brain utilizes 25% of the body's oxygen supply), and protects the blood against anaerobic bacteria. Cancer cells cannot exist in the presence of oxygen.

Wheatgrass is also the courier of many other benefits:

- It restores alkalinity to the blood. It has been used successfully to treat peptic ulcers, ulcerative colitis, constipation, diarrhea, and other complaints of the gastrointestinal tract. (see section on Alkalinity in "Kitchen Sink Farming Volume 1: Sprouting", pg 112)
- It increases red blood cell count and lowers blood pressure. It cleanses the blood, organs and gastrointestinal tract of debris. Wheatgrass also

stimulates metabolism and the body's enzyme production. It also aids in reducing blood pressure by dilating the blood pathways throughout the body, removing plaque build-up in the blood vessels and the sources of plaque.
- It stimulates the thyroid gland, correcting obesity, indigestion, and a host of other complaints.
- It is a powerful detoxifier, and liver and blood protector. The enzymes and amino acids found in wheatgrass can protect us from carcinogens like no other food or medicine. It strengthens our cells, detoxifies the liver and bloodstream, and chemically neutralizes environmental pollutants. Wheatgrass rejuvenates aging cells by cleansing the blood and helps slow the aging process. It will help tighten loose and sagging skin.
- It fights tumors and neutralizes toxins. Recent studies show that wheatgrass juice has a powerful ability to fight tumors without the usual toxicity of drugs that also inhibit cell-destroying agents. It neutralizes toxic substances like cadmium, nicotine, strontium, mercury, and polyvinyl chloride (PVC).
- It contains beneficial enzymes. Whether healing a cut or dissolving fat while you exercise, enzymes do the actual work. The life and abilities of the enzymes found naturally in our bodies can be extended if we help them from the outside by adding exogenous enzymes, like the ones found in wheatgrass juice. We can only get the benefits of the many enzymes found in grass by eating it uncooked. Cooking destroys 100 percent of the enzymes in food.
- Applied to the skin, wheatgrass juice can help eliminate itching almost immediately. It will soothe sunburned skin and act as a disinfectant. Rubbed into the scalp before a shampoo, it will help mend damaged hair and alleviate itchy, scaly, scalp conditions. It is soothing and healing for cuts,

burns, scrapes, rashes, poison ivy, athlete's foot, insect bites, boils, sores, open ulcers, tumors, and so on. Use the juice (or wet pulp) as a poultice and replace every two to four hours.
- It works as a sleep aid. Put a tray of living wheatgrass near the head of your bed as you sleep - it will enhance the oxygen in the air and generate healthful negative ions to help you sleep more soundly.
- It sweetens the breath and firms up and tightens gums. Just gargle and swish the juice before you swallow it.
- Because of its powerful oxygenating properties, it can turn gray hair back to its natural color and greatly increase energy levels when consumed daily. It can also decrease or remove body odor, which is bacteria putrefying on partially digested wastes excreted through the skin and built up in places without much air flow, like armpits. In much the same way it can combat halitosis, or bad breath.
- One enzyme found in wheatgrass, SOD, lessens the effects of radiation and acts as an anti-inflammatory compound that may prevent cellular damage following heart attacks or exposure to irritants.
- Studies have shown wheatgrass can restore fertility in women and increase lactation.
- This is one of the very few juices that can actually remove heavy metals from the system. Regular consumption will greatly help to prevent Alzheimer's disease and any other mental problems.
- It can double the red blood cell count just by soaking in it. Renowned nutritionist Dr. Bernard Jensen found that no other blood builders are superior to green juices and wheatgrass. In his book *Health Magic Through Chlorophyll from Living Plant Life* he mentions several cases where he was able to double the red blood cell count in a matter of days merely by having patients soak in a

chlorophyll-water bath. Blood building results occur even more rapidly when patients drink green juices and wheatgrass regularly. Wheatgrass has been shown to build levels of iron in the body and thereby relieve anemia. It also helps balance blood sugar.
- The high anti-oxidant content helps neutralize free radicals and oxidation that find their way in the body. It helps reduce the harm caused by air pollutants like carbon monoxide or cigarette smoke.
- Health experts believe wheatgrass is effective in treating arthritis. Chlorophyll is thought to benefit arthritis and wheatgrass contains tons of it. Chlorophyll fights inflammation, which is associated with joint pain.
- When experiencing fatigue, the body is deprived of oxygen and has a weakened immune system. Chlorophyll helps to increase oxygen supply in the body's cells and tissues, contributing to cell regeneration, healing the body and reducing fatigue symptoms.
- The fine chlorophyll and beta-carotene obtained from wheatgrass juice is beneficial in fighting and preventing cancer. A variety of flavonoid compounds found in this grass are powerful anti-oxidants and anti-cancer agents. Studies have indicated at least a 40% risk reduction in cancer development.
- The anti-bacteria effect of wheatgrass creates an unfavorable environment for yeast and harmful bacteria (those that live without the presence of oxygen). Regular consumption of this juice will help to prevent further yeast (candida) and bacterial growth.

Nutritional Benefits

The most outstanding feature of wheatgrass juice is its very high content of chlorophyll, about 70%. This alone makes it a superfood that has a highly energizing and alkalizing effect.

But wheatgrass has many vitamins and minerals, and is an excellent source of vitamin C, E, K and B complex (including B12). In the minerals department, it is rich in calcium, cobalt, germanium, iron, magnesium, phosphorus, potassium, protein, sodium, sulphur, and zinc.

This miracle grass also has a long list of amino acids – about 17 types of them and about 80 known enzymes.

Why Cleansing is Important

Early 20th century French biologist Dr. Alexis Carrel was fascinated by the aging process, and hypothesized that cells could live much longer in a clean environment. In an experiment which began in 1912, Carrel took cells from an embryonic chicken heart and suspended them in a saline solution of the proper pH, temperature, and nutrient balance. He changed this fluid daily, and the cells, which would normally die after a few months, lived for 28 years. The experiment was stopped because the results were conclusive: "The cell is immortal. It is merely the fluid in which it floats which degenerates. Renew this fluid at intervals, give the cells what they require for nutrition and, as far as we know, the pulsation of life may go on forever." – Dr. Alexis Carrel, winner of the Nobel Prize in Medicine for this experiment.

The cleansing and waste removal systems of our body: the digestive system, bloodstream, liver, lymph, lungs, skin, and others, become clogged with toxins over time, impairing the normal functioning of all body processes. Short-term cleanses that target each of these systems are an important aspect of over-all health and well-being. But the most powerful and effective cleanse is the one that happens every day, in every cell, in every system of our bodies; the purification and rebuilding that our bodies do automatically when given the proper nutrients. I came across the Alexis Carrel experiment when I was very young, and I've been doing cleanses for most of my life. In addition to a diet and lifestyle fairly well free of toxins, I've done all the organ and system-specific cleanses I could find. Having my body is the only thing that's certain throughout my life, and its condition is the number one factor that effects my happiness. So I try to take better care of it than redneck does his truck. We don't assume that our cars will fix themselves if we ignore a clunking sound or flat tire, but our bodies are such powerful machines of cleansing and regeneration that's just how we treat them. The most powerful cleanse I've ever done, or rather experienced, is the one that happened when I started eating only living foods. There are subtle shifts and pendulous swings one notices when doing a cleanse: no appetite giving way to ravenous hunger, almost overwhelming amounts of energy cycling with wanting to sleep for 12 hours a night, laser-like focus alternating with an impenetrable mental fog. These symptoms in the presence of top-quality nutrition and mechanisms of detoxification are a sign that the body's innate wisdom sees an opportunity to get rid of accumulated toxins, which were formerly rushed out of the bloodstream and into the safety of fat deposits to be dealt with only if a healthy opportunity presented itself. When I started on nutrient-rich living food that I grew myself, these cycles continued for about 6 months, in a slowly spiraling upward trend towards a newfound vitality that I had previously only wistfully imagined. More energy and better sleeping, fresher breath and a more positive outlook, brighter eyes and skin; the benefits that are commonly associated with cleansing were just the beginning. And it was health problems that made me make the change, not already glowing health that I was fine-tuning. It's as if I was building an entirely new body, optimal vehicle for my life force given my age and genetics.

I'll wrap up the section on cleansing with one more quote, credited to Eubie Blake, jazz and ragtime pianist who lived from 1883 to 1983:

"If I'd known I was going to live this long, I would have taken better care of myself."

Take care of yourself.

FURTHERMORE

As in the Dr. Hagiwara quote above, trying to understand a single nutrient, even one as potent as chlorophyll, is limiting in scope. The ICP (inductively coupled plasma) spectrometer, an imaging device about the size of a pickup truck, shows us that food nutrients are more varied and numerous that we ever imagined. A grape, for example, contains over 5 million compounds. Modern science has barely scratched the surface of comprehending or even naming these nutrients, let alone understanding the seemingly infinite interactions between them. And while single nutrients are important and we have to go with the info that we have when treating disease or discomfort, it seems silly to rely on such a fractured approach to nourishment. The best vitamins are whole, living foods, pulled directly from the dirt, or vine, or branch, that have been proven for centuries or millennia to repair and maintain vibrant human health.

How to Grow and Enjoy Grasses

To grow grain seeds into cleansing and nutritious grasses, they must be soaked, sprouted, then taken one step further. After they've grown a small tail, they are transferred onto a tray of growing media, where their little roots have an opportunity to take hold and support the development of bright green blades, they will shoot upwards like, well, grass. For this, you'll need a couple of extra tools: dirt or a dirt substitute, and something to hold it in. We'll also be discussing light, plant food, and because we're growing it for 2 weeks or more, pests in the form of molds, fungi, and bugs.

Dirt, New and Used

"Growing media" is the name of the various things seeds can be planted in, and serve three purposes: holding the plants up, retaining moisture, and most importantly, providing nutrients to the growing plants. Supporting most grass and micro-greens is easy; in fact, in just a couple of days many plants will quickly create their own thick mat of interwoven roots. With 2 or 3 daily waterings, the plants can stay moist enough, but when I tried many times to grow grass this way to try and save my apartment-bound readers the extra effort of dealing with dirt, the grass was always weakly and eventually taken over by mold and fungus. When planted on dirt, however, the same sprouts yielded strong, bright green blades of healthy and darkly emerald juice. Even though it's possible to grow a bed of grass or micro-lettuce without any more support than its roots and neighbors provide, I recommend using growing media of some kind, the practical varieties of which are described.

Dirt

As the weeds growing up through cracks in a city sidewalk will maintain, any soil will work for growing grasses and micro-lettuce. Organic is always better, and some retail soils contain beneficial microbes which will create an environment of more available nutrients for your plants. Most store-bought soils don't have these microbial helpers or advertise the microorganisms they do contain, so a sterile soil will yield a more reliable growing material. Obviously, dirt is also available for free in most of the world. Composted cow manure or earthworm castings make a dark, loamy soil full of nutrients for your grass to thrive on, and is often given away by gardeners and farmers. It's also the stuff underneath the grass in city parks. I don't know your local laws (heck, I don't even know mine) but I recommend you check them before you head to the park with a shovel. For growing grasses, dirt can be used only once, as the afore-mentioned root matting will turn it into a solid carpet. For most micro-greens, which have a less tenacious root structure than grass, soil can be turned over, fertilized, and used again for another crop. Then compost the whole thing or take it back to the park or woods you got it from, and with the addition of your organic fertilizer and plant matter, the returning soil will be better than you found it. Choose soil from out-of-the-way places, avoiding places that are walked or peed on if possible. The base of a tree is bound to have nutrient-rich, biologically active soil, as the tree roots protect it from both mineral erosion and pathogens.

Dealing with dirt in an apartment

Soil is great because it is (or can be) free and renewable, not in the grand scheme of things but in your own yard or city park, but it's also the only growing medium that has its own built-in nutrients and for this reason it's my #1 choice. Dirt is a living, breathing thing, and supports more life within than on top. No two molecules of humus, completely broken-down soil, are or will ever be alike, like snowflakes or boy bands. Yes, it can be slightly messier than the surgical sterility of perlite or clay pellets, but if I have my way, earth underneath the fingernails will be a badge of honor in the near future.

> Sterilizing Soil at Home
>
> When using "found" soil and you're unsure about the benevolence of its community of microorganisms, sterilizing your soil will remove concern about mold growth or pathogens. Influence by unfriendly bacteria, molds, or fungus shouldn't be a major source of distress, as we're cutting the grass or green above the soil line and influence of these critters, but if you don't want a culture of fuzzy growth marring the beauty of your indoor garden, or you have pets or kids in the house, you may want to utilize one of these four methods to remove unknown factors from your soil.

Oven Method - Spread soil not more than four inches deep in non-plastic containers, such as seed flats, clay pots and glass, pyrex, or metal baking pans. Cover each container tightly with aluminum foil. Insert a meat or candy thermometer through one of the foil covers, and into the center of the soil. Set the oven between 180° and 200° F and watch the thermometer. Heat the soil to at least 180° F and keep it at this temperature for 30 minutes. Do not allow the temperature to go above 200° F - higher temperatures may produce plant toxins. Then cool, remove containers from the oven and leave the foil in place until ready to use. The heated soil will give off an odor somewhere between pungent earth and caramel.

Microwave Method –Microwave soil for 90 seconds per kilogram (2.2 pounds) on full power. Don't use metal containers and aluminum foil when using a microwave.

Use quart-sized plastic containers with lids, such as yogurt cups. Check the rims of the containers to make sure there is no aluminum of any kind; eradicate any trace of metal or foil seal. Fill the containers with very moist soil and cover. Poke a hole through the plastic lids with a nail for steam ventilation; a plastic temperature probe goes half way down into the soil through this hole in one of the containers. In a carousel-type microwave oven, heat the soil to 200°F and maintain that temperature for 20 minutes, varying the cooking program as necessary. In a large microwave, up to 7 quart containers can be sterilized at a time, making this a very efficient way to sterilize soil. Allow the container to cool and put a piece of tape over the holes in the lids to keep the soil sterile until you're ready to use it.

You can also use a zip-loc gallon freezer bag; wet soil, leave the top open and place in the center of your carousel microwave. Treat for 2.5 minutes on full power (about 650 watts). After treatment allow the soil to cool and close the top of the bag.

> Not a bad idea for cleaning soilless media in between hydroponic usages, which are susceptible to algal growth.
>
> **Steam Sterilization** - Pour about an inch of water into a large pot. Fill containers that will fit in the pot (like loaf pans, baking pans, or glass canning jars) with leveled, loosely packed soil. Cover each container with aluminum foil. Stack the containers, if possible, to allow steam circulation. Leave the bottom container empty, or put the filled containers on something to keep them above the water. Cover the pot and bring the water to a boil. When steam begins to escape, continue boiling for 30 minutes at the lowest setting that will still produce steam. Turn off the heat and replace the lid. Remove the soil when cool.
>
> Make sure that your sterilization stays below 200° F – heavier soils and soils containing large amounts of organic matter may release compounds toxic to plants when heated too long or at a too high temperature. These toxins can cause poor seed germination or weakly plants. The toxicity is caused by an accumulation of ammonium compounds (see pee warning above), soluble organic compounds (the breakdown of which increases with heat, making the soil too rich for growing food), or high-temperature activation of salts. If there's a really convenient place for you to get you soil but it's yielding strange results, use a simple test to determine if the sterilized soil is toxic to plants: sow a few lettuce or other seeds with a high germination rate in both the treated and untreated soil and see what happens.

Because soil is only lacking in the easiness and cleanliness departments, I've devised a couple of techniques to make it just as easy to work with as the more futuristic and expensive options. The standard planting trays that are 20" by 10" take a little less than a gallon of dirt. Organic soil is available from nurseries and hardware stores in sizes starting at 8 quart bags, or 4 gallons. Take some gallon-sized zip-loc bags to the store with you, and in the parking lot, scoop the soil into 4 baggies (or however many you get out of the bag you bought.) Leave a little room in there; and keep it loose - if you pack it too tightly you'll end up with not more than a trayful. Then go back in the store and throw the bag away in their garbage and wash your hands. Back home, you can store your bags in a plastic tote or an unused drawer in the kitchen, but if you're putting it somewhere that you don't want dirt, make sure you put it in a garbage or plastic grocery bag for safety. Then when you're ready to do some planting, dump the dirt into your tray, turning the bag inside out, and put your hand in the inside, formerly the outside (and more importantly the clean side), and use it like a mitten to smooth the dirt. Turn the bag right-side out and zip it (now the dirt is on the inside again and sealed), storing it for the next time you go to the store. Larger bags of soil are obviously cheaper than smaller, so if you have the storage, I recommend buying 40 lb. or 32 quart bags and filling up 7 or 8 gallon zip-locs per , respectively.

The second technique skips the bags and instead stores dirt directly inside a lidded plastic tub, which range in size from mouse coffin to garrison. They're sold at storage and discount stores, and are often available with wheels. They can be filled with soil and a plastic cup or scoop kept inside, the lid doubling as a work table when it's flipped over and laid across the top of the open bin perpendicularly. Very easy. Like most things in the book, these two techniques require a little bit of simple prep, but then actually doing them is a breeze.

Soilless Media

Several options are available if you don't want to deal with finding or using dirt. **Rock wool** is a combination of rock and sand, spun into matted fibers that are formed into many shapes and sizes. It's made in a similar way to cotton candy, and was originally used as wall insulation until its best virtues were discovered. It retains both moisture and air very well but is only usable once, and buying a new mat for every tray of grass at $4 or so, while still far cheaper than buying shots of wheatgrass at your local juice bar, is not the best option. Same goes for **baby blanket**, a thin organic pad sold in foot-wide rolls, **Tencel**, an eucalyptus-derived polymer, **coconut fiber**, a waste product of the coconut industry made from powdered husk, and **sphagnum**, a matted moss, and **peat moss**, which takes so long to grow that it's just not sustainable. **Coarse sand and clay**, if they're available to you, are good options for root support, though they will quickly dry out and don't hold nutrients for very long. Either one can add drainage to soil if your source is too dense and holds too much moisture. **Perlite** is a volcanic mineral that when heated to over 1600 degrees pops like popcorn and cools full of tiny air bubbles. The soft beads now resemble pearls, and have the unique ability to expand to 20 times their size when soaking up water. For this reason, they're an excellent addition to soilless growing mediums like sand that don't retain moisture well. Perlite is also pH-balanced, and can stabilize the acidity or alkalinity of the medium you choose.

Though the cost of soilless media is the main deterrent (with a consideration to the environmental impact of packaging, marketing, and shipping) most of them retain moisture longer than dirt, which can be handy if you have less time to water or are going out of town for a few days. In an area of medium humidity, soil-based plants require watering about once a day at the beginning (with water needs increasing as the plants get bigger). If I'm going out-of-town for a few days to a week and don't want a lag in my grasses or greens, I'll start them in a moisture-retaining soilless medium like rock wool or coconut fiber, which I have for just this occasion, pre-soaked in fertilizer and water for a full day before they're planted. I'll leave 1/8" of the water sitting in the bottom of the tray for the medium to wick upwards as needed. I cover the tray with a clear greenhouse dome or plastic wrap and say a little prayer to the water gods. When I get back I'll give them a good watering, and I'm often pleased to return to hardy little plants, rebelliously growing happily without my care.

The above are materials commercially-labeled as soilless media, but anything that will hold moisture in and plants up will do. Ground Styrofoam packing peanuts, window screen, sea sponge; these and much more are viable options, depending on what's abundantly available to you.

Sprouts still have a rich food source to draw from, like an egg, but once they've doubled in size, they need to be given another source of food. Soilless media require fertilization, because unlike dirt, they don't have any of their own built-in minerals or soil-based organisms to continuously transform the plant's wastes into fresh, usable raw materials for healthy growth. More on this later, but keep in mind when choosing a medium that sowing a seed in the ground and keeping it moist is just *allowing* the earth to obey the inscrutable mandate of its nature, and create new life from old: the decaying plant and animal matter that makes up soil is transformed by an invisible microbial workforce into nutrients that feed adeptly sprouting seeds in millions of processes that science will never fully understand. Saying "this plant needs such and such nutrients to grow" sequesters a growing procedure from the mysterious and miraculous process that begot and continues life on Earth. Certainly, buying seeds online with PayPal, having them shipped across the country, germinating them in a jar and spreading them in a tray in your windowsill isn't exactly a shamanistic approach to honoring the elemental forces that sustain life, but we do what we can. If it's growing wheatgrass in a Hello Kitty lunchbox under a reptile light you found in a dumpster or nothing, I'd obviously recommend the former. Just like a blade of grass can't be recreated in a lab, there are aspects to soil and plant nutrition that we don't understand and therefore can't duplicate artificially. So if you have a choice, and it's not so tedious or messy that it will keep you from your grass, natural, organic soil is best.

Containers

The standard receptacle for growing grass is a nursery tray, black or terra cotta-colored plastic rectangles about 20" by 10" by 2" deep with holes in the bottom for drainage. They're available online or in hardware, nursery or hydroponic stores for about $5 each. They are often sold alongside deeper trays that can catch drips, and high, domes clear plastic covers that retain moisture and turn the setup into a mini greenhouse. You only need 2 or 3 of these little kits, and in my opinion the price is low enough to curb more creative options. The shallow trays have thin channels running long ways along the floor of the container, and for some reason, the holes are always on the higher level of the bottom, in between the channels, allowing a good deal of water to sit in the tray. This can cause rot and mold. I recommend adding lots of holes to the lower-most surface of the tray by poking and twisting with a sharp, pointy knife, leaving an open circle that's big enough to let water drain out but small enough to keep dirt in.

Putting the 2" holed tray into a deeper tray not only collects the water that will continue drip out, it both allows for air circulation underneath your plants (important if you live in a tropical place or are growing in a humid season), and keeps moisture in for those that live in arid regions. Experiment with the clear cover, if you opt to use it, for moisture retention. It's also a visual indicator of moisture: you'll want to have a fine fog on the inside of the plastic; if the inner surface is dry there's not enough water, and if whole drops are collecting and running down the walls, it's too wet.

If you're getting the same kind of mold every time you grow, for example, a white fuzz that looks like fluffy cotton, you might want to try using the cover to protect your crop from airborne spores. Keep the clear cover over the plants anytime they're exposed to outside air. Remove the cover, water and drain it in a protected place, like your shower, then replace the cover before you put it back in the windowsill or outdoors. Mold isn't actually a big deal; just cut your grasses above the unwanted growth and rinse them before use. Sprouting and growing grasses is such a short-term endeavor that many pest problems that plague vegetable gardeners can be ignored or dealt with in a quick and superficial way.

There is no limit to what can be used as a growing container; if you don't want to spend the money for the prettily matching tray setup, you can use any vessel you have lying around. Cracked Tupperware containers, clay planter dishes, cookie sheets, the plastic clamshells that salad greens come in, old shallow bowls - anything that will hold dirt will do. If there aren't any drainage holes, you'll have to either punch some in the bottom (you can line it with coffee filters if your container comes pre-holed or cracked, or you were too enthusiastic with your hole-making) or you can just hold the growing medium and seeds in with your hands and tilt the container so that as much water as possible drains out. Many seasoned wheatgrass growers use trays with no drainage holes and use the tilt-drain technique; there's no shame in no holes.

Light

Plants require full spectrum, or "all color", light if they are to develop chlorophyll. Grasses grown without a good light source will be pale yellow, thin and sickly. There are two options: sunshine and artificial light. In the same way that modern science doesn't fully understand how microbes in dirt compost waste into a myriad of nutrients, we have only a very basic knowledge of the effects of natural and artificial light on plant and animal growth.

Sunlight, when shined through a prism, will break up into the colors of the rainbow. This is the visible spectrum of electromagnetic energy, a tiny fraction of the wavelengths that make up light. Infrared (less than red) and ultraviolet (more than violet) light are the two wavelengths that bookend visible light and, though we can't see them, are essential to life. Infrared frequencies provide heat, without which life would be impossible, and ultraviolet light is responsible for chemical reactions such as those that help us create vitamin D, which helps us use calcium, regulate insulin, and power up our immune system.

Artificial light doesn't produce an even amount of each wavelength, but has peaks and valleys throughout. Sometimes this is the best that can be done with the type of bulb being used, and sometimes it's based on the manufacturer's preference. If you think you can choose the kind of light you use based on the amounts of each wavelength and your growing needs, consider this: when John Ott, of the Time Lapse Research Laboratory, studied the effects of artificial light on pumpkins in the mid-seventies, he found that the female pumpkin-producing flower withered and died under pinkish-white light, and consequently didn't produce fruit. When more blue was added to the spectrum to remedy this, the female buds produced bountifully while the male buds shriveled and fell off. In these artificial light conditions, reproduction could not take place.

Artificial light does just affect the different sexes of plants; the animal world is also adversely effected by variances from natural light. In an experiment conducted to see the effects of different kinds of light on animals, 1000 mice were divided into three groups, each with its own light environment. Those receiving natural daylight produced an equal amount of male and female offspring; those under white fluorescent bulbs produced 70% females and 30% males; and those under pink fluorescent bulbs produced 30% females and 70% males. For some reason we still don't understand, the latter group wasn't as healthy as either of the two other groups. All those exposed to the pink light quit breeding two months earlier and died one month earlier than those in the other groups. Humans are also affected by exposure to artificial light. In countries with long winter nights, it's been noticed that girl reach sexual maturity months or years younger than their grandmothers did. Assuming no change in diet or lifestyle (improbable, but it was their experiment, not mine. See pg 49 for effect of diet on hyper maturation), it was concluded that their normal rate of maturation is adversely affected by the introduction of artificial light.

The allure of artificial light is tempting, and appliance-like machines are available that can grow veggies and herbs from a dark corner with packets of plant vitamins and robotic precision. Under artificial light apples will grow larger than their natural counterparts, but will never ripen, a fact that's easy to miss when growing non-flowering, non-fruiting plants such as grasses or micro-lettuces. When choosing a spot for your grass, and all of the food in the next chapter that needs light to thrive, I strongly encourage you to seek out natural light, whether through a window, or on a porch or rooftop. If the eerie examples above inspire you set up a complex network of mirrors or knock on your neighbor's door with an offer to build a plant hammock or dumb waiter between your two apartments, then I've done my job, but if you've maximized your available natural light (quite easy to do in apartment and city-living), by all means supplement with artificial. I've just harped on the difference to curb lazy, unnecessary, and expensive glow-light set-ups. That, and it's fascinating.

Keep in mind that grasses don't need much direct light, and too much will burn and dry them out. Diffused or filtered light is best, for about 14 hours a day, though an hour or two of direct light and 8-10 hours of filtered light also produces good results. Experiment, and pay attention to the following factors: depth of green color (how much chlorophyll is being made), thickness of the blades (juiciness), and speed of growth (in the natural world, less light usually follows colder temperatures, and thinking it's winter the plants will grow more slowly).

If you've done all you can to pipe all of the available natural light onto your little patches of garden, artificial light may be necessary to supplement the sun or extend the day. When I lived in sunny Southern California, I was in hilly, dense woods and only one window got any appreciable amount of outside light, which was indirect for most of the day. So I built shelves on that window (a rolling wire shelving unit would have worked just as well, but this place was so tiny that my shelves were made of clear Plexiglas and fold down when they're not in use), each of which has a T5 glow-light mounted to the bottom. The lights are daisy-chained together, and are moveable so that, if I was nearing harvest time on a flat of wheatgrass and it's a rainy day, I could move all 4 lights to one shelf. I moved my flats outside onto my stairs on the mornings that I'm home, but my grow-lights and timers, set from 7 AM to 9 PM, made it possible for me to enjoy fresh, nearly free wheatgrass juice every day. It also adds bright, full (visible) spectrum light to my apartment from the vicinity of the windows; not a bad thing. The shelves were packed up and went with me to Portland, where they're quite useful.

Fertilization - Feed Your Soil, Not Your Plants

We can't use the minerals in soil directly. To our metabolisms, they are just tiny rocks. We need a plant to uptake the nutrients and add an atom of carbon, thereby turning them into nutritious and delicious vitamins and minerals. In the same way, plants can't use nutrients directly from other plants and animals, which is why kitchen compost and animal wastes can't be added directly to the soil for instant plant food. It first has to be digested by microorganisms, who lovingly start the cycle over again.

A century of soil depletion has left our food nutritionally empty. Modern agriculture has discovered that plants need 3 nutrients to do the basic process of growing and bearing fruit: potassium, nitrogen, and phosphorus. There are over 100 minerals in healthy soil, and though different plants need different nutrients to be healthy, it's usually in the 50-100 range. With the 3 basic nutrients, plants are weak and sickly. They have no immune system of their own, and millions of tons of new pesticides are dumped on the world's farmlands every year. If it's not in the soil, it's not in the plant. These nutrient-deficient "foods" have no flavor - it's like eating a picture of a tomato – it may look like a tomato, but it doesn't taste like a tomato, nor (most importantly) does it nourish like one. Our grandparents can tell you what food tasted like before the mass depletion of nutrition from the soil. There are plenty of carbs in modern veggies, basically sugars linked together to form chains, but not much else. One of the greatest things about growing your own food is that you can increase the nutrients your plants are getting. If it's not in the plant, it's not in us, and by taking responsibility for what's in the soil, growing medium, and water (in the case of sprouting) of our Kitchen Sink Farms we can become want we want to be.

As mentioned above, when growing on soilless media it's necessary to fertilize your crops. Grass seeds will quickly use up the nutrients packaged into their hulls, and like a marooned spaceship will soon send out tiny probes in search of moisture and food. Even when growing in freshly composted, nutrient-rich soil, additional trace elements can only help. There are two types of fertilizers (we'll only be dealing with organic ones here, for what I hope by now are obvious reasons): those that are added to the germination and watering water, and those that are added to the growing medium. Though there are many options for each, I recommend only two for grass and micro-greens, and both are of the first variety. Grasses, as I've mentioned, are a relatively quick crop, and all the great nutrients in soil additives go largely unused. We'll come back to them when we discuss container gardening, but for now we'll stick to liquid fertilizing. Both liquid kelp fertilizer and ocean-based mineral solutions utilize the sea's inherently full spectrum of elements to provide your plants with all the nutrients they can use. Both are incredibly concentrated (dilute them with water 700:1 and 100:1, respectively) so one $15-$30 bottle lasts so long that it might just get passed down to your grandchildren. They're also really easy to use; just soak and water with the diluted solution like it's regular water. An easy and cheap source of nutrition, and you might want to leave it at that.

In the Kitchen Sink Farmer tradition, however, it is possible to make one's own fertilizer, traditionally called a "compost tea". A sprout bag or nylon stocking filled with a cup or two of blended compost is submerged in a gallon jar of water in a bucket. A teaspoon (1/2 oz) of unsulphured molasses is added to the brew as a food source for microorganisms. Cover it if gathering bugs will bother you, otherwise open is fine. In about 2 weeks you'll have your very own nutrient-rich and biologically-active compost tea, which will be diluted and added to your sprouting soak water and sprayed onto your plants; a light mist every day for grasses and microgreens, and a thorough watering once every week or two for container plants.

The same method can be used for "manure tea" if you have access to organically-fed livestock. "Hu-manure" can be processed in the very same way, and though we cringe at the thought in civilized society, I'm sure that future apartment farmers, who eat only pure, organic food full of healthy microorganisms, will appreciate the opportunity to live in a closed-system, creating no waste and being totally self-sustaining by resourcefully recycling everything.

H, P, and That Sneaky Little O: Hydrogen Peroxide

Another additive to consider is Hydrogen Peroxide, H_2O_2. As you can see from the chemical formula, Hydrogen Peroxide, or HP, is just water with an extra atom of oxygen. Oxygen is a very unstable element, and can be easily transferred from one molecule to another as it does in the upper atmosphere, where hydrogen gas (H_2) snags an oxygen or two from ozone (O_3), making both water and HP. Both will fall to the earth as rain, and the HP will keep its extra O unless it comes into the presence of a molecule with unstable atoms, like pollution, which will steal away the extra oxygen in an effort to stabilize itself. When HP can survive long enough to fall on plants, it adds extra oxygen to their life processes and neutralizes fungus and harmful bacteria in the soil.

The instability of oxygen is quite a lucky accident, because the beneficial bacteria in fermentation and digestion are aerobic, or oxygen-loving. "Bad" bacteria, with whom we don't have a symbiotic relationship and can make us sick if they overgrow, as well as fungi, molds, viruses, and cancer cells, are anaerobic – they can only survive in an oxygen-free environment. A single oxygen molecule, a beneficial free-radical, will separate from the HP molecule and destroy an anaerobic cell. This reaction can be seen if HP is poured onto a cut; the foaming, bubbling reaction is the oxygen splitting off from what is now non-reactive water (this isn't recommended for first aid, however, as some body tissues are anaerobic and will be damaged). HP both stimulates our crops' growth and targets harmful microorganism, leaving the good guys healthier than ever. Like sending poisoned pork to a concentration camp.

HP is also produced inside the body. Vitamin C fights infection by stimulating the production of HP, which fires off the extra oxygen to destroy the foreign cells. The probiotic cultures in our digestive systems produce HP to protect themselves (and us, consequently) from the growth of harmful yeast, fungus, and bacteria.

HP is essentially an oxygen supplement. Using it during the germination and growing of plants will help them stay disease-free, and can make them grow twice as fast. Just

drip some food-grade 30% or 35% solution into the soak water, and dilute it about 1 part HP to 10 parts water for watering. While you're at it, the same dilution ratio works great as a fruit and vegetable wash, facial toner, hand sanitizer, or kitchen and bathroom disinfecting cleaner. The solution can be added to baking soda for an old-school

---

Everyday Algebra

When using HP on the skin or in the mouth it's a good idea to be a bit more exacting with the 3% concentration. If 3% isn't available, or you buy 35% to save money or space, the dilution formula is Volume 1 times Concentration 1 = Volume 2 times Concentration 2, or $V_1(C_1)=V_2(C_2)$, with the concentrations being what you're starting (1) and ending with (2), and volumes being what you're trying to figure out (1) and what you want to end up with (2). It's actually really easy; use it once or twice and you'll have it down.

So if you're starting with 35% and want a liter of 3%, it's:

V_1 times 35% = 1L times 3%

> V1 times 35 = 3
>
> (divide both sides by 35 – starting to ring a bell?
>
> V1 = 3 divided by 35
>
> V1 = .0085L, or 85mL (you could also start with V2 as 1000mL)
>
> In your liter jar pour in 85mL of 35% HP and fill the rest with water. Presto, you're a mathemagician. How you figure out 85mL is up to you (canning jars have 100mL marks on the sides, a kitchen scale is also handy, or use a dropper - about 10 drops equals 1mL.)

whitening toothpaste, and used full strength is a non-toxic laundry bleach or energizing bath additive, adding oxygen and scavenging bad bacteria wherever it goes. When I travel, I carry a 3.4oz (100mL, the maximum allowed in carry-on luggage) plastic dropper bottle of 35% HP and an empty spray bottle with a mark where it should be filled to. I can fill the spray bottle (with UV-sanitized water if I'm in a developing country) and use it for sanitizing my hands, toothbrush, dishes, toilet seats, ears after swimming, and anything else that has a ticket to my insides, as a facial toner and of course, sprouting accomplice.

Doin'It

Now that we've thoroughly covered the basics, we'll go over the actual recipe for growing wheatgrass and micro-lettuces like sunflower and pea.

Sprout 2 C. (8 oz) of seeds in the normal way. Remember that seeds with hulls, such as sunflower, will float, so they must be submerged or weighed down as described in the sprouting section. When the tails are about as long as the seed, they're ready to be planted.

Spread the growing medium in a tray, and pour the seeds evenly over the surface. There's no need to bury the seeds; the tails will root down and we'll keep them in the dark until they've got a solid foundation. Cover the seeds with a paper towel and water them thoroughly. The paper towel keeps the seeds from moving while they're watered and also block out the light so that they think they're underground – they won't be very enthusiastic about growing if they think they could be disturbed at any moment. Block out the rest of the light by covering the whole thing with a towel, or keep them in a dark place, such as a shower floor in a dark bathroom, closet, or a covered plastic storage container.

Keep them moist by spraying the paper towel a couple of times a day, and in a couple of days the roots that started when sprouting will spread and bury themselves, with little white points shooting straight up from the seeds. These are the infant grasses, and they're ready for the light. Put them under filtered sun, artificial light, or a combo of the two. It's quite remarkable how quickly they green up, and a new tray of grass is always a source of entertainment and wonder for this reason.

All that's left to do is water - one daily watering is enough if you live in a humid jungle, three may be necessary if you're in a bone-dry desert, but two waterings, in the morning and evening, is just right for most of us. I take my shallow dirt-filled trays out of their deeper drip trays, put them on the floor of my shower, and spray them thoroughly with my chlorine-filtering shower handle. After they drip fairly dry, I put them back in the drip trays.

When the grass is 6-8 inches high, it's at the peak of nutrition and ready to be harvested. I start cutting when the grass is about 4 inches so that by the time I reach the end of the tray it's no more than 8. If the grass is growing out of control, feel free to cut it all, put it in a zip-loc, suck out as much air as possible, and stick it in the fridge. It's better to use it freshly cut, though. To cut it, you can use clean scissors, holding a tuft of grass and snipping it just above the seed, or saw it off with a sharp or serrated knife.

Easy enough

How to Juice Grass

There are specific juicers just for wheatgrass that crush the grass by means of a turning screw. The dry pulp comes out one hole, and the bright green juice comes out another, right into your cup. They're powered by hand or electricity, and if you drink a lot of straight juice, one is probably a good investment (they start at $40 and go up to a couple of hundred). Grass juices can go from a sweetish just-mowed lawn flavor (wheat) to bitingly bitter and acrid (barley), so many people like to mix it with other flavors. I'm one of them, and I don't have room for a grass juicer, so I use my high-speed blender. Drop a large handful of freshly-cut grass into water, vegetable or apple juice, kombucha, kefir, or whatever you prefer, and blend the grass on high for 30-45 seconds. This will heat up the blender's contents, so some ice can be thrown in at the end if you like your juice cold. Ice can be water or fruit juice, by the way.

Your concoction is ready to drink, pulp and all, right out of the blender. If you wait a minute or two, though, all the pulp (indigestible fiber) will float to the top, and tilting the blender will pour out only the liquid, leaving the pulp behind. We all know the benefits of fiber for digestion and aging, but maybe just drinking a superfood that you grew yourself is enough right now.

If you don't have a wheatgrass juicer or high-speed blender, a regular juicer won't really do. All that yummy pulp will quickly gum up the screen and you'll be left with a wet mess. A regular blender or food processor isn't the best choice, but if that's all ya got, here's what you do. In the blender, pulverize the grass as much as possible; just beat it up like it stole your girlfriend. Then dump it into a sprout bag, clean panty hose, or other sieve-like fabric, and squeeze out as much juice as possible over a bowl. You won't get as much liquid this way than if you were to use a fancy machine, but it's a lot better than nothing. And if you know you're only going to get 2/3 the amount of juice out of a tray as your friends, plant another tray and you'll have 1/3 more than them. Now who's fancy?

My favorite grass in the wheat family is Kamut. It's never been hybridized or genetically modified like common wheat, has never seen a chemical pesticide or fertilizer, and its big fat seeds yield thick juicy grass. It's also a lot more nutritious than the common wheat all juice bars sell - another reason to grow your own. Spelt is my second choice (see "Kitchen Sink Farming Volume 1: Sprouting", Appendix A – Sprouting Seeds for more on kamut and spelt). Spelt is slightly more expensive than kamut and takes a few more pre-soak rinses to come out clean. It is, however, sweet and delicious, and far preferable to modern wheat.

Micro-Lettuces, Shoots and Greens

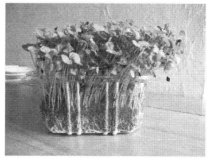

As I mentioned in the first paragraph of this section, any leafy green sprout can be grown into a micro lettuce or micro green. It's as simple as sowing your seeds into a soil or soilless medium-filled tray and keeping it moist. The process is the same as grasses, though the germination (soaking and sprouting) phase happens right in the dirt. Seeds grown into micro lettuces are always quite small, so soaking is a cinch – your wet paper towel will keep the seed buried and moist, so that's all there is to it. Also, microgreens are much less light sensitive; just 3-6 hours of diffused sunlight is plenty, though pale and leggy plants grown in a lightless bookshelf wouldn't be the end of the world. This is also a great first-dirt project, because you'll only have to keep them alive for a couple of weeks, tops.

Choosing your plants

Each micro-lettuce will grow at a different speed in different conditions. Some greens are ready in 1 week, while others can take 3 weeks. For this reason, I recommend starting out with mono-crops, planting for example, a tray with arugula, one with alfalfa, and one with broccoli, and as some grow quickly and some take their sweet time, you'll always be in the micro-greens. The other option is to use an organic micro-greens mix, which has been put together to compliment taste and growing time. It's also a good way to try things you wouldn't (or can't) buy and plant separately, like Cherry Belle Radish, Beet Bulls Blood , Pak Choy, Cabbage Red Ace, Kohlrabi , Swiss Chard Lucullus, and others, commonly found in mixes but pretty much impossible to find on their own. Seed packets are also quite inexpensive at $2-3, and because we're growing them past the sprout stage a little goes a long, long way.

Watercress micro lettuce

It should be no surprise by now that my favorite option is to DIY and make my own mix. After you can identify individual varieties of micro-lettuces and combine them in appetizing ways, it's quite easy to buy a few grams of each and sow 'til your heart's content. I'm slowly discovering mild, tangy, Provencal, and Asian mixes that suit my palate. I buy the organic seed packets and dump them all together into a small, dry bottle, ready to be sprinkled onto a fresh bed of dirt.

The last step in sustainability in micro lettuces is to harvest your own seeds. This would mean growing a few micro-lettuces into a larger container, and letting them go to seed; collecting, drying, and saving the seeds for future plantings. Buying packets of organic seeds online or at the local natural foods store is a luxury and in the event of a disaster, natural or otherwise, the person who is already living in a self-sufficient manner is going to be eating much better than those that have to scramble to get set up.

Another important difference between growing micro-lettuces and grasses is that the lettuce won't mat the soil with a resolute root system, allowing most of the growing medium to be used again. For this reason, it's fine to plant in a deeper container, pulling out the roots of your last harvest and tilling the soil (that means turning it over to mix the nutrients, for you city folk) with a fork. Deeper containers include plastic clamshells that spinach and herbs are sold in and

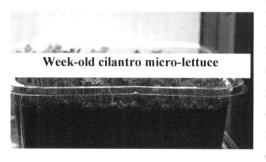
Week-old cilantro micro-lettuce

restaurant Styrofoam to-go containers. Punch ¼" holes in the bottom every 4-5 inches, and use the lid of the container as a drip tray. Fill it with soil, leaving ½" of space at the top so that watering doesn't overflow the container, and moisten well. Sprinkle your seeds on the soil and cover with a paper towel or 1/8" more dirt, and spray that with a little water to get them germinating.

Keep the top layer of soil moist but not wet. When the sprouts start pushing up the paper towel, remove it and put the container in the sunniest window you've got. The micro-lettuces can be harvested after a week or two; the best time is right before the second set of leaves opens. The first leaves are called "seed leaves", and the second "true leaves", and when these come about the plants gets ready for the long haul, trading in tender deliciousness for increased nitrogen uptake, causing a tougher texture and more bitter flavor. Unlike grass, the cut lettuces won't grow again, because they're still technically sprouts.

Start a new batch when your current crop is a week in, and you'll have micro-lettuce salads all year round.

Shoots

Larger seeds such as legumes and shell-on sunflower can be grown into larger veggies. Like grains grown into grasses, they must first be soaked and sprouted a little before they're sown on a growing medium, which allows them to be germinated evenly without having to be sown underground, bringing up the dirty dirt with them as the grow. The seed will rest on top the dirt, the root will go down, and the clean stalk and leaves will go the opposite direction. A legume will quickly shoot up a tall, straight stalk, and small leaves will begin to develop when it's 3 or 4 inches tall. This is called a "shoot", and should be harvested soon after the first pair of leaves open, 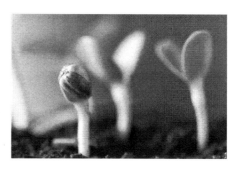 or it can get tough. If the second set of leaves open before you can cut them, they will be quite un-chewable, and their best use is one that utilizes the high-speed blender.

Sunflower Lettuce

One of my favorite greens, sunflower lettuce is cheap and easy to grow into thick and crunchy double-leafed tendrils. They are cultivated the same way as grasses and legumes, but their deliciousness deserves a special mention. Also, their shells require a slightly different technique during both soaking and harvesting.

Sunflower seeds in the shell will float,

Sunflower micro-lettuce

staying dry, if left to their own devices. Put them in a jar with a screw-on lid and fill with clean water. The seeds will stay on top of the water as the level rises. Continue filling until the seeds are above the lid but not quite falling out, then screw a lid on to push the seeds down into the water, submerging them completely If there's still an air bubble, just shake the jar a couple of times during the soaking to rotate the dry seeds. . If you don't have a canning jar, they can be imprisoned in a sprouting bag and held down by rock in any water-filled container. Then sprout them for a day or so until a little turtle tail pokes out of the shell, and spread them on some dirt or other growing medium.

The other thing that's unique to sunflower lettuce is that the shell won't stay earthbound, but will slither upwards on top of the sprout, protecting the leaves until they're ready to come out. In 5-8 days the shells will begin dropping off as the pair of succulent green leaves swell and spread. It's great fun to listen to the seedpod dropping to the shelf or ground; it's how I imagine a jungle to sound. I like to eat them as soon as possible after this rite of passage. It feels, nutritionally speaking, that with luminous vitality they've shed their adolescence and are straightening themselves with a new and fresh adulthood, and stepping into the sunshine with their faces deliciously raised. That's when I bite down. Hey, it's a cruel world.

They can also be gently pulled off by hand. Notice the difference between leaves that were forced into maturity and those that came into it on their own. Try to do it with one hand without pulling the root up, and you've got yourself a game more fun than Operation, and with a much better prize at the end. Sunflower micro-lettuce is great wherever sprouts are used: sandwiches, warps and burritos, as a garnish for soups, in veggie juice and salads. In fact, sunflower greens have such a mild, crunchy, and fresh flavor that they can be the only lettuce in a salad, either kept whole or chopped.

Container Gardening

Outdoor Growing

It's quite feasible to grow herbs, any vegetable, even tree fruits like citruses, pears and apples from a small city apartment amongst sirens and smog. With attention to water, fertilization, light, and warmth, any balcony or landing can be made into a lush growing area that can feed you and your family or friends daily. On the 3 ½ foot square landing at the top of my stairs I'm growing 3 kinds of peppers, tomatoes, mint, 3 kinds of basil, tarragon, peas, and strawberries. I also have a large Meyer lemon tree that supplies me with a lemon or two per week, year-round, and months of the most heavenly scent imaginable. Container gardening can afford more flexibility than a traditional garden: move pots to follow the sun, bring them inside on frosty nights, or hang pots or bags above the tongues of hungry wildlife. It's also a good way to recycle containers and use found vessels: buckets, lined baskets, bathtubs, and vintage high-heeled shoes will all hold dirt, and therefore the roots of food. Just make sure they have a hole or holes for drainage.

Dirt and soilless media was covered at length in the last section, and all of that info holds here as well, with a thought towards longer-term plant needs. While the dirt used for a week of growing grass is quickly composted and forgotten, the growing medium that will nourish and sustain your plant and you for months or years requires a sustained-release nutritional support. Dirt purloined from a garden or park won't drain quickly enough for a container, so a soil mix is necessary. Your plants need a mix that holds some moisture, but drains well, and contains a generous supply of nutrients to get the crop started off right. Though different types of plants have different moisture and nutrient needs, a good basic potting soil is one part dirt from the ground, one part sand, and one part composted soil or worm castings. If you live in an arid climate, less sand may be necessary; the opposite is true if your local earth has a lot of clay. A handful of perlite (see pg 285) will retain just the right amount of moisture, lighten the soil further, and help neutralize the pH. We'll need to re-fertilize at intervals – more on this a little later.

Light

This is the first thing that must be considered when planning your garden. It's a good idea to map out your space by the amount of sunlight each area gets. Small city spaces can have widely varying amounts of light in sections of rooms right next to each other, from several hours of full sun to only sparsely reflected light. When looking at your space this way, it's easy to start seeing the amount of food that can come from even the shadiest windowsill and teeniest patio.

Full Sun

If you're lucky enough to have a large window or patio with full sun, you'll have no problem growing fruit trees, berries, and all kinds of vegetables. Fruit, including fruiting vegetable such as bell peppers, eggplant, tomatoes, cucumbers, etc. need 4-5 hours of full sun a day, preferably more, and a few more hours of indirect or reflected light. Your main concern will be lack of space, and you'll have to consider temperature and humidity, but sun is usually the scarcest resource for most urban apartment dwellers so it's best to make the most of what full sun you have. If you have an outdoor area with plenty of light, I recommend focusing your container gardening efforts here, and once this space is maximized, branching out to the other possible growing areas in your home, office, and neighbor's places.

Medium Light

Plants that require less light energy are those with smaller fruit, like cherry tomatoes and chili peppers. Squash is easy to grow, but its size can be prohibitive in containers. Try a smaller variety like zucchini, which is even more versatile in the kitchen as it is the garden. Slower-growing varieties of legumes, such as bush peas and bush beans, require less sun than their more common counterparts, the "pole" varieties, which ultimately produce larger crops over time, and are a better choice if you have the light.

Possibly the most efficient use of medium light conditions is to grow plants for their seeds. Amaranth and quinoa, for example, produce huge clusters of nutrient-packed tiny seeds, which can be collected and sprouted for a very large amount of actual food from one plant, much more than can be harvested in fruit or vegetable mass.

Low light

The last place to spend your gardening energy can still be a very effective growing space. Root vegetables like beets, turnips, potatoes, and carrots can do very well with only a few hours of reflected light. Root and tuber plants are quite cooperative with Kitchen Sink Farming by storing most of their energy underground in the part that we harvest for food, so it's less important how much light they receive daily and more important how much sun they soak up over the entire season. Therefore, letting them go as long as possible before harvest will yield the fullest, juiciest roots. But all root vegetables can be harvested and eaten small, so even scraggly plants grown in paltry light can produce a delightful crop of baby root vegetables.

Lastly, leafy greens have fairly low light requirements than plants that we want for their flowers or fruit. Full sunlight may actually burn many plants that have evolved large, wrinkled satellite dishes for collecting scant illumination. They can be grown year-round in many climates, and many varieties can even be started in the fall for continuous winter salads. Beet and turnip greens, lettuces, kale, collard greens, arugula and spinach can also be defensively started inside, in front of a window or under a glow light then placed outside when they're a little more established. For the same reason, many ground-covering herbs like mint, rosemary, and tarragon can thrive in low light conditions.

Garlic is a quick-growing low light plant, whose shoots (chives) are just as delicious as the bulb-roots themselves. Stick a clove or two, point down, in dirt-filled plastic containers like yogurt cups and put them anywhere you want. Garlic will make the soil unusable by other plants so it's best grown alone, its bedding composted after the roots are harvested. Even the tiniest apartment will have more room for garlic than the tenant has appetite. Same goes for green or spring onions, which can go from ghostly white to deep purple in color, and pungent to sweet in flavor, so much so that some varieties are delicious eaten washed and raw. I made many meals of the wild onions that grew on the banks of the large river by my childhood Ohio home, cursorily cleaned in the swirling rapids. Today, a spring onion or two goes in just about every dressing and soup, providing the perfect multi-cylinder sharpness and fresh bite.

Maximizing Sun

If you're lucky enough to have no buildings blocking out the sun for some of the day, you'll want to think in three dimensions to maximize your amount of sun-sweet, chlorophyll-rich food. Terracing and vertical gardening are ways to keep plants from blocking each other and maximize precious floor space. Put taller trees, trellised vines, and peas, beans and corn closest to your wall, leaving a few inches for light to reflect onto the backs of the plants. You may also cover the wall with used aluminum foil, those silver tanning blankets people lay on at the beach for the same reason, reflective car sun shades, thermal emergency blankets, or anything else that will maximize your light in an otherwise unexpected direction. Medium height plants such as broccoli, cabbage, cauliflower, cucumbers, and tomatoes come next, with shorter plants like herbs and flowers in the front row. Arranging crops by height is called terracing, and is a simple technique used with great benefit for thousands of years in hilly farmland. If your crops aren't widely divergent in height, you can produce this effect by making steps, whether by building them out of scraps of plywood to fit your space, or stacking crates or plastic boxes to create the same result.

Now comes 3D-thinking to maximize space in the vertical axis: upside-down growing. This technique allows the ceiling of a patio to be used almost as efficiently as the floor. Baskets and bags are hung from hooks in the ceiling along with tumbling vines of tomatoes, peppers, strawberries, herbs, or baby vegetables like patty pan squash or Persian cucumbers. Not as pretty than wire baskets or store-bought grow bags, but possibly more effective because of their dark, sun-sucking color, are DIY grow bags made with those reusable grocery totes with doubled plastic grocery bags or plastic trash can liners on the inside. A few well-placed horizontal slits on the front surface of the totes (put a cutting board inside the bag and cut the tote and liners at the same time with a utility knife) will make pockets for your berries or baby zucchini to be planted in. Fill the bag half full with potting soil, place the roots of your seedlings in through the slits, and after seeing if its handles need to be reinforced, hang it from a strong hook screwed into a joist (2x4 running underneath the surface of the ceiling. Find them, and learn which direction they run, with a stud finder or by knocking with your knuckles and listening for a higher-pitched, solider sound than the surrounding area). The color of tote or bag is an important consideration; darker will absorb as much warmth as possible, great for starting seeds and cooler months, but will require more water during warmer seasons, possibly 2 or even 3 times a day at the height of summer. Potting mixes are generally lighter than soil and are recommended to keep the bag from being too heavy. If your bags hang over a walkway or sitting area, make sure to check the integrity of the bag more frequently and diligently.

Plastic bags, especially the larger-sized, thick black liners can also be used instead of pots by simply poking some drainage holes and filling with soil and a single plant, or using the slit-pocket method described above. They can expand or shrink depending on the season by regulating the amount of dirt inside, and are (unfortunately for landfills) surprisingly durable. They can also be closed with a twist tie and laid on their sides, with slits cut into what is now the top and like a low, wide, flexible pot. This makes for a compact and easily moveable garden, if a sunny space is being used temporarily or without implicit permission. Plants can also be grown this way in a hammock slung between two balconies or posts.

PVC piping can also be used as an effective and versatile growing device. Drill or cut holes at least 1 ½" wide all around a length of PVC tubing, scraps of which are always available for free at lumber yards. There's also a pocket-cutting technique described in the "Growing Wall" section that's even better. You'll need to buy the right-sized cap for the bottom, and a chain or strong rope to attach to the top for hanging. Drill lots of small holes in the bottom cap and attach it to the pipe; you may want to glue it in place if the fit isn't snug, as it will be holding a lot of the weight of the soil and plants. Drill two more holes at the top of the tube to feed the chain, wire, or rope through (this will be getting wet so a synthetic, waterproof material is best) and hang it from a sturdy hook, preferably attached to a ceiling joist or other structural beam (see 2 paragraphs up). The end a hose can be left in the top to be turned on for a minute or two every day. If you have a spigot, setting up a drip system on a timer may be the best option for multiple hanging tubes, and the whole system can be made in an afternoon, the rest of a gardener's time free for sipping fresh strawberry margaritas and reading my blog (but if you're considering this set-up, check out the "Growing Wall" plans first).

Choosing Crops

When deciding what to grow, you have two options when conforming to the natural laws of space, light, warmth, etc. You can choose to grow a variety of fruits and vegetables, giving you and your family and friends varied nutrients and flavors. You can also grow a larger amount of fewer kinds of plants – finding the type and variety of plants that will net you that maximum food for your space. The latter route has two benefits. The first is that it will take less time, both in learning the different needs of your diverse garden and in tending. Much quicker to water everything at once, feeding all simultaneously with the same fertilizer, and dealing with pests with the single Hammer of Judah instead of the many pebbles of David. As most Kitchen Sink Farming projects are limited not by space but by time this can be a very big difference.

If you live away from people, or at least like-minded people, growing a myriad of different plants may be the way to go, but trading bushels of beautiful tomatoes for future vegetables of a different sort, or honey, milk, or anything else one person might have an abundance of, including services, is the best description of community I can think of. There's an African proverb that asks how someone can eat a fish for a year – the answer is that they divide it amongst their neighbors, who then share their food.

I started a non-profit in Portland called GardenAngels.org which turns the excess organic produce from overgrown gardens and public domain trees into non-perishable, raw foods like zucchini breads, fermented apple butter, and kale crackers, and distributes them to the needy. The gardener is repaid with prepared foods unless they'd like to donate their portion. Again, hunger is not a supply problem, it's one of distribution, as LA's sidewalks strewn with rotting oranges and downtown littered with hungry people attests to.

Indoor Growing

Many plants will do much better in indoor containers, a boon for the average urbanite who has much more indoor space than out. The inside of a window allows light that's almost as good to stream in to a temperature-controlled environment, and options for trapping heat and humidity abound. Some plants, like ginger root, do better indoors, where the tropical conditions in which it thrives are recreated more easily than outside. Clear or wire shelving units are essential for growing grasses and micro-lettuces, and if there's still room, leaf and small-fruit plants that can utilize a slightly less powerful light should take up residence.

Self-Watering Containers

This simple and cheap development in container gardening is so easy to make and use it's just amazing that they're such a recent development. The advantages are several. They assure proper soil moisture at all times, eliminating thirsty plants, but also taking care of problems from over-watering, which can also starve the plants of precious oxygen or dehydrate them, as roots can't take in water when the soil's moisture is over 40%. Soil that's too wet can also contribute to many diseases such as root rot and mold. The layer of air at the bottom of self-watering containers increases oxygen to the roots of the plants, which breathe just like we do. They also strengthen the root system by inspiring them to reach down to get at the water, the way plants in nature grow, while top-fertilizing stimulates a second system of roots more toward the surface of the soil. This double-layer root system creates faster-growing and higher-yielding plants, which can often out-produce plants grown in the ground. The most important argument for self-watering containers, however, is that by essentially watering themselves from a back-up reservoir, you may be able to cut your container gardening efforts to once a week, freeing up time for other things. Not many farmers can go to Cancun in the middle of a growing season.

The underlying idea behind self-watering is a reservoir of water with a "wick" that draws moisture up into the soil. There are a few ways to do this, and after the couple of examples that follow the resourceful Kitchen Sink Famer will be able to easily create custom containers to suit their own purposes.

Simple Self-Watering Devices: "the spike" and "the holey bottle"

The Watering Spike

You'll need:

A 2-liter plastic bottle and a foot long piece of PVC that's slightly larger than the mouth of the bottle.

Cut the bottom of the PVC at an angle, and drill holes in the sides, the size of which will be determined by the plants' water needs. Fill the 2 liter bottle with water and turn it over onto the PVC. This allows not only for the soil to regulate its own moisture level, but for the water to be delivered directly to the plant's roots. The spike will fill with soil when inserted, so it doesn't water as heavily as it would seem.

A plastic soda or water bottle can also be buried in the soil and filled with water; the size of the holes poked around the bottom of the bottle will determine the speed of flow.

The Self-Watering Bucket

Step One: Assemble your materials

These are:

A bucket,

A soil barrier,

Fabric wicks,

A watering tube,

A utility knife,

And soil.

Bucket – this could be a five gallon bucket and lid, or any two buckets that fit inside of each other, available from hardware stores, restaurants, nurseries, recycling centers, and many other places for cheap or free. Be careful not to use a bucket that's had paint or any other chemical in it, which will almost certainly end up in your soil, plant, food, and liver. My top choice is soy sauce buckets from Japanese restaurants for their cool labels, though many foods are packaged this way. You can also use a pretty plastic pot, or even a terra cotta one, for a more presentable planter. Any big enough container with no holes will do.

Soil barrier – something round that's small enough to slide inside the bucket but too big to go all the way to the bottom. If using a 5-gallon bucket, this can be the middle of the lid, cut out for this purpose (save the outer ring for step 3), a plastic planter tray, or an entire other bucket, if the bottoms are 4 far enough apart to leave room for the water reservoir. Make sure you can cut or drill holes in whatever you choose in the soil barrier. If the soil barrier doesn't leave enough room between the two (think 3+ inches, more if you want a bigger reservoir and less frequent refilling), a rock or block of wood can be put in to hold the bucket up higher. If you're using a tray-type soil barrier, make sure that there's still a tight fit around the edges because we can't let dirt fall through gaps into the water. The soil barrier will need to be stiff and strong enough to hold up the weight of the soil and plants.

Fabric wicks – We'll use a few foot-long, 1-inch-wide strips of cotton cloth; an old towel works well. The basket-wick described in the next plan uses soil to bring up water. This system requires a little bit more work but is also more effective.

Watering tube – This is how we'll fill the reservoir, bypassing the soil. The rigid tube needs to be a few inches taller than the bucket, and can be PVC pipe, plastic (including clear for sneakiness), bamboo or metal (like copper water pipe, cheap and lovely), depending on availability, cost, and aesthetics. I have faith in you.

Step Two: Cuts and Holes

1 - Place your soil barrier into your bucket, and drill or cut a few small holes about an inch above the bottom of the soil line around the side of your bucket. It's easier to do this from the inside of the bucket with the barrier in place. Sounds obvious, but I've seen plans that include complex ways for finding out where on the outside to drill. These holes allow oxygen in to the roots, creating faster-growing, hyper-producing plants, and btw this 30-second procedure should be done to all growing containers. Cut a larger (1/4" or so) hole an inch below the soil line; this will be the overflow hole to let you know the reservoir is full. If you're using a terra cotta or clay container (again, no holes at the

bottom) use a ¼" glass and tile drill bit, sprinkling water over it as you drill to keep it cool.

2 - Cut 3 small holes in the soil barrier, just big enough to pull the fabric wicks through.

3 - Cut a larger hole at the edge of the soil barrier, just big enough to fit the watering tube into. If it's not a really snug fit, cover the hole with a round piece of burlap or other coarse, thick fabric that's much bigger than it, and cut a small "X" in it for the tube to go into to keep soil from falling into the reservoir.

4 - Cut the bottom of the watering tube at an angle to allow a free flow of water when it sits on the bottom of the bucket or pot.

Step Three: Assemble your planter

Tie large, loose knots in the middle of your fabric wicks. Insert the wicks through the top of the holes in the soil barrier, until they reach the knots. Slide the soil barrier into the bucket, pushing down evenly on the edges until it's flat. Insert the watering tube into its hole and fill the bucket with pre-moistened, un-fertilized soil, leaving a couple of inches of room at the top.

If you'd like to use a moisture barrier, lay it over the top of the soil and attach the remaining outer ring of the lid, assuming you cut out the inside for your soil barrier. If you don't have a lid, tape works. A black plastic garbage bag is fine, though many other products are available. Cut X's in the barrier and insert your plants. Fill the reservoir with the watering tube, stopping when your overflow hole goes into action. Top fertilize every two weeks. Then hit Travelocity.

The Self-Watering Garden

This is a larger-scale project, because it's hard to grow much food in a 5-gallon bucket. The concept is exactly the same (not repeated here so read the above first), but the details are a little more conducive to food growing. A large plastic tote, discarded bathtub basin, or kiddie pool are all perfectly acceptable containers, and again, having two of them that fit inside each other will make the process much easier. Otherwise, the lid is the next best option for a soil barrier, the edge cut off to form a tight fit and saved to hold down a moisture barrier, even more helpful with all the soil surface area you're about to have. You can also use two large plastic garbage bags with a rigid flat surface or lattice, and blocks or bricks to hold the inner one up. The watering tube is the same, but depending on the size of your garden you may want to use several, and you also might want to secure them to the sides of the container with a hot glue gun, bailing wire, duct tape, or a bolt. As mentioned above, the wick is going to be slightly more complicated, but also much better at distributing water evenly through soil, because the wick itself is made of soil.

The soil wick, or foot, is a plastic kitchen strainer, a "fish and chips" basket that seafood and sandwiches are sometimes served in, or a plastic bowl, small plastic planter, or other short fat container, with enough holes poked in it to resemble a basket.

If you're sticking with the 5-gallon bucket container because of its size and easy transportability, you may want to use a soil wick as well. Find a yogurt cup or similarly-shaped container and poke several dozen holes all around it. Pack it tightly with moistened soil and insert it into a hole cut in the soil barrier, small enough that it doesn't go all the way through.

Fertilizing

Non-organic fertilizers promise massive bright red tomatoes and watermelons the size of Volkswagens, but their allure quickly fades when you take of bite of the tasteless fruit. Organic fertilizers are tremendously more effective, better for everyone, and nearly free if you make them yourself. Every two weeks or so (more when your plants are producing), top-fertilize by adding compost tea to water and pouring it evenly over the dirt, or adding worm castings or freshly composted soil to the top of the soil and pouring some water over it to mix it up.

See "Plant Nutritional Deficiencies" on pg 377 for specific nutrients needed by less-than-vibrant plants and where to get them.

Furthermore

Aside from light, dirt, fert, and water, the only thing left to discuss on the subject of growing food in a container is the stalk-by-stalk specifics of each plant's need. And this is probably the most important. Which is why I'm going to skip it.

There are piles of wonderful books, blogs, and local experts about your specific climate and what you want to eat, and I couldn't possibly cover it all here. So I'm going to leave it up to you to educate yourself, suggesting you start with one plant, maybe a citrus tree if you have a warm sunny spot, an herb or two if not, and think of them as houseplants 2.0. Add a plant or two to your patio or windowsill farm whenever you've gotten the hang of the last ones.

Hooked on 'Ponics: Hydroponic and Aeroponic Gardening

Sprouts grow quickly and, drawing nutrients from water, can increase 30 times in size. Next, we have micro-lettuces, that with a little bit of dirt can do even better. But if you want to grow a large amount of food, whether for your family or neighborhood to eat, barter, or sell, you'll need to know about hydroponics (from the Greek "to labor with water"). You've probably heard about hydroponics, a system that floods plants' roots with a nutrient-rich water solution, and aeroponics, which suspends plants' roots in an environment made humid and delicious by constantly or intermittently spraying them with a nutrient-water solution. Both have their benefits and drawbacks, and this section will go into more detail about their differences so you can make an informed decision about which is best for you.

Hydroponics and aeroponics are based on the fact that dirt serves only two functions – to hold the plant up and supply it with water and nutrients. Both hydro- and aero- grow plants without soil, which are held up by a soilless medium and fed with nutrient-rich water. The main difference is how that solution is fed – hydroponics washes the roots with a flowing current of water while aeroponics keeps the roots hanging in a constantly misty environment and sprays them with nutrients. Aeroponics is thought to be superior for several reasons, but hydro does have two advantages.

First: The Similarities

Plants grow much more quickly and produce more in a hydro or aeroponics set-up, because they're being spoon-fed readily usable nutrients; instead of having to spend energy growing roots and digesting what they find. They can put all of their effort into producing food. Because of this lack of hardship, their fruit isn't going to be as hearty and full of flavor as food grown in containers or the ground, but again, there's going to be a lot more of it. Also, because the roots aren't inspired to grow very long the pots stay small and closer together, making the system more compact than container or ground growing. But because the kinds of nutrients the plants are given directly affects the stage of growth they can enter - fruiting, flowering, seeding – the timing of all of these stages can be regulated. This means that if you're growing basil, which is an annual and seeds and dies at the end of the year, you can stick to the vegetative nutrients and stay in the pesto indefinitely. You can also grow, for example, a few amaranth or quinoa plants, which produce huge amounts of seeds, and keep them in the seed-production business just to have seeds to sprout to large quantities, potentially the most effective growing setup for feeding large numbers of people. I believe that having hydroponic "seed factories", then sprouting those seeds, both with home-made liquid fertilizer, to yield potentially thousands of times the amount of food that can be produced by growing a plant in a pot, will be the large-scale urban farming of the future, capable of feeding entire apartment buildings from the roof with an unending chain of week-long growing seasons, or the answer to the distribution issue of global hunger. Enough food can be produced to feed everyone in the world, many times more if we were all to become vegetarians. But the difficulty in *getting* the food to the people that need it is what keeps them hungry. "Sprouting seed factories" can be localized and many, and could be an answer.

Hydroponics and aeroponics are both beneficial to the environment because their carefully controlled growing environment makes chemical fertilizers and pesticides completely unnecessary. They both use less water and fertilizer than in-the-ground gardening, take up much less space (especially with the growing wall and bucket systems discussed later), and can be used anywhere, from underground basements and caves to space stations.

Now: the Differences

Of the two, aeroponics will yield about 25% faster results because the roots aren't suspended in water, and are therefore have access to more air. Plants' roots need oxygen to absorb nutrients, and carbon dioxide is a necessary factor in photosynthesis, another way plants feed. Hydroponics uses a mineral solution that can become infected with algae, parasites, and bacteria over the two-week period it's used. In aeroponics, the infestation of plants is minimized because each 15-minutes-apart nutrient spray is fresh and sterile. Contact between plants is also minimal in aeroponics, thereby preventing the spread of diseases. In aeroponics, gardeners have greater control over the growing environment, and properly maintained plants will be totally free from diseases and pests, while hydroponics cannot be so precisely controlled.

Aeroponics another edge in that it uses less water and only a quarter of the nutrient supply. It does require more electricity, however, because the pump that powers the misters is constantly going, as opposed to intermittent pumping in hydro. And because aeroponics is such a finely-tuned system, the result of a power failure is catastrophic; the plants will begin to wilt and starve immediately if the power goes out or more than one or two sprayers get clogged. For this reason, aeroponics requires more attention than hydro, which once established, can be left on its own for days or weeks. Many aeroponics growers that depend on the food they grow actually have a back-up hydro system in case of power failure.

Because there's a fairly constant water level in an aeroponics system, some people raise edible fish in the reservoir, which will raise the heat in the system (better for the plants) and fertilize the water. This called "aquiponics", and can be a completely self-enclosed system, with fish waste feeding the plants, the plants filtering out the waste (which is toxic to the fish), and algal growth feeding the fish. It's possible make an aquiponic set-up with the fill-and-drain of hydroponics, but the reservoir would have to be really big to keep the fish happy.

So when choosing between hydro and aeroponics to feed your family or community, it really comes down to two things: electricity and attention. A vacation home or remote greenhouse in an area with high-priced power or a just few solar panels? Hydro it is. A community garden or teen center with many hands and eyes and an abundance of free energy from wind, sun, or hydroelectric sources? Free to be aero. Your situation is most likely somewhere in between these two extremes, so your decision won't be quite so cut and dry. The good news is that both systems require the same amount of skill to build (e.g. – not very much) and will allow you to pretty much grow as much food as you want, being more limited by your time and passion than by your space and funds.

The Plans: Hydroponics

Hydro has one more advantage that wasn't mentioned earlier, the ability to build a system out of just about anything. While aeroponics can be conceivably carried out with a spray bottle and a whole lot of free time, it's a finely-tuned system that needs to be set up in a conscious way. Hydro, however, can be pretty much be slapped together from trash, and though it always incorporates a pump to flood the system, one could potentially just dump fertilized water over the plants' suspended roots a few times a day, collecting it as it drains, forego all fanciness and call it hydroponics. Conversely, to make a well thought-out and efficient system only requires a small pump ($5) and plastic tubing ($1.50), and it's quite possible to build the rest entirely out of found objects – discarded plastic tubs, 2 liter soda bottles from the recycling center, roadside gravel as a growing medium, etc. This section will teach you how to make compact, efficient, and automated systems that can be left alone for weeks at a time, customizable for your space, lighting requirement, handiness, and number of plants, and money-saving variations will be left up to your imagination.

But first, a note about algae:

Algae - which can be green, red, or brown - are a form of plant life that is a natural consequence of exposing nutrient-rich water to light. Algae aren't given a second thought by container growers but it can be a concern in hydroponic set-ups. They're actually non-toxic to your plants and can even supply extra nutrients, but as they bloom, die, and decompose they will rob your plants of valuable oxygen. They can also propagate on roots, limiting or cutting off their supply of nutrients. If algae grow out of control they can also block tubes and fittings. Though there are some natural water additives that can inhibit the growth of algae, namely grapefruit seed extract and hydrogen peroxide for more established plants, prevention is always the best medicine. Blocking as much light from the inner workings of your system is an effective means of algae control, as they can't live in darkness. In single-planter systems (like the small-scale set-up below), the planters can be covered with light-proof film, plastic, or aluminum foil, with holes poked out for the plants. Make sure that the growing media, tubing, and reservoir are either wrapped or in a cabinet, or placed inside of commercial anti-algae bags.

Four sets of instructions follow: 1 and 2 - the small and large scale set-ups, 3 - bucket and drum growing, and 4 - the growing wall, or vertical garden. The smaller set-up consists of individually flooding containers, can be put together in a couple of hours with a single trip to a hardware store, and are a low-commitment and small-space way to get started with a few herbs, tomato or strawberry plants. The larger system will utilize a large "bath" that plants can easily be put into and taken out of, and will be more expensive (though still under $100) and require more handiness, but if you're serious about growing food and have the space (for two plastic totes, which can be stacked on top of each other, so not super huge), I recommend you jump right into this one. Bucket and Drum growing are a little more industrial and do best in a greenhouse situation, or at least a large room that gets flooded on at least 2 sides with sunlight for several hours a day. Same thing with the Vertical Garden, though if you have the light (natural or artificial) it will turn a wall into a breathtaking cascade of greenery and nutriment. The important thing here is that the simple concept of flooding and draining roots with nutrient-rich water is the same, and if after reading through all the plans you want to hybridize them or create a system that's completely your own, more power to ya.

Small-Scale Set-Up

This system is designed to go in front of a window. If you don't have adequate light for fruiting plants (if that's what you're going with), your window space is already being used for grasses or micro-lettuces, or you'd just like to put the system elsewhere for esthetic reasons, check out the section on artificial light. It's very quick and easy to get up and running, and finding sources for the equipment is by far the most time-consuming part (but I've tried to help you out in "Resources").

What you'll need: (unless you have a friend who works at a hydro store, it's cheapest and easiest to get everything but the bottles online, but the stores that would carry the individual things are listed for your convenience)

Recycling center or neighbor's garbage:

3 or more 2 liter soda bottles with caps. The bottoms will be cut off, the bottles turned upside down, and the opening will hold the plant.

Pet Store:

Aquarium pump, 1 psi or the smallest/cheapest you can find

1 ft of ¼" air tubing

Hardware Store/Lumber Yard/Nursery:

2 ft of 3/8" vinyl or plastic irrigation tubing, add a foot for every extra soda bottle planter

A number of 3/8" barbed plastic "T" adapters, 1 for every bottle, minus the last one. Also called barbed hose fitting, and available in nylon.

1 - 3/8" barbed plastic elbow, see above

13 feet of 1x4 lumber – 1 @ 32", 4 @ 28", and 4 @ 3 ½"; the lumber yard can cut them for you if you don't have a saw, for 25-50 cents per cut, though if you ask nicely they may waive the fee

1 - Piece of plywood or melanine, 32" x 28". This is the front cover and is just for looks, so can be skipped or made as pretty as you like. I'll leave it up to you how you want to attach the cover; anything from just leaning it against the legs, to a loose nail that can be pushed in and out, to hinges that allow you to swing open your apparatus and wow your book club, will do fine. The sides can also be covered for noise reduction and looks – add more material as needed.

24 - 2" drywall screws

(Hydroponics store or internet):

Growing Medium (See chapter on soilless growing mediums, but there's one extra thing to think about when choosing one for your project: density. The more air there is in your medium, the more water you'll need to fill it up, and the larger your reservoir tank will need to be. Pea Gravel is a good solution for hydro growing: cheap and packs tightly.)

Plants and nutrients

Tools:

A tube of silicone caulk

Utility knife

Measuring tape

Drill with a screw bit and 7/32, 3/8, and 1-1/4 inch bits. I cringe at the thought of you buying a drill for this project – you'd have to grow a lot of tomatoes before you came out ahead. Maybe you know someone who has one you can borrow or trade for sprouts.

Drilling and cutting:

Drill 3/8" holes in the center of all the bottle caps, and an additional 7/32" hole in one (for the reservoir). Make sure to leave room for the threads of the bottle when it's screwed on.

Cut the ends of the tubing at angles to make it easier to stick them through the holes.

Cut the bottoms off of all the 2 liter bottles but one (the reservoir). Poke multiple holes in the bottom and invert it inside the bottle to hold the growing medium. Depending on the size of the growing medium you're using, you may also want to use a plastic produce bag with many holes poked in it, and the opening rubber banded or paper clipped to the opening in the bottle. [Side Note – Sunlight Dishwashing Liquid comes in bottles that are smaller than

2 liters but have nipples underneath the pop-out dispenser tops that fit 3/8" tubing perfectly. If you'd prefer growing a larger number of smaller plants or can't find barbed connectors and have a source for these bottles, go for it.]

Drill 1 ¼" holes in the 32" piece of 1x4, 5 ½" inches from each end and 4" apart. This will give you 5 holes.

Quick and Easy Assembly

Apply silicon on all wet connections

Screw 1x4 pieces together to form the case as shown

Feed about a foot of the 3/8" tubing and an inch of the ¼" tubing through the top of the cap of the reservoir bottle, the one with two holes

Place elbow and "T" connectors through bottle caps and screw onto bottles.

Invert bottles through holes in cross-beam, the one with the elbow connector at one end

Connect the bottles together using 3/8" tubing with enough length so they won't pull on the connectors, but short enough so as not to form a "U" in between connections. The elbow connector is on one end, the "T" connectors are in the middle, and the reservoir is on the other end, standing on the ground.

Connect the reservoir and aquarium pump with the ¼" tubing

Getting It Going:

Rinse your growing medium until the run-off it clear, and put it in the planters with a plant. If you're using a potted plant, gently rinse off any soil with in a sink or with a hole. Put a layer of growing medium in the bottom of the planter, then hold the plant in place with one hand while gently sprinkling in the rest of the medium until the plant is secure.

Make some nutrient water, and while putting a kink in the 3/8" tube between the last planter and the reservoir (you may want to bend it and cinch it with a rubber band or have a friend hold it) fill the planters to just below the top of the growing medium. Then take out the kink so that the water drains into the res. This is the best way to make sure you have the right amount of water. If the reservoir fills up, there's too much water in the system and it could back up into the pump, which will ruin it. See if you can use a denser, or less, growing medium. About half to three-quarters full is a good level. Time how long it takes all the water to drain out.

Plug in the pump. The air fills up the reservoir and pushed the water up into the planters. Time how long it takes to do this, then unplug the pump and time how long it takes to drain. The two times added together are one cycle, probably around 2 minutes. Set the timer to 3-5 cycles per day, if you're using one. If any water or air leaks out, drain the system and use the silicon on the offending openings.

Large-Scale Hydro Set-up

The idea behind this system is the same as the last: nutrient-rich water washes over the roots of growing medium-suspended plants at pre-ordained intervals. The difference is that instead of having a few-inch-in-diameter planter for each plant, the large-scale set-up uses one large, shallow basin as a shared planter, with room for dozens or hundreds of plants. You'll notice that the list of supplies and steps to assemble is about the same size in both recipes.

What You'll Need:

2 Plastic Tubs…

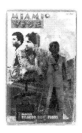 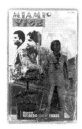

…just kidding

They should be at least 1 ½ ft by 2 ft, and if one has a lid, and the other is half as deep or more (at least 7 inches) and can sit on top of the deep one, so much the better. The deep lidded one will be the reservoir and the shallow one on top will be the growing tray. If you're going the stacked, small footprint route, make sure that the lid can handle a hundred pounds of weight, and that you can handle a hundred pounds when you have to move the growing tray to get to the reservoir, like when you change the water every two weeks. Otherwise, cinderblocks or a sturdy shelf or rack can hold the growing tray up higher than the res.

A Submersible Pump

This is the heart of the system. Get one that's rated at least 200 Gallons Per Hour (GPH). There are two other things that matter: "x-feet head", and "psi". The "head" tells us how far the pump can pump; if it's less than 4 feet, the length of our tubing, it might be the little engine that couldn't so play it safe and get the stronger model. If you want to expand in the future, you will be glad you did. Acceptable models start at $20-$30.

An Aquarium Air Pump and Air Stone, or Bubbler, with tubing.

This will oxygenate your nutrient water to prevent settling and stagnation, and are often available as a unit. This item isn't absolutely necessary, especially if you can create a splash when the upper tub drains into the lower.

2 Elbow Fittings, called "*Plastic Mushroom Head*" or , "90 degree through-wall fittings"

These are "*barbed*" so that tubing can be attached, are plastic, nylon, or brass, and they come with a nut on the other side so they can be secured to the wall of your tray. Try to find the same size barbs as your submersible pump so that the tubing will fit

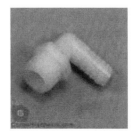

without an adapter, but if you can't it's an easy fix.

Tubing, 4 kinds:

1 - For your aquarium pump, if it didn't come with

2 – 5 feet, to go from your barbed fittings to your submersible pump. If they're not the same size, get an adapter or resizing tube that will allow 2 different-sized tubes to be connected together.

3 – 5 feet, twice the diameter of the above tube

4 - 6 inches of stiff plastic tubing with the end of the tube covered with a wide-mesh screening material (like window screen) and rubber-banded in place

A Timer, Growing Medium, Nutrients, and Plants

Tools: a drill with a 3/8" bit, and a tube of silicone caulk

Assembly

Drill 2 holes in the shallow growing tray, just wide enough to fit the barbed fittings through. They should both be in the center of one end of the tray; one as close to the bottom as possible (but make sure you leave enough room to screw the nut on the fitting) and the other 6 or 7 inches up. It's easier to drill through thin plastic if you hold a board or piece of wood against the other side of the wall.

Insert the fittings into these 2 holes so that the barbs are on the outside pointing down, apply silicon to both sides, and screw on the nuts.

Drill 3 holes in one end of the lid of the bigger container; 2 for tubing and one for power cords.

Insert the stiff plastic tube into the lower fitting from the inside. This will keep debris out of the reservoir, and will assist drainage (by the "capillary effect"; the surface tension created by liquids in thin tubes adds extra suction which even allows water to flow uphill, and this will keep liquid from pooling at the bottom of your growing tray. You've seen this cool phenomenon when soaking up water from a countertop with a paper towel; tiny pores in the fabric "wick" up many times their weight in liquid. This was the subject of Einstein's first paper.)

Connect the submersible pump to the upper fitting, running the tubing through one of the holes in the lid. Connect a piece of tubing from the bottom fitting and run it through another hole in the lid. Run the power cord of the submersible pump through the third hole in the lid, and put the pump in the reservoir tub. DO NOT PLUG IT IN YET.

Put everything you've constructed so far where it's going to live. Make sure that the place you choose can support a few hundred pounds. If you're not putting the growing tray on top of the reservoir, put it on a sturdy shelf or platform that's at least as high as the top of the reservoir.

Rinse your growing medium until the run-off it clear, and put it in the growing tray, about 6" deep.

Put a kink in the drainage hose, clamp or rubber band it, and fill up the growing tray until the water is about an inch below the surface of the growing medium. Record how much water it took to do this. Un-kink the hose and let it rain.

Because your growing medium was already wet, you know how much water is in the reservoir, and therefore how much nutrient solution to add to it. If you lost track, you can measure down from the rim, empty the water out, and fill it back up to the mark, taking note of how many gallons you've used. Add your nutrient solution. In the future, you may want to make your own solution, but with different nutritional needs at different stages, for different plants, and in different climates, I recommend you get the hang of hydro first. Here's a great resource when you're ready for it: www.motherearthnews.com is a great database for homemade nutrient solutions – search "hydroponic nutrients".

Plant your plants! If you're using starters that were formerly in soil, gently rinse it all away, then bury the roots in the growing medium. In hydroponics, plants can be put much closer together than in soil - you can plant them half the recommended distance apart.

Plug in the submersible pump. The pump sucks water in from the reservoir and pushes it into the grow tray. Time how long it takes to do this, then unplug the pump, and time how long it takes to drain. The two times added together are one cycle, probably around 20-30 minutes. Set the timer to 5-8 cycles per day. Watch your plants to see if they droop (not enough water) or turn yellow (too much water), and adjust accordingly.

If you're using the aquarium pump, it will sit outside of the system, so run its tube through one of the holes and plug it in.

With a powerful enough submersible pump and a "T" fitting in the filling tube, this system can easily expand to two growing trays and beyond.

The Growing Wall

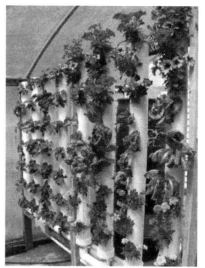

Both the Growing Wall and the Barrel Garden, which follows, require more technical skill than the smaller hydro set-ups, though only about half as much as putting together a bookcase from IKEA. For the Growing Wall, each of the 3 main steps: 1) assembling the wooden frame and PVC planters, 2) assembling the lower pipes, 3) setting up the irrigation tubing and pump, are separated into their own section, each has its own materials list and assembly instructions. It's best to look through the entire plan before you get started, then buy all materials for all 3 steps at once.

Step 1 - Frame and Planters

Step 1 Materials:

2-3" tape; masking, painters, duct, whatever.

Marker or grease pencil (a different color than the PVC)

A heat gun or powerful hair dryer

Saw, circular or hack (see Cutting the PVC, paragraph 2)

Nice but not necessary:

A spray bottle with water

PVC:

About a foot of 1.25" PVC (1.5" will also work)

4 – 57'" lengths of 4" thin wall (Schedule 20) PVC (buy 2 - 10' lengths, available in white or black; do you want your wall garden to be ninja or samurai?)

[Note – you need to be able to reach the top of the tube, and if you're a shorty and don't want to use a stepstool, plan ahead. The tubes will start at 2 feet from the ground, so measure how much higher than that you can reach and cut the PVC accordingly. Then read and understand these instructions so you'll know what other mods to make before you start.

Note 2 - If you don't own a saw or don't feel like cutting, you can buy 3 - 96" 2x4's and 2 - 10' lengths of PVC and ask them to cut them to the appropriate lengths for you. I'd keep a measuring tape with me and use it (you can borrow one from the store while you're in it) to make sure the cuts are accurate, or to inspire the cutter to make them so.]

Wood for the frame:

2 – 80" 2x4's

1 – 43" 2x4

1 – 40" 2x4

If you'd like to give the frame a coat of paint or other finish, now's the time.

Step Assembly:

Cutting the PVC

We'll be staggering the planting holes so we can fit more of them. Run a piece of tape that's 2 or 3 inches thick from one end of the tube to the other. Lay your measuring tape on the tape and make a mark at 2". Make a mark on the other side of the tape, 6" away from the first mark. Continue to mark every 6", alternating sides, until you have 9 marks. [One side of the tape: 2", 1'2", 2'2", 3'2", and 4'2". The other side of the tape: 8", 1'8", 2'8", and 3'8"]

Repeat on the other 3 PVC tubes, and remove the tape.

Next, we'll be cutting slots horizontally in the tube when it's standing up (crosswise), with the mark we just made in the center. Measure and mark or eyeball 2 ½" lines on the marks, and cut them with an electric circular saw or hack saw. The latter is much easier to control if you're not tool proficient, but will take a little longer. It's even more of a chore, but if you don't want to spend the $15 for a hack saw you can just buy a blade, make a handle by wrapping a rag around one end, and hold it while you saw. If you're using a circular saw, use a plywood blade turned backwards, so the teeth don't catch the surface. Then set the base plate to allow 2 ½", front-to-back, of the blade to stick out. Wear eye and face protection to keep smoke or shards out of you.

The end of the PVC pipe that has a slot 2" away from the edge is the top, and the end with the slot 8" away from the edge is the bottom.

Making the planting pockets

With your glue gun or hair dryer, heat one of the slots in an oval, about 3" wide and 5" high. Keep moving the heat so that the PVC doesn't brown or smoke. Keep heating until the PVC is soft and pliable. It will be hot so use something to poke it besides your finger.

By sticking your 1.25" or 1.5" piece of PVC into the slits, make pockets by pulling the bottom lip out and pushing the top lip in. Work the PVC into the pocket and firmly pull it towards you like a lever to position each lip properly. Make sure the pockets are hanging straight out from the surface of the PVC, not at a jaunty angle. Wait for it to cool down; spraying it with water will speed the cooling. Repeat on the other slots, making sure that they're oriented the right direction. If you mess up, the pocket can easily be re-heated and re-formed.

Keep the heat away from the very ends of the tubes so they don't deform. It's not easy to get them back in shape.

Step 2 - Assembling the lower pipes

Step 2 Materials:

PVC glue

4 - 4" to 2" PVC reducers with schedule 20 (thin wall) to schedule 40 (thick wall) adapters. (Some reducers have the adapters built-in, if you don't find those just buy 4" thin-to-thick adapters separately and glue them in the 4" opening of the reducer.)

2" PVC:

4 – 2" PVC at 2" long

2 – 2" PVC at 3" long

2 – 2" PVC at 10" long

3 – 2" PVC "T" fittings

1 square foot of plastic "cut your own" air conditioner filter

2' Plumbers strap

Step 2 Assembly:

Attach 2 of reducers to the "T" fittings. Connect the 2" side of the reducers to the "T" fitting by sliding the 2" long piece of 2" PVC into both openings. Make sure that the "T" and reducer touch, if not, shorten the 2" piece until they do. When everything fits together well, take them apart, glue all touching surfaces, and put them together permanently.

Repeat with the other 2 reducers and the "L" fittings. Glue the 10" lengths of 2" PVC into the openings of the "L" fittings.

Cut 4" round circles out of the air conditioner filter material by laying the 4" bell of the reducer n top of it and cutting around it with a utility knife. The round filter pieces goes inside of the 4" bell of the reducers. This will keep the growing medium in the planting tube and out of the water reservoir.

Lay the "T"s and "L"s down flat on a surface. The "T"s go in the middle and the "L"s go on the ends, with the openings towards the middle. There needs to be 11" in between the fittings, center-to-center, so insert the end of the 10" long 2" PVC from the "L" into the "T" fitting, marking it at the appropriate distance and cutting if necessary. Glue them together and quickly align the reducers so they're pointing the same direction. One way to do this is to put the 4" bells down on a flat surface and make sure both the top edges of the bells touch all the way around. You now have one "TL" assembly. Make another "TL" assembly with the other "T" and "L" fittings.

Glue the 3" pieces of 2" PVC into the other end of the "T"s, so you can attach the last "T" fitting in between them, this time pointing the exact opposite direction. This will be the drain. You'll have to do this by eye. Make sure that, as before, the middle "T"/reducer assemblies are exactly 11" apart, center-to-center, cutting the 2" PVC if necessary.

Attach the finished reducer assembly to the frame

Lay the frame down with the horizontal 2x4's on the ground. Position the finished reducer assembly against the lower 2x4, with the 4" bells up and the bottom edges of the bells resting on the top of the 2x4". Wrap a length of plumbers strap around the reducers so that the ends can be screwed into the 2x4, holding the assembly in place. The strap can be cut to the proper length with shears or bent backwards and forward several times until it snaps off. Attach the strap to the 2x4 and put 2 screws in each end, as these straps will be holding the weight of the planters, growing medium, and plants, then put a screw as close in to the corner as possible to tighten it down.

Insert the 4" planting tubes into the reducers, making sure that the front (where the tape was) is pointing straight out. When you like the fit, glue it.

The top of the planting tubes should be even with the top of the wood frame. Make sure that the tubes are 11" apart all the way up. Put a screw through the inside of the tube into the top horizontal 2x4.

Step 3 - Setting up the irrigation tubing and pump

Step 3 Materials:

15' of ½" black irrigation tubing

½" electrical conduit brackets (black plastic cuffs with nails sticking out that we'll use to attach the irrigation tubing to the wood frame.)

1/8" tubing poker (in the irrigation section of the hardware store)

Growing medium. Can be scavenged roadside gravel, coarse sand if you're by a beach, or pumice (spongy lava rock) if you live near a volcano, but perlite (pg 285) is recommended because it's very light and cheap. Vermiculite, pea gravel, and clay pebbles are also good options. You'll need 90 quarts of medium, which, just to give you an idea, is 30 pounds of perlite ($30-$40).

Submersible Pump with at least a 7' lift, which will be 150-600 gallons per hour of flow.

You'll also probably need an adapter so your pump can connect to the 1/8" tubing, as they usually as designed to fit a garden hose.

Choosing a pump - how high it can pump the water (the head) is much more important than the volume of water it can pump (the flow). Sometimes, the head isn't listed, but you should be safe with at least a 200 GPM pump. These start at around $35 (check eBay), but pumps with better warranties and similar specs can go for over $300. If your cheaper pump croaks, you'll have to water by hand until your new one comes. Worth the savings I think.

Drill and a 3/16" bit

Breathing mask

Step 3 Assembly:

Turn the frame and PVC assembly around so that the back of the horizontal 2x4s and the smooth side of the PVC is facing you. Leaving a few inches of the ½" irrigation tubing sticking out to the left, attach it along the underside of the top horizontal 2x4 with the ½" electrical conduit brackets every foot or so. When you get to the right side, you won't be able to put a 90 degree angle in the irrigation tubing without kinking it, so just go as far as you can and then start attaching it to the back of the vertical 2x4 on the right.

The tubing will go behind the upside-down "T" fitting in the middle of the "LTTTL" assembly and into the bucket, so make sure when you attach it that there's room for both corners, without kinking.

To cap off the open end of the tubing at the upper left, kink it at the edge of the wood and fold it back on itself. Use 2 nylon zip-ties to attach it to THE PTHER TUBE so that no water can spray out of that end. Trim the ends of the zip-ties and turn the thing around to face you.

Using your 1/8" tubing poker, poke 2 holes in the ½" irrigation tubing in between the planting tubes and one on each side of the far right and left tubes. The holes can be evenly spaced for esthetic reasons. Cut 8 pieces of 1/8" irrigation tubing about a foot long. Cut the ends at 45 degrees so that they won't seal against the back of the larger tube and block the water flow; it also makes them easier to insert. Put them into the holes you poked.

Drill 3/16" holes in both sides of all the planting tubes. Position the drill bit about 1 or 1 ½" from the top and start to slowly drill. When the bit catches, move the drill so that you're drilling down at about 45 degrees. Insert the free ends of the 1/8" tubing into these holes, so that each planting tube has 2 water inlets, just in case one gets clogged.

[During Use: Check the pipes every so often by pulling them out of the PVC and confirming that they're squirting water out at the normal volume. If they're not, pull the other end out, turn it around, and reattach it, so that reversing the direction of flow will blow out the clog.]

Fill the planting tubes with your growing medium. It's a little dusty, depending on your medium, and messy, depending on your pouring skills. It's best to do this as close as possible to where your wall is going to live, but if you have to fill it outside and have a friend help you carry it in, take a picture of yourselves negotiating the elevator and send me a copy.

[On choosing a spot: if the wall is going to be inside next to a real wall, it can be screwed though the top 2x4 to hold it up. It can also be held upright in this way on the outside of a building, or against an eave or tree (though maybe you can use a rope instead of a screw). If it is to be free-standing, attach 3 foot 2x4s to the legs as a base, with angled 2x4s or upside-down shelf brackets, or angle irons to brace it. Make sure to secure the wall somehow if it could be hit by a gust of wind. If your bucket is going to be in the sun, be careful that it doesn't heat up too much. Putting something reflective around it will help keep it cool, but putting up a shade screen is even better, and of course, you'll want to cover it to keep dirt and bugs out.]

The easiest way to fill the tubes is to prop the Growing Wall at an angle, fill a bucket with the medium, and pour it into the tubes. Make sure you're wearing a breathing mask. When you've filled the tubes as much as you can at an angle, straighten the wall and top them off.

Put your wall in its final destination. Fill the 5 gallon bucket with nutrient water and put it underneath the drain "T". The drain can be run elsewhere if your growing wall is a work of art, and you don't want the bucket in view. Use a reducer and 2" PVC to drain the water wherever you want, making sure that there's enough downward grade in the pipe for the water to drain. Put your bucket in a box on the side of the wall, around a corner, or even through the wall behind it into a closet, which will minimize the sound as well.

Connect your pump to the 1/8" tubing, with a clamp if necessary, but don't plug it in yet. Gently place it onto the bottom of the bucket, plug it in, and say a little prayer. If you've done everything correctly, you will hear a gurgling, feel a slight vibration in the wall, and in 15 minutes will find dampness in the topmost pockets. As things go on, watch the level of your bucket; depending on the growing medium you've chosen, you'll have to add more nutrient water to the bucket to keep the pump submerged. In an hour and a half, you should be able to find wetness in all the pockets, and the water level in the bucket will stay steady as the all the medium has become fully saturated.

The Growing Wall is ready to be planted. (Or maybe, now that you're a pro, you'd like to build a few more walls first.)

Planting the Wall

With a blunt object, like the handle of a paintbrush or screwdriver, make a hole in one of the pockets by pushing the medium out of the way in all directions. Take the plant's roots (all the dirt rinsed off if you're using plants started in soil) and gently put it into the hole, letting its roots spread out as much as possible. Fill in any gaps with more growing medium (you can steal it from the top of the tube) and you're all set. Be careful when planting in the bottom pockets that you don't disturb the filter.

Barrel and Drum Gardening

Materials:

A Barrel

Medium Marker

Straight Edge as tall as your barrel

Measuring tape

A way to cut out slits in the barrel, whether a circular saw, utility knife, router, or something else, but a circular saw with the plate adjusted for a 4" cut is the fastest

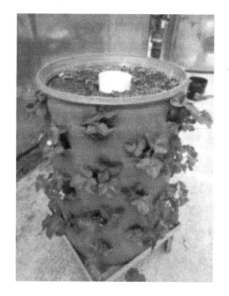

Choosing your barrel

Size Options:

Any size barrel can be used, and the biggest that will fit your space is recommended. If the barrel might need to be moved, it can be put on a garbage can roller. A 55 gallon barrel has room for 80 plants plus a 4 foot square area on top, a 5 gallon 25 plants, a little less than 1 square foot. 300 gallon barrels are also available.

If you decide to go with a used barrel, keep in mind what it was used for. No pesticides, paint, or other chemicals. Food use is best.

Remove or cut off top and clean off the edges with a knife. Cut the lid off down from the top as opposed to from the side, to keep the strong ring that runs along the top of the barrel just below the upper edge.

We'll be making growing cells 4" apart all over the barrel, which is too close together for most plants. When we discuss planting in the barrel, we'll be skipping cells vertically to allow for more room for roots, either every other cell for strawberries, lettuces, peppers, etc, or every third cell for larger plants like squash, larger tomato varieties, and cucumbers. 4" apart is fine for herbs and non-fruiting plants like that. We're making planting cells in this way to allow for the most flexibility in choosing and planting plants, but if you know for sure that you're only going to be using your barrel garden for larger plants, save time by making the rows 12" apart.

Measure around the barrel and top to bottom to find out how much surface area you have to determine how many rows, columns, and total planting cells you're going to have. For example, a 55 gallon drum is 36" high and 75" in circumference. If you use cells 4" apart, you'll have room for 7 cells in a vertical column and 18 in a horizontal row, 84 total. Now you know how far from the top and bottom to make your cuts, at least 4", and in this example, exactly 4". Make sure there's an even number of marks in a horizontal row.

Wrap a measuring tape around the top of the barrel and mark every 4" with a dot. Using a vertical seam in the barrel, a straight edge, or a level, mark the bottom row of cells even with the top. Then, using your straightedge top-to-bottom or a pre-marked piece of string pulled tight between the top and bottom rows, mark the barrel every 4". Go around the barrel this way until you run out of room, and you will have a hive of intercrossing diagonals If it's not perfect, don't worry about it, because as long as there's maximum room for plants, the rest it just aesthetics.

Now, connect the dots. Draw a line between two dots in a horizontal row, then skip, then connect the next two, going all the way around like this. Because there's an even number in each row, we won't be left with a long space or a long line. Then do the next row down, but STAGGER the lines from the top so they don't line up vertically, like rows of bricks. This will give your plants' roots extra room. Keep connecting dots this way to finish this row, then continue down the barrel, staggering every row. If you're confident in your abilities, you don't need to connect the dots with marker, you can just cut away. But one daydream and you may end up with uneven rows. If you're super sneaky, you can make half as many marks in each row and center the saw blade when cutting.

Cut the slits. If you're using a circular saw, adjust the plate so that only 4" of blade is exposed, front-to-back. This way, when you put the front of the saw against the barrel's surface and lower the back down to cut the slit, you won't have to move the saw at all except for this downward motion. Heat and open the slits in the same way as in the growing wall instructions above, focusing more heat on the bottom lip than the top. It will take about 45 seconds to a minute to heat it, and the same to stretch and cool it. If you have 84 slits you're looking at an hour and half to two hours, so consider putting on a movie or getting another heat gun and a friend to help. It will speed things up as well if you make wedges out of 2x4s cut in half long ways and at an angle to stick though the heated slits, to hold them in place as they cool.

Nearly any plant can be grown with an aeroponic growing system. Aeroponic plants grow faster, yield more, and are healthier than soil-grown plants. Aeroponics also requires little space, making it ideal for growing plants indoors. No growing medium is used with an aeroponic growing system. Instead, the roots of aeroponic plants are suspended in a darkened chamber, which is periodically sprayed with a nutrient-rich solution. One of the biggest drawbacks is affordability, with many commercial aeroponic growing systems being quite costly. That's why many people choose to make their own personal aeroponic growing systems.

DIY Aeroponics

There are actually many ways to create a personal aeroponic system at home. They are easy to construct and are by far less expensive. A popular DIY aeroponics system makes use of large, storage bins and PVC pipes. Keep in mind that measurements and sizes vary depending on your own personal aeroponic needs. In other words, you may need more or less, as this project is meant to give you an idea. You can create an aeroponic growing system using whatever materials you like and whatever size you want.

The following is instructions for a simple aero set-up, using a plastic tote container. The system is so simple that it can be easily modified to work with another container. An aeroponic hybrid of the Growing Wall, using vertical or horizontal PVC, is a simple modification.

The Aero-Tote

Materials:

A Heavy Duty Plastic Tote Container with Reinforced Lid. Make sure the lid has raised edges so any water overspray won't run off.

A Fountain Pump, 200 GPH (see pg 141 for more info on pumps). [A smaller cheaper pump might work as well, but the backpressure may become an issue]

4' - 1/2" Poly Tubing that's the same size as your pump's fittings, or adapters

3 - T-type Poly Connectors

6 to 12 - 360-degree misting or fogging Spray Nozzles with 1/4" fitting

4 - 8 1/4" poly tube extenders.

Hose Fitting to attach pump to 1/2" tube.

12" - Clear Vinyl Tube (this will be the water level indicator)

Angle connector, Misc connectors and Rubber Washers for Water Level Indicator.

30 to 40 2" Plastic Net Cups

30 to 40 - 2" Neoprene collars for net cups. Only about 35 cents each, but these can also be homemade.

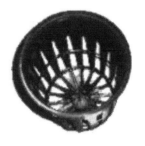

Growing Medium, Plants, Organic Fertilizer (bat guano mixed with kelp or seawater is good)

Optional:

EPDM Weather Stripping (to help seal the lid to the base, a good idea if the unit will be kept somewhere that can't get a little wet.)

Plastic Spring Clamps (Optional)

If your unit will drop below 60 degrees, add a small aquarium heater to the reservoir.

Tools Needed:

Drill with a 2" Hole Saw, Wire Brush Bit, and an (approx.) 5/8" bit

Sharpie for marking.

2 channel lock pliers to tighten fittings

Serrated knife or box cutter

Zip Ties

Assembly

Step 1 - Prepare the Plastic Lid:

Using the 2" hole saw and drill, cut as many holes as you can without cutting through the structural ribbing. You'll be able to fit more holes (and therefore plants) if you mark all of your holes first to make sure they are evenly spaced. [Make sure to keep the left-over plastic "doughnuts" - you can use these instead of the neoprene collars by cutting a slit from the center hole to the edge.]

Our final pattern looks like this. We end up with 40 holes this way.

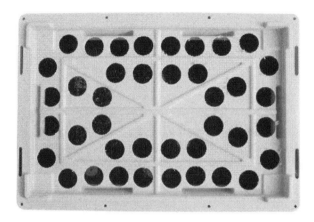

Use the wire brush to clean up the holes and remove the burrs. Don't use it too long in one spot or you'll melt the plastic.

Step 2 - Prepare the Water Level Indicator

The Water Level Indicator lets us know how much water is in the reservoir without having to remove the lid to check.

Cut a small hole near the bottom of the reservoir. The size will depend on the thread size of the connector pieces you have, ours was 5/8".

Attach the fittings with a rubber washer on the inside.

Attach the clear vinyl tube and secure it by drilling 2 small holes in the handle of the reservoir and securing it with a zip tie.

Step 3 - Tubing, Pump and Nozzle Assembly

The exact sizes for your tubing will depend on the size of your reservoir. Measure the inside of your container length times width, subtract 4" from both the length and width of your containing, and multiply the two numbers together.

Use the Hose Connector and T fittings to create an "8" that is 4" less than the both the length and width of your container. The fitting are compression fittings, so no glue is required. Use a downward-facing T-fitting in the middle of the center tube to attach the pump, with enough vertical tubing that the "8" sits several inches above the water line. The pump will be completely submerged with several inches of water above it.

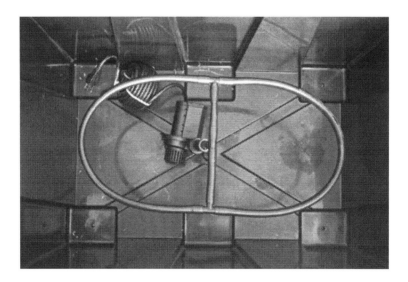

Attach the Spray Nozzles evenly around the "8". Insert the heads into the 1/2" Poly-tube by punching a small hole then threading on the heads. Direct the heads so that the spray will cover the entire area.

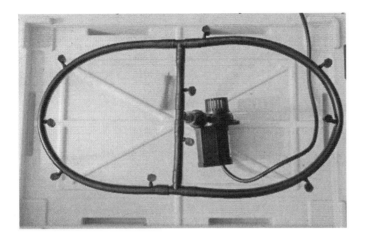

If your pump is unstable and wants to tip over, attach it to a plastic pot base by drilling two small holes and using zip ties to secure it.

Step 4 - Testing the system:

Clean the reservoir well. Any bits of plastic or dirt may clog the pump or spray heads. Fill the Tank with water, enough to cover the pump by a few inches.

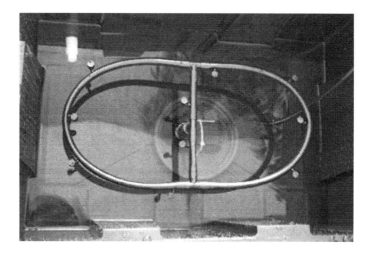

Plug the pump in and look for any areas that don't receive spray.

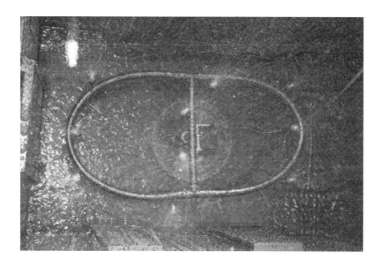

Step 5 - Assembly

Weather Strip the containers edge, if desired. Clean the lid, and run the weather stripping around the rim of the container. This step will prevent overspray from dripping down the sides of the unit.

Cut a hole in the side of the res to allow for a place to run the power cord, slotting the lid if necessary.

Secure the lid down with the spring clamps.

Insert your Net Pots and Neoprene Collars or Plastic Donuts. Pull out that Sharpie and mark your water level on the clear tube.

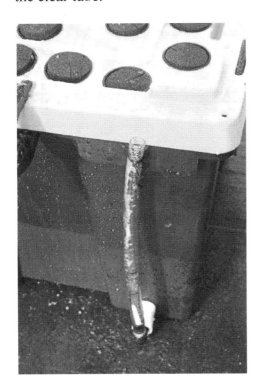

Step 6 - Operation

Test the unit one more time with the Net Cups in place, and see if they're getting wet. If you have a few dead spots, added a few more spray heads, to get full coverage. Spinner-type heads may give the most thorough watering.

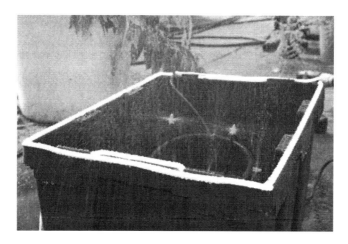

Fill the net cups with growing medium and add your plants. If they are coming from dirt, rinse the roots completely. Add fertilizer to the water. The unit will need to be cleaned with hydrogen peroxide or diluted bleach after each cycle to prevent algae, fungus, and bacteria.

Composting and Worm-iculture

A forest is the ultimate self-sustaining garden. I grew up in the rural Midwest, and was lucky enough to have a backyard bordered by many acres of mucky woods. I spent a lot of my childhood back there amongst the living mud, crumbling branches, and moldering leaves, and often thought about the difference between the dirt there and in our yard-locked garden, just a hundred feet away. Have you ever noticed the dark, rich, and loamy soil in the woods? And how cracked, dry, and blonde a recently abandoned garden will become? No one needs to water or fertilize the woods.

Decay is La Différence. A forest floor is covered in decomposing matter: leaves, the spongy trunks of fallen trees, the fur, feathers, and bodies of dead animals and bugs. Microorganisms and worms in the ground recycle this and any other formerly-living matter into stable soil capable of feeding the next generation of growth. The tree canopy shields the forest floor from harsh sunlight, sprinkling it with a soft green glow. Exactly the right amount of moisture is retained for the native flora. If I would have taken a cactus and tried to plant it out there, it would have taken in as much water as possible, planning to store it for the next dry spell which would never come, and it would burst. A jade houseplant would have rotted with too much water. Likewise, plant a maple tree in a mountain pine forest, where the trees have developed tiny needles to gather sunlight and retain moisture, and it will wither and die while the plants around it will continue to thrive in their own way.

A forest can even purge itself of toxins and harmful chemicals. The composting process can neutralize volatile organic compounds (VOCs), bind heavy metals and render them inert, and even eliminate wood preservatives, pesticides, hydrocarbons, and explosives. I was once walking in the woods in Maryland and found a section along an ancient trail that was littered with old glass jars from before my time. This was early spring, the trees were slowly waking up from their winter sleep and the ground was still thawing and barren. But inside of every one of the jars the green leaves of little plants were unfolding alongside bright emerald mosses and delicate mushroom caps. I imagined that these unlikely terrariums found springtime before the rest of the forest every year, protected from the cold winds and enjoying sun-warmed, moist air. These plants must have grown too large for their containers and found their way out of the opening while the rest of the forest was just beginning to BLOOM, adding moisture to the forest climate and extending early invitations to animals and birds that would add their valuable influence to pollination and fertilization. These jars had in fact extended the growing season of this arboreal garden by a few weeks, and allowed for that many more fruits, seeds and grams of compost to be produced. The forest had found a way to deal with the most toxic influence of all, that of inconsiderate humans, in a way that added to its communal prosperity and evolutionary advantage.

In the same way, permaculture, the approach to designing agricultural systems that mimic nature, is sometimes whimsically called "lazy agriculture" by its practitioners. This isn't a jab at modern hippiedom but an appreciative awareness that if Nature is given a toehold, it will seize command. Once we establish a garden with even the slightest opportunity for sustainability, natural law will take over and very little effort is required by us to keep it "growing".

There are several different ways to put nature to work for you in making luscious new soil for your food-producing plants, and which you choose will depend mainly on your living arrangements. If you have yard space (and city ordinances allow it) then a traditional, low-maintenance compost heap is your best bet. A store-bought or homemade compost tumbler can go on a patio, balcony, or rooftop, and its sleek design and tight-fitting lid will keep its purpose and smell out of the minds and noses of neighbors, landlords, and pests. If you only have indoor space to work with, you can use what might be the most effective composting method of all: vermiculture, or worm composting. These guys will not only reduce the amount of food waste that goes into the garbage, they will also make a most delicious (to your plants, that is) fermented compost tea.

Even if you're more of a sprouter and fermenter and have little need for good dirt, keeping your kitchen scraps out of landfills and spreading your homemade soil in a local park or community garden is a very good deed. In a landfill, your kitchen wastes (which accounts for an average of a quarter of what people throw into the garbage, according to the EPA) decompose anaerobically (without oxygen), making methane, a greenhouse gas that's 72% more destructive than carbon dioxide, the gas that comes from burning coal and petroleum products. In a compost pile, the food and yard waste break down aerobically, producing a fraction of the methane. Since the 1700's methane in the Earth's atmosphere has gone up 150 times, while CO2 has increased "only" about 35 times (we know this from testing air bubbles in glaciers – very cool). Landfills are by far the largest source of atmospheric methane, with developed countries accounting for most of the production. Also, methane will be produced for years after a landfill is closed, as anaerobic decomposition of living matter is a much slower process than what happens in nature.

First, let's discuss how composting works. Layered compost piles mimic what happens on the forest floor, creating the ideal conditions for quick, natural breakdown. The process requires 4 ingredients: living matter, soil organisms, water, and air. During decomposition, bacteria, nematodes, and worms in the soil break down living matter into its simplest parts. This produces <u>fiber</u>-rich, carbon-containing **humus** with inorganic nutrients that plants can use.

Living matter is the main ingredient in the home compost heap, and it comes in two kinds:

1) "Green" - food scraps, lawn clippings, and fresh manure from vegetarian livestock, if you have access to it. Pet manure is fine if you make their food yourself or know exactly what goes in it. Seaweed, tea bags, and coffee grounds are great sources of supplemental nutrition to your pile, and attract a host of beneficial organisms. Meat, dairy, and oil however, are difficult to digest for a passive or new compost pile, and can create unpleasant odors. They're best added to a well-established, hot and oft-turned heap. Putting them through a blender or food-processor first will speed their decomposition, though some sources say that to avoid vermin in outdoor set-ups, meat and dairy should be skipped altogether. If any part of you is motivated to compost because of environmental factors, however, you may want to look into the negative global impact of raising animals for meat and forgo your bratwursts altogether. Crushed egg shells, however, are great additions in new compost piles.

2) "Brown" – dead leaves, newspaper, cardboard, pine needles, junk mail, dry straw and hay, and paper grocery bags. Greens have plenty of nitrogen while brown has more carbon, two essential nutrients for a thriving compost heap. The best ratio is 2 parts brown to 1 part green; a pile of dead leaves can take years to decompose without the heat of nitrogen, and a pile of kitchen scraps (or a jack-o-lantern in November) without the drying carbon of brown matter will quickly turn into wet goo. A varied diet results in varied sources of plant matter to your compost, which will result in varied nutrients in your finished soil and food.

The following shouldn't go into your compost pile:

- **Diseased garden plants** - They can infect the compost pile and influence the finished product.
- **Invasive weeds** - Spores and seeds of invasive weeds (buttercups, morning glory, quack grass) can survive the decomposition process and spread to your plants when you use the finished compost.
- **Charcoal ashes** - toxic to the soil microorganisms.
- **Pesticide-treated plant material isn't great** – though it's an unreasonable requirement that food waste that goes into your compost heap be 100% organic, pesticides are harmful to the compost organisms and some types may survive in the finished compost. This especially applies to the particularly virulent ones that have been outlawed in America, and so are sold to developing countries and used on the fruit and produce that's then shipped back to us. Assuming the chapter on commercial farming did its job and you don't use conventionally-grown produce, if your less informed or more frugal neighbors donate their locally-grown kitchen scraps to your compost pile, then at least they stay out of landfills.

Soil microorganisms need water to live and oxygen to function. At the outset, dry brown matter should be thoroughly wetted, like a wrung-out sponge; afterwards the pile will generally take water out of the green matter and maintain its own moisture level that way. An exposed compost heap has easy access to air; prettier composting breathes well because of a good bin structure.

In an "open air" compost bin, made of wood pallets, chicken wire, or anything whose sole purpose is to keep out pests, respiration goes both ways and there will be an unpleasant smell. These structures are best in the corner of a yard, which obviously requires permission if you're in an apartment, condo, or rented house. Wood pallets are often available for free at any store that sells a lot of something:

Home Depot, Sam's Club, Target, Wal-mart, etc. Just go around back of the store and ask for some; they might tell you to come back at a certain time, after a delivery, but the big stores get several deliveries a day, so you'll probably get lucky. You'll need a minimum of 4, for a 4-sided bin, but if you have the space, you can add another 3-walled bin for every stage of the process: one for fresh material, one for partially composted matter, and the last for finished compost (10 pallets in all). Just dig a shallow square hole as wide as your structure, line 3 pallets up as walls and either screw them together or use bailing wire on the corners. Then use latch bolts on the fourth pallet to make a removable door, or just use more wire to make hinges and a twisted lock. If you're in a dry climate, you can speed up the compost process by stapling plastic sheeting around the inside of the bin with a separate sheet for the door, to keep in moisture.

This technique is known as passive composting, where the ingredients are piled up and nature is allowed to take its course. After the initial set-up the only effort required is removing the finished compost from the bottom and adding more food scraps on top, though the entire pile can be "harvested" at once if left to cook long enough. "Active composting" requires a little bit of daily effort, but is much faster and allows for an enclosed structure that mitigates smells. Whether it's tediously turning with a pitchfork or simply turning crank on a sleek tube depends on the bin.

 A simple active outdoor composter can be made from an old plastic or metal trash can with a tight-fitting lid. Drill holes every few inches around the sides and bottom or punch them in with a hammer and nail to allow for ventilation. Then put the can on top of cinderblocks or paving stones to allow draining, especially important if you're using a rustable metal container. Layer in your 2 parts brown matter to 1 part green, making sure that the moisture level is like a wrung-out sponge. Put the can on its side and roll it back and forth for 30 seconds or so, until all its corporeal contents are thoroughly mixed, and put it up on the blocks. Repeat this every few days to a week, adding fresh material as desired.

It will take about 4-6 weeks for the compost to be finished, so choose the size of your can accordingly: 20-40 gallons is about right for a family.

If you don't have the yard space for Donkey Kong and need to keep your barrel in one spot while mixing, you can buy a compost tumbler for a few hundred bucks, or you can make your own in a couple of hours for less than $50.

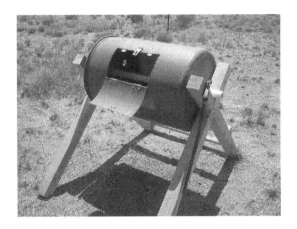

DIY Tumbling Composter

Get:

A plastic drum of 20-55 gallons (metal will work to, if you have to skills and tools to cut and drill it). All measurements in this recipe will deal with a 55 gallon drum, so alter the sizes to fit your barrel.

A 4' PVC pipe (a foot longer than your barrel), 1 ½ - 2 inches wide

5 pieces of metal rebar, 20" long

5 - 36" 2x4's (15' total board feet)

2" Drywall screws

A non-toxic epoxy that will bond PVC and metal

Tools: a utility knife, a drill with a ¼" bit, a bit the same diameter as the rebar, and a hole saw the same diameter as the PVC

Do:

Using the drywall screws, build 2 X's out of 4 the 2x4's, crossing them at right angles, and connect them halfway down one leg with the last piece of wood so they make a stand for the barrel on its side. If the tumbler is going to sit on a hard surface, cut the bottom ends of the X's so they're flat against the ground.

If your drum held anything potentially harmful to your compost, like cooking oil, wash it thoroughly. Don't use a barrel that held anything toxic like paint or petroleum.

Drill small holes all over the barrel, every few inches or so. (If you go with the "X" aesthetic theme mentioned below, you may want to drill cris-crossing bands of holes to form thick "X"s – purely cosmetic.)

Drill holes in the exact center of the lid and base of the barrel the same size as the PVC

Drill holes in the PVC just a bit smaller than the rebar, so that the metal rods sit snugly in place, even before they're glued. Drill a hole an inch from each end and 3 more holes evenly spaced that will be inside the barrel.

With the barrel on its side, cut a 3-sided flap in the side of the barrel about a foot and a half long (with the barrel on its side) and a foot tall. This will be the door. Attach a handle of some sort so it can be easily opened from the outside: an extra block of wood screwed on from the inside or glued, an old cabinet handle, whatever. You can also cut out all four sides and re-attach the bottom with hinges. If the plastic is so thin that the door pulls inside of the barrel, make the handle overhang the top edge of the flap so that it catches on the barrel and acts as a stop. Or get fancy and attach a "hasp" to the flap. This is a $1-2 piece of hardware with a loop on one side, and a flat piece of metal with a hole in it that goes over the loop on the other, often found on utility shed doors.

Insert the PVC in the hole in one of the round sides of the barrel. Insert all of the rebar through the holes in the PVC, inside of the barrel, except for the one an inch from the end. Epoxy the dead center of the rebar, and center the PVC so that the rebar sticks out evenly on each side. Put the other end of the PVC through the hole in the other side of the barrel, and epoxy the last pieces of rebar in the holes in the ends, outside of the barrel. These will be your cranks, turning your nouveau-pitchforks with ease. You only need to turn one crank at a time, the other one just keeping the end of the PVC outside the barrel. If you have a lot of compost mass, however, it helps to have two people turning, and this is a great way to involve a kid.

Lastly, instead of having a single rod as a crank, 2 rebars in the shape of an "X" on either side looks pretty cool and industrial, like a pirate ship's steering wheel or the hatch in "LOST", matches the "X"s in the wooden stands, and is slightly easier to turn. Totally up to you. Also, if you're not comfortable having a crank made out of potentially sharp, metally metal, you can make one out of PVC with 2 elbow fittings and 2 pieces of tubing, one at 12" and one at 6", standing with your side to the tumbler and grasping the short tube with two hands, turning it like an oar in a Viking longship. Cover the terminal end if you like with a PVC pipe cap or skip the short PVC and instead use a broken rake handle for the full Norse experience.

Your tumbling composter is ready to be filled with brown and green matter, wetted, and tumbled every few days.

If your tumbling will be conducted on a balcony or in a shared space and the earthy perfume is a concern, the device can be vented. Get a few feet of galvanized metal ducting from a hardware store, cut a hole to fit in the top of one or both sides of the barrel, and screw it on with a square plate fitment. Then (and this is the tricky part) buy some replacement filters for a home air purifier that have activated carbon. The expensive purifier appliance just pushes air through what really does the work, which is the inexpensive activated carbon. Stuff some of these sheets into the duct tubing, and you've made an apparatus for a few bucks that will drastically reduce the composting smell. Coffee grounds in the compost will also help.

Worm-i-culture

The most efficient composting, especially for apartment dwellers, is accomplished by worms in a cooperative procedure called "vermiculture". They will do all the tumbling and aerating, removing the need to turn compost by hand, and they will work year-round, making compost that's even better than that from an outdoor heap. Worms add their castings to the compost and make a dark and rich soil, and their work creates a nutrifying fertilizer called "worm tea", used as a fast-acting soil supplement. Many people balk at the thought of having a box full of wriggling bait in their living rooms, but it's very easy to make their lair quite inconspicuous, and the slightly earthy and rich smell they create is pleasant to some and non-offensive to most.

> "From food all beings are born,
>
> By food they live and into food they return."
>
> - Taiitiriya Upanishad 3.2

Choosing a Worm Bin

The first thing you'll need to think about is size. Estimate the weight of a week's worth of food scraps, and plan on 1 square foot of surface area for every pound. A 2' x 4' box, for example, is large enough for eight pounds of kitchen scraps a week. The container will need to be 8 to 12 inches deep. A few small bins will be lighter and might be more manageable than one large one, but you'll have to feed the worms new kitchen scraps every few days so make sure not to have more bins than you can support.

Commercial bins are available in wood or plastic. Plastic tends to hold too much moisture, and while wood "breathes" and maintains the proper humidity, it is subject to rot and termites. Also, treated wood is toxic to worms, and many "found" wooden containers, which we'll discuss next, have questionable finishes. The best solution is to use redwood, hemlock, or untreated pine finished with 2 coats of non-toxic varnish. Wood is also a great insulator and will help to keep your bin the proper temperature, above freezing and below 80° Fahrenheit.

Buying 2 plastic totes, one inside of the other and one of

the lids underneath to protect the floor, is an easy and inexpensive solution. Discarded barrels, dresser drawers, or trunks work great too, and are not only free, they can also have way more personality that garish plastic totes or minimalist commercial worm bins. In fact, an entire dresser is an awesome worm bin with its multiple boxes (aka drawers) which are already covered by the drawers above. Holes are drilled through each drawer except the bottom one, which isn't filled with worms and dirt, but covered in plastic sheeting or painter's drop cloths to catch the worm tea. It looks like furniture (on account of that it is) and your guests don't need to know the slithery secret therein. Depending on the size of the dresser, the drawers can become quite heavy so look for a good sliding mechanism. Also, it's not a bad idea to put your worm bin on wheels or casters before you start.

You can also have a main bin outside or in a basement (great because it's warm, dark, and dry) and a mini-bin conveniently placed right in the kitchen, dumping the too-foody contents into a bigger bin and scooping a few inches of new dirt and dirt-makers before it's taken back to the kitchen counter.

Preparing your bin

Whatever container you choose, it must have adequate ventilation and drainage. Drill a few ¼" holes per square foot in the bottom to allow air to circulate in the underside of the biomass, and to allow drainage of the tea. If the material becomes too wet, drill some more holes up from the bottom. Put the bin on bricks or wooden blocks to allow air in, and put something underneath it, like a large tray or a plastic sheet with the edges laying over something to raise them up. The sides can then be gathered like a Santa Claus bag to remove the liquid fertilizer. The container needs a cover to keep out light and conserve moisture. If your bin is indoors, the darkness and seal provided by sliding a drawer in or closing the lid of a trunk is ideal. Otherwise, a piece of burlap thrown over the top is fine. An old coffee bean bag will make the worms very happy, and add a nice coffee smell to your earthy loam. If your bin is outside it's best to seal it up in such a way as to keep out pests and rain – but remember that worms are animals and need to breathe, so make sure your bin has adequate ventilation.

The bedding materials are the same for worms as for compost with one exception – a couple of handfuls of sand or dirt will provide the grit worms' digestive tracks need. Add your brown matter and wet it to the consistency of a wrung-out sponge. It should form a ball when packed in the hand. Your bin is ready for worms and scraps.

Acquiring worms

The two types of worms best suited to vermiculture are both of the red variety: red wigglers (*Eisenia foetida)*, and the less common *Lumbricus rubella.* They are found in aged manure and compost heaps. The cheapest route (and best story) is to go to a horse stable or farm and get permission to harvest them from some manure. Another way to gather redworms is to put a large piece of wet cardboard on your lawn, garden, or local park at night. The most virile worms will crawl upwards to feast on the wet cardboard. Lift up the cardboard in the morning to gather the your new co-gardeners. They can also be purchased from bait stores (but be careful of the species you're getting! Red wigglers are also called manure worm, red hybrid, striped worm, and fish worm, but night crawlers et al will not work) and online. Two pounds of worms can handle a pound of kitchen scraps daily, or a four square foot container. Worms can be pretty expensive at $20 per pound (about 1000 worms) but they will quickly multiply. Breeding worms can lay two or three cocoons per week which will hatch in 21 days, each cocoon producing two or three worms that will mature in 60 to 90 days. A worm population eventually stabilizes at a level that can be supported by the amount of food and space. If you're starting with a small Mayflower of pioneering wrigglers, start them slowly on small snacks until they're populous enough to decimate a (vegetarian) Thanksgiving dinner.

Care and feeding

Every meal to every few days, dig a little bit into the bedding material, bury your scraps and cover it over. Try to use a different spot each time to distribute the food evenly. Worms especially like melons, lettuce, and apples but you can feed them any vegetarian scraps, like fruit cores, rinds and peels, vegetable scraps, grains, or bread. Coffee grounds are much beloved, as well as the filters. Try to give them a variety of foods, and only a little bit of citrus so that the pH stays fairly neutral. The smaller you cut up your food scraps the faster they'll disappear, so high-speed blender and food processor waste is great. Make sure to cover the pits and peels with an inch or two of bedding; if you leave wet green matter uncovered it may attract fruit flies or smelly yeasts and molds. Otherwise, if you have a good ratio of worms to food scraps to area, your bin will manage itself for the 2 – 6 months it will take for the brown bedding material and all of the food scraps to be converted into chocolate-colored, homogeneous and glowingly fertile earth. This material is called "worm castings", and my favorite worm species, the "dirt pooper", sums up the process nicely. The end result will have majorly reduced in bulk, as the elemental particles have settled and compressed. It's important to be aware of this moment (which shouldn't be hard, as you're in there at least every few days, right?) as the worms will begin to die with nothing left to eat. They need to be separated from the castings and given a new home, and though there are complicated contraptions in commercial worm bins that let the soil fall out the bottom sans worms, there's a simpler way. Push all of the new soil to one side of the bin, and put a new batch of bedding in the open space. It's a great time to alter the bedding material, as different raw materials equals different nutrients, both for your worms and you plants. Start putting your food scraps in the new bedding and in a couple of weeks, the worms will flock to the new bedding like gay high-schoolers to traveling Broadway auditions. The soil can then be diluted to 1 part worm castings to 2-3 parts regular soil and used in your wheatgrass trays or to replace settled dirt in your container (the same settling has happened there as in the worm bin), saved in plastic bags, or just stored right there indefinitely. For container gardening, including grasses and micro greens, use. If you put your used soil in the bin with this end ratio in mind, you'll save yourself one more step. Full strength castings can be directly to the soil as a top fertilizer in pre-existing container plants.

If you want the fresh dirt immediately, want to check out the number of your worms, or want a fun project for the kids, you can just turn the bin over onto a garbage bag and remove the worms by hand. Watch for the lemon-shaped worm cocoons (or "capsules") that contain between 2 and 20 babies. They're actually much tougher than the worms themselves, but worth their weight in gold and easy to miss.

I leave you with two thoughts on either end of the spectrum. One deals with poop. The wasted manure and compost of your community: your police horses' droppings, your fields of cow pies, your neighbors' pet's poop tentatively scooped and sequestered into the illusion of sanitary little plastic bags. I guarantee that most of the best waste in your neighborhood is going to waste. I'm not suggesting you pick through piles of manure you find in fields (though one of our presidents didn't think it beneath him; in fact he found more joy in that endeavor than most others *see quote below) though I'll applaud you if you do, but what's to stop you from supplying your neighbors with a lidded bucket and a promise of weekly collection? Or setting up a "soil from soil" station at the local dog park? Just keeping those neatly tied sacs of droppings out of landfills is enough of a reason; the local gardeners that will clamor for the sweetly fragrant soil that you've carefully composted outdoors, and the boxes of free veggies *that* will bring, is just a bonus.

The other is a kind of prayer, the poetic offers of two guys passionate about earth. Not "the Earth", that vague and vast network of systems, each with its own politics and dogma, but *earth*, the actual stuff that land-dwelling animals daily quantify between their toes as home in the universe. These men were, I hope, far ahead of their time and not eulogizing the single force that creates, sustains, and destroys, building the very bodies of newborn babies from the rotting death of the millennia.

"In making experiments upon the varieties of Soils and Manures... you will find as much employment for your interest and as high a gratification to your good taste as in any business of amusement you wish to pursue. The finest productions of the Poet or Painter, the Statuary or the Architect, when they stand in competition with the great and beautiful operations of Nature, must be pronounced mean and despicable baubles." - John Adams, 2nd President of the US

and

"Behold this compost! behold it well!

Perhaps every mite has once form'd part of a sick person—Yet behold!

The grass of spring covers the prairies,

The bean bursts noiselessly through the mould in the garden,

…

The summer growth is innocent and disdainful above all those strata of sour dead.

…

Now I am terrified at the Earth! it is that calm and patient,

It grows such sweet things out of such corruptions,

It turns harmless and stainless on its axis, with such endless successions of diseas'd corpses,

It distils such exquisite winds out of such infused fetor,

It renews with such unwitting looks, its prodigal, annual, sumptuous crops,

It gives such divine materials to men, and accepts such leavings from them at last.

Walt Whitman – from "This Compost". When our world finally celebrates its worms and nematodes and soil bacteria, this will be their anthem.

Appendix A - Plant Nutritional Deficiencies

Macronutrients

Calcium (Ca)

- **Symptoms:** New leaves are deformed or hook-shaped. The growing tip of a leaf turns brown and dies. Contributes to blossom end rot in tomatoes, tip burn of cabbage and internal browning in plants like escarole and celery.
- **Remedy:** Crushed eggshells sown about 2" down, Lime, or Gypsum (which should be used only in alkaline soils).
- **Notes:** Too much Ca will inhibit other nutrients, and is often a "transpiration" issue, that is, the plant is exhibiting the symptoms of a Ca deficiency not because of a shortage in the soil but because its roots can't breathe either from root-lock or too much moisture in the soil.

Nitrogen (N)

- **Symptoms:** Older leaves, generally at the bottom of the plant, will yellow. Remaining foliage is often light green. Stems may also yellow and may become spindly. Slow growth.
- **Remedy:** Manure is very rich in nitrogen, and can be sown directly into soil. Earthworm castings are wonderful, as are coffee grounds (acidic, add to alkaline soils only).
- **Notes:** Nitrogen is hugely important to plants, kind of like protein is important to weightlifters. Growing plants build themselves out of it, all the way down to their DNA. Be vigilant, because many forms of nitrogen are water soluble and wash away.

Magnesium (Mg)

- **Symptoms:** Slow growth and leaves turn pale yellow, sometimes just on the outer edges. New growth may be yellow with dark spots.
- **Remedy:** Compost, or Mix 1-2 teaspoons of Epsom salts per gallon of water until condition improves.
- **Notes:** Needed for photosynthesis, as the magnesium atom is central in the chlorophyll molecule. All plants can be deficient in magnesium, but tomato plants and apple trees are particularly prone.

Phosphorus (P)

- **Symptoms:** Small leaves that may take on a reddish-purple tint. Leaf tips can look burnt and older leaves become almost black. Reduced fruit or seed production.
- **Remedy:** Chicken manure (no need to compost it, just put it right in the soil), rock phosphate, ground-up bones (if you have any handy) or bone meal.
- **Notes:** If your soil pH is above 7.3 or below 5, there may be plenty of phosphorus but it's been fixed and the plant can use it. Consider a pH amendment instead. Phosphorus must be mixed with water to be usable, so dissolve it first or water heavily after applying.

Potassium (K)

- **Symptoms:** Older leaves may look scorched around the edges and/or wilted. Interveinal chlorosis (yellowing between the leaf veins) develops.
- **Remedy:** Wood ash, which raises pH; potash magnesia is usually sold as "sul-po-mag", which also contains magnesium and sulfur, often absent alongside missing K.

    Notes: Needed for strong stems and disease resistance.

Sulfur (S)

- **Symptoms:** New growth is stunted and/or turns pale yellow while older growth stays green.
- **Remedy:** Mix 1-2 teaspoons of Epsom salts per gallon of water until condition improves.
- **Notes:** Sulfur plays an important role in root growth, chlorophyll supply and plant proteins. Just like iron, S moves slowly in the plant, and hotter temperatures will make S harder to absorb like iron. But unlike iron, S is distributed evenly throughout the plant which is why both new and old leaves are affected.

Micronutrients

Boron (B)

- **Symptoms:** Poor stem and root growth. Terminal (end) buds may die and immature flowers may fall off. Resembles Calcium deficiency (see Notes)
- **Remedy:** Treat with one teaspoon of Boric acid (sold as eyewash) per gallon of water. Can be applied as a foliar spray (directly to the leaves).
- **Notes:** Aids in cell division and protein formation, important in keeping calcium soluble and available to the plant. The most common deficiency in non-organic, over-worked soils; is a problem organic gardeners rarely encounter. Lucky us.

Copper (Cu)

- **Symptoms:** Stunted growth. Leaves can become limp, curl, or drop, and their tips can become blueish-green. Stalks can become limp and bend over.
- **Remedy:** Copper chelate, at about ¼ of the recommended rate
- **Notes:** Cu is influenced by soil pH and organic matter. Copper is unavailable above a pH of 7.5; peaty and acidic soils are most likely to be deficient. Unfinished compost can make copper unavailable in the soil.

Iron (Fe)

Symptoms: Young yellow leaves with green veins, symptoms which are often confused with nitrogen deficiency.

Remedy: Compost is best and quickest. Adding sulfur to the soil, which will turn into sulfuric acid and lower the pH, will make the existing iron more available. This will take a while.

Notes: Essential for plants to make chlorophyll, plays a role in the synthesis of plant proteins, and helps plants fix nitrogen. Fe deficiency is usually the result of too alkaline soils; at a pH above 6.8 Fe is fixed in the soil. Can also be caused by too much manganese…

Manganese (Mn)

- **Symptoms:** Growth slows. Younger leaves turn mottled, or spotted, yellow, often starting between veins. Veins may stay green. May develop dark or dead spots. Leaves, shoots and fruit diminished in size. Failure to bloom.
- **Remedy:** A handful of dolomitic limestone per gallon of soil.
- **Notes:** Helps enzymes break down for chlorophyll and photosynthesis production, as well as it works with plant enzymes to reduce nitrates before producing proteins.

Molybdenum (Mo)

- **Symptoms:** Older leaves yellow, remaining foliage turns light green. Leaves can become narrow and distorted.
- **Remedy:** Dolomitic limestone provides a tiny amount of Mo, but is effective in raising the soil pH, which is most likely the problem. **Notes:** A very rare deficiency. Acts as an enzyme co-factor to metabolize nitrogen they take up from the soil, so is often confused with nitrogen deficiency.

Zinc (Zn)

- **Symptoms:** Yellowing between veins of new growth. Terminal (end) leaves may form a rosette.
- **Remedy:** Manure, which decomposes quickly. Leaves and stems often fail to grow to normal size.
- **Notes:** Though a rare deficiency in organic plants, corn, potatoes and bean are the most susceptible.

Recipes - Why Living Foods?

None of the recipes or preparations in this book cook the food you've sprouted, grown, or fermented. Heating fresh foods past 110° F or so destroys a lot of the nutrients (carbohydrates become caramelized and unusable, vitamin C levels decline dramatically[16], etc), and all of the probiotics, but perhaps most importantly, the food's *enzymes* perish when the food is cooked. This is the temperature at which proteins denature and unravel, no matter if they're in bacteria, enzymes, or our bodies, which is why a high fever can cause brain damage.

Enzymes are the tiny chemical catalysts for change in the body, from healing a cut to breaking down a hastily-chewed porterhouse. When foods are consumed that don't have their own enzymes, they must be supplied by the body. Neither vitamins, proteins, hormones, nor any other

---

[16] "Vitamin C levels declined by 10 percent in tomatoes cooked for two minutes—and 29 percent in tomatoes that were cooked for half an hour at 190.4 degrees F (88 degrees C)."
Thermal Processing Enhances the Nutritional Value of Tomatoes by Increasing Total Antioxidant Activity; Veronica Dewanto , Xianzhong Wu , Kafui K. Adom , Department of Food Science and Institute of Comparative and Environmental Toxicology, Stocking Hall, Cornell University, Ithaca, New York 14853, *J. Agric. Food Chem.*, 2002, *50* (10), pp 3010–3014, **DOI:** 10.1021/jf0115589, Publication Date (Web): April 17, 2002

food can work without them. Enzyme-deficient meals put undue strain on the organs that produce enzymes, and takes their energy away from the things they really should be doing, like cleaning out toxins and re-building old or damaged cells. A diet rich in enzymatically-active foods leads to an abundance of resources and energy to make the body the best it can be. Plentiful energy, beautiful skin, perfect weight, ample strength and flexibility, and I dare say, inner peace, are the natural state of affairs in a healthy person. Giving the body the nutrients it needs and *adding* energy instead of taking it away with unconscious or uniformed diet and lifestyle choices is the surest way to get these benefits and countless others.

Western science is fantastic at isolating the ingredients of life; from cataloguing the 3 billion pairs of codes that make up DNA to measuring the "nutrients" in the ashes left behind when food is burned. But still glaringly missing from the focus of most microscopes is the electrical impulses that make everything *happen.* If the body is a clock, enzymes are the winding that put those countless gears in motion. The human body somehow loses 21 grams at the moment of death[17]. Living cells have an electrical field; dead cells do not.

> "The food enzyme concept probably has more to offer as a permanent contribution to those seeking health than any system yet proposed. It points out the basic and underlying causes of the killer diseases and seeks to eradicate these causes... It is reckless and almost dangerous for the human race to abruptly remove food enzymes from its diet."
>
> – Dr. Edward Howell,
>
> Early 20th century physician and enzyme researcher.

Enzymes are of three types: 1) food, which come from fresh foods, 2) digestive, which are made by the pancreas to help digest cooked and processed food, and 3) metabolic, which do all the other healing, cleansing, and rebuilding in the body. The cool thing about enzymes is that they can easily change from one type to another, becoming whatever you need them to be. That means that if you eat a food with an over-abundance of food enzymes, like sprouts, whose

---

[17] Based on experiments conducted by Dr. Duncan MacDougall in 1907

enzymes are all geared up to grown the little sprout into a big plant, all the extra enzymes not needed to digest the sprouts will turn metabolic and start mending broken bones, getting rid of toxins in the bloodstream, or make you wake up earlier and more refreshed.

There are different types of food enzymes; each digests a particular kind of food, protease digests protein, amylase digests starch, etc. The other cool thing about food enzymes in whole, uncooked foods is that the different types of enzymes exist in perfect complement with the nutrients present in the food. This means that the exact amount and type of enzymes required to digest the food are *in* the food, in its whole, raw form. I'm sure there's a perfectly scientific explanation for this, like: when amino acids organize themselves into proteins, the enzymes that catalyze the process stick around in the peptide bonds that hold everything together and are released when the structure is broken down. This is another one of my half-baked theories of why living food so perfectly invigorates us, but I'm also completely comfortable accepting that it's magic, and that the universe is just a benevolent place.

I used to think that a raw, vegan, whole food diet meant that breakfast was a cucumber and lunch a bell pepper, both eaten like an apple (which would be dinner), but there is actually a universe of delicious menus. Sun-dried tomato pesto over olive-oil tossed raw zucchini noodles (pg 432), cinnamon-spiced warm corn and yam salad (pg 431) wrapped in a corn-hemp flatbread tortilla (pg 510), and a silken chocolate tart with a sprouted almond-maple kefir crust (pg 522) are delicious examples of living whole foods, proving that taste or boredom can never hold someone back. When we sit down to a meal, there are two options when choosing foods: those that add energy and life to the body, and those that take it away. Sometimes our digestion is weakened by life and we need the help of cooking to break down a food into an easier-to-digest, though less nutrient-rich form. But in general, living foods are a pretty safe bet.

You like how I snuck the "vegan" in to that last paragraph? More on that now: the ethics of a life-for-my-lunch aside, a meat-based diet is simply disastrous on our bodies and ecosystem. Simply put, it takes more energy to digest meat than we get out of it (this includes *all* animals, for those that consider fish a vegetable), and its connection to heart disease, cancer, and all around feeling yucky can't be logically refuted. As far as the rest of the world goes, the addiction to eating animals is incredibly irresponsible, **as a 2006 United Nations report summarized by calling the meat industry "...one of the top two or three most**

significant contributors to the most serious environmental problems, at every scale from local to global." The report recommended that animal agriculture "be a major policy focus when dealing with problems of land degradation, climate change and air pollution, water shortage and water pollution, and loss of biodiversity." It takes 17 grams of plant protein to make 1 gram of meat protein. That's it from me, but there's loads more info on both of these topics in the books found in the "recommended reading" section.

That being said, there's a lot of fanaticism about raw food and it's sometimes hard to separate fact from enthusiasm. No two people will find homeostasis in exactly the same place. 100% raw is not, in fact, for everybody, as it requires a powerful digestive fire and should be eased into for this reason. Everyone can benefit from some living food, and as I said at the beginning of this section, we're not cooking any of our lovingly-grown crops in the following recipes so we can get as much out of them as possible. When I carefully nurture a strawberry, watching it go from a little green lump at the end of a dying flower to a ripe, juicy bright red fruit weighing down the branch with a delicious and explosive life force, the last thing I want to do it throw it in a processed white flour pancake (how did that kind of cake slip into the list of acceptable breakfast foods, anyways?) and fry it up with rancid oil in a greasy pan. If all you get out of this guide is a way to grow boatloads of tomatoes that become your Grandma's marinara instead of getting pesticide and chemical fertilizer-laden 3-D tomato photocopies shipped from the other side of the world, that's certainly a good thing. But I'm greedy. I want my food to have all its nutrients intact. And I'm lazy. I want my food to energize me, not the other way around.

The dogmatic way some people approach a "raw diet" can do more harm than good – eating unsprouted seeds and nuts isn't much better than eating them cooked, enzymatically-speaking, and just because agave syrup hasn't been heated past 110° F doesn't make it good for you. Living foods' enzymes, which help with a lot of metabolic processes like cleansing and energy production, are all for naught if your guts go into overdrive to digest a sprouted, unfermented soy bean– hard work for any being with only one stomach.

The digestive fire will also fluctuate. Congestion, fever, travel, winter, emotional trauma, decrease in exercise, and disease will all change the body's ability to digest, absorb, and assimilate. You may notice more gas when eating apples when you have allergies, or that you can eat twice as much of the same food trekking in Mexico as ice fishing in Canada.

As they say, the proof of the pudding is in the eating, and only by objective observation can each of us find out what's best for our bodies, which changes from place-to-place, season-to-season, and for the keen observer, even day-to-day. Make sure that, when you think you've lit upon a working method for optimal health, you don't broadcast it to friends and family as a new self-righteous identity, and for god's sake don't write a book about it, until you're firmly established in your diet with receptive humility and the awareness that no one else shares your precise path.

Fermented foods are a totally different story, however, and should be aggressively enjoyed daily by everyone.

Also, please remember that though a piece of chocolate cake at Grandma's house might not be so great for your physical body, you may one day find that it is the perfect medicine for your emotional one. Listen to your body, heart, and mind, and learn to discriminate between good and great: mindlessly filling a short-term emptiness or mindfully choosing long-term wellness. Sometimes (ok, lots of the time) this means flexibility, gratitude, humility, and acceptance.

One of the great things about preparing living food is that there are no complicated chemical reactions using so much baking powder and having to cook an egg at so many degrees for a specified amount of time. There's no too much or not enough oil, overcooking pasta or undercooking chicken. There's just vibrant food in yummy combinations. You can take any flavors that are good together, like vegetables and curry powder, or cacao, almond sprouts and bananas, and do whatever you feel like with 'em.

Make sprouted hemp-corn tortillas with chili and lime and fill them with sunflower-cherry tomato kefir cream cheese, avocado, sunflower sprouts and chopped cilantro.

…Or make sprouted sunflower-cherry tomato chips and crunch them over a pureed soup of sprouted hemp, avocado, chili, cilantro, lime, and lay a fresh sunflower sprout on top as a nutritious garnish.

…Or add some sprouted flaxseed to make doughy corn-cilantro samosas, stuffed with sprouted hemp seeds and garlic-sundried tomatoes and an avocado-lime dipping sauce. OOOOR… See? The same ingredients combined any way you can think of. The possibilities are endless with fresh food that's been chopped, sliced, pureed, juiced or dried into flatbread, bars, cookies, chips, granola… the list goes on. The only limit is your own curiosity and creativity. The following chapters will give you valuable information, techniques, and time-saving tricks, and hopefully soon you'll only need this section to remind and inspire new combinations and preparations that you'll plagiarize, adapt to your own taste and crops, and run with. As you learn, you're nourishing yourself completely, vivaciously, so even as a bitter bite or weird flavor combo gives you pause, the way you'll feel will encourage you on the next attempt.

On Measuring:

After the integrity of ingredients is established, the only important factor is taste. If a recipe calls for 1 cup dry garbanzo beans and ½ cup peas, it doesn't really matter if you switch the amounts. The numbers, and ingredients, really, are just general guidelines, or for people that like to know they've mastered the fundamentals before they try something on their own. I never measure anything, and I taste a lot as I go, waiting for the magical, irreproducible moment. Having a little knowledge about how flavors go together will help fill in the missing level of taste, or balance out a too-obvious characteristic. Sometimes it's that magical pinch of honey-dried orange peel, thought of halfway through the meal, that makes that quinoa salad melt in your mouth.

Food is always a work in progress. My rule is: when I want to devour the entire batch as-is, it's done, or ready to go into the dehydrator, freezer, or whatever the next step is. And because fresh food can taste different at different times of year, or day-to-day, or even hour-to-hour as millions of molecules wondrously mature and change, you can't re-create that mystical moment of singing flavors you created in a dish the year before. I used to experiment a lot to capture that "perfect" recipe, so next time I could just go on autopilot and wake up in deliciousville. But it just doesn't work that way. Now, I add salt slowly and check in frequently. I try to taste the whole ingredients first to get a bead on their flavors, sugar and water content, and alter recipes based on what I found.

Curiosity is king. Change is the only constant. Living food never stops changing, and neither does your taste. Both are dependent on season, weather, company, time of day, age. Stay engaged, and always think about what you can do more deliciously, more easily, or more whimsically. If you're preparing food for an important occasion, like the third-date picnic on your living room floor (btw- good luck), try a test batch first, get it in your bones, and then see what you'd change. I think nothing's sexier than preparing and eating food with abandon, and your new friend might agree. There's only one universal rule in preparing living food: more yum, less yuck. The following recipes are all simple concoctions. The focus here is to give you ideas to springboard your own creations, wherever you fall on the culinary skill continuum.

The Blessing of Bad Food

If you can't quite get it down; if you're struggling with balancing flavors and textures and keep finding bitter or over-herbed runny glop on your plate, I urge you to keep it simple. Don't be afraid of boring; all we're trying to do here is enhance the innate wonderfulness of fresh, whole-flavored produce. While it's true that some fermented foods can occasionally teeter between robust and unpalatable and are better on those occasions as a condiment or flavoring, most of the foods in previous chapters are great eaten in simple, equal-parts combinations.

Humans are incredibly adaptive, and when we choose foods with our logic and intuition instead of our emotions and instinct (which is ok sometimes), we quickly adjust to getting as much or more pleasure from a handful of ripe blackberries, dripping bright juice down our forearm, than we used to get from that slice of greasy pizza. I've often noticed that the amount people take pleasure in or complain about their lives depends not on how much money, success, marriage, free time, or whatever they have; when one or more of those things change they soon shift their level of satisfaction to what they do or don't have now. When we get dumped or fired, we think it's the end of the world, until we get a new job or relationship or grow as a person, and think it was the best thing that could have happened. Similarly, if we win the lottery or get a new toy, we're happy for a little while but quickly grow used to the new circumstance and start lamenting our lack of something else. Most of the pleasure we get from things is rooted in our beliefs about them, and studies show that when people are given wines of the same value and told that they come from $10 or $100 bottles, different centers of the brain are active, and they actually enjoy the wines different amounts, chemically. It's hard to argue with someone enjoying or despising something on a neurological basis but they, and we, still have a choice. And if your attempts at the gourmet art of "not" cooking are valiant yet wanting and still *you stick to it*, you'll enjoy slightly better food like it's your tenth birthday cake. So get a deep understanding of the benefits of eating this way, and you'll soon get more enjoyment from your simple meals than anyone scarfing down a Neanderthal feast of charred rib eye and boiled potatoes swimming in butter and sour cream. Trust me. I did, and I do.

Helpful Tools for Preparing These Recipes

A good knife – In my humble opinion it's much better to blow your wad on one good knife than spend the same amount on a block with a bunch of knives you may never use. I used to only have a really great 8" Japanese chef's knife that I inherited from my brother (my latest and most treasured hand-me-down, so far. I'm still eyeing the early 80's Oldsmobile he won in a poker game). I did everything with it: chopping, opening young coconuts, delicate paring, peeling, julienning, and so much more. I now have a big heavy Chinese cleaver for those 'nuts, a mandolin slicer, and a paring knife and mandolin slicer for elegant garnishes when I really want to impress someone, which is not often. So I really recommend that knife.

Sharpener – A sharp knife is a safe knife, because it minimizes slipping off of food and into things you'd prefer to keep whole. I like the hand-held sharpener with two angled tubes that you scrape the knife down on, one side and then the other. With any sharpener, it's all about technique, and it should only take a few swipes to keep your blade keen.

Another option for cutting is a **Mandolin Slicer** – a tool with a flat surface that has a blade going across it. Fruit and veggies are dragged back and forth across the surface and perfect little slices fall out the bottom. Food can be shaped beforehand so the slices come out like half or quarter moons (slice a circular veggie down its length once or twice, stopping before you get to the end), stars, cherry blossoms, or many other shapes. My Benriner Japanese Mandolin Slicer comes with 3 blades, is infinitely adjustable and nearly indestructible, $25 on amazon.com.

Cutting Board – I like the hard plastic roll-up ones, about $5 for 3, which can be folded and drawered, or stuck to the side of the fridge with a magnet. I like to try and minimize dishes by cutting on the plate I will then eat on or use a mandolin slicer to drop pieces where they're going, but if I'm making food in any quantity I find it's safer and faster in the long run to use the right tool for the job.

Spiral slicer, Spirilizer, or Saladacco – This is a very fun and inexpensive tool for making very long noodles or strips out of veggies. You put one end of a beet, for example, against a spike on the cutter and the other end on a crank. Then you turn the handle and out of the other end come feet of fettuccini, spaghetti, papardelle, or many other shapes and thicknesses. When I'm making a veggie pasta for myself, I just cut thin, flat strips with a mandolin, but this tool is great for entertaining.

Dehydrator – Opens up another galaxy in the universe of raw cuisine. Dehydrated food isn't as good as fresh food, but sometimes you have more of something than you can possibly use, and drying it will extend its usability for months or years. Also, it's really fun to make breads, crackers, cookies, pie crusts, leathers, low-temp roasted veggies and mushrooms, and countless other things, concentrating flavors and creating otherwise impossible textures. The best brand on the market is the "Excalibur", which varies the temperature of the air to keep the food a consistent temp. The Excalibur is available in 4, 5, and 9 tray sizes, with basic and deluxe options. The only difference between these two is a timer. My first dehydrator was the basic 4-tray, to which I added $5 plug-in timer, though I only turned it off when I go on trips, as I seem to be dehydrating things all the time. After I ran that one over during a move (though I'd planned on replacing it anyways as I'd cracked the top with fermentation jars) I bought a vintage nine-tray deluxe model from eBay for almost the same price as a new one. But because the technology was the same (great customer service, btw) and it was so much sturdier, with a see-through door and wood grain exterior, I snatched it up. An oven on the lowest setting, an open door, and periodic temperature-taking can be used instead, though I'll bet the utility bills will soon outweigh the cost of a dehydrator. If you don't want to buy a dehydrator, the sun is free, and I'm sure the interweb abounds with plans for a sun-oven. Temperature regulation is close to impossible, though I for one would forgive the source of all life on the planet for inadvertently squishing some enzymes.

Thermometer – a candy thermometer is $2-3 and goes from way colder than you'll ever need to way hotter, unless, I suppose, if you're making candy. I use a laser thermometer, which you point at a surface like a laser pointer, push the button, and get a pretty accurate reading. These are more expensive and less accurate, but they give an instant reading and more importantly don't touch the food and therefore never have to be cleaned. Also, I break candy thermometers. You'll want to monitor the temperature of warm sauces and soups being heated up in a high-speed blender (more on that machine in a minute), to make sure they don't get above 110°. I'm usually successful. It's also handy to check that fermentations are at the optimal temp.

Kitchen Scale – really handy for all sorts of things, from measuring ingredients for recipes, to weighing tea and sugar for kombucha, to doing ratios for concentrates like fertilizer or hydrogen peroxide. I never use cups or measuring spoons anymore, just the graduated measurements on the sides of mason jars for liquids or seeds, and the ones on a sprayer, for things like fertilizer. I got mine on eBay for $20, and it's also useful for weighing letters and packages to print out postage at home, which, by the way, come with free tracking.

Sprouting bags, which you hopefully already have for the myriad uses mentioned throughout these pages, are great for straining and separating pulp from juice, too.

High-Speed Blender - Most professional kitchens, smoothie bars, and serious home chefs use a high-speed blender called a Vita mix. Though they can be pricey, a high-speed blender is an invaluable tool. These aren't your average little $20 margarita-mixers, these are powerful, professional quality blenders that can liquefy fruits and veggies, grind grains and dried foods into flours and powders, and can actually boil soups and sauces because of the powerful friction of the blades moving through them. I'd heard of the Vita-Mix for years but didn't understand just how versatile and very useful it could be until I got one. Now, I use it several times a day to juice whole vegetables, grasses, and fruits, emulsify sauces and dressings, make creamy and rich hot soups, grind nut butters, sprouted flours, and cookie batters, pates and so much more. If these recipes seem out-of-reach to you now, you'll quickly learn that with the help of a high-speed blender, it's almost as easy as throwing a bunch of stuff in and turning it on. With subtle changes in the container material, the lid, etc, the Vita mix has been made the same way for decades. It's the most expensive thing in my kitchen, by far. These run $450-$600, depending on features, extra containers, and accessories. Refurbished models can also be snagged for $379 on the Vita-Mix website, which come with the full 7-year warranty. I put off buying one for many years and finally paid $275 for a barely used ten-year-old one on craigslist. If you use it several times a day like I do, the quiet motor, ease of use and several-year warranty make it all worthwhile. It totally changed the way I eat, making fresh whole food much easier to incorporate into my diet. After the warranty expires, they'll refurbish a unit for $150 and give it a 6-month warranty, so a used one that's under $150 is a good buy.

There are a few different tiers and price-levels for high-speed blenders, and Blendtec, K-tec, and a few others are just below Vita-Mix in quality, though the price is about the same. These companies put more money into extra features (which some feel are unnecessary): LED screen, timers, settings... I just like to be able to turn it on and adjust the speed manually, though I would like a thermometer option, and have considered attaching one of those stick-on aquarium thermometers to the outside of the container. They're not super accurate though, and an auto-shut-off when the liquid reaches 110– now that is something I could get behind.

Next are the $200 models, available online and in department and discount stores. I recently bought one of these for a family vacation home that seemed to have all of the features and power of the Vita-Mix, but there was a noticeable difference in ease of use, and it started smoking after a week. Exchanged it and the same thing happened. With most products that aren't top-of-the-line, however, there are quite a few discounts available on quality high-speed blenders if you look. My mom found a $179 Jack Lalanne High-Speed Blender at a department store sale for $15. Why she didn't buy them all I'll never know. Coffee shops and juice bars going out of business will often sell their commercial models at a huge discount. Check eBay and craigslist, and if you do go with a Vita-Mix, the company will honor the 7-year warranty even if you bought it second-hand. If you don't have $300 to spend or this way of eating is new to you and you want to see how it goes for a bit, I'd recommend going with a $35 food processor, which is a little more versatile than the average blender.

Soups and sauces can be pureed then heated in a sauce pan, stirred continuously, and taken off the heat when they begin to steam.

Routine

On creating a routine that supports happiness:

"The chains of habit are too light to be felt until they're too heavy to be broken." - Bertrand Russell

It's hard to get a boulder moving, but once rolling it's hard to stop. If you implement just one new idea a week, in a few months you'll have sprouts, krauts, crackers, kombucha, fermented seed cheeses, all kinds of things going like your own little garden of deliciousness. Bread takes about a week both to make and eat, so, when a loaf comes out of the dehydrator, start another one a-sproutin'. Similarly, it takes about a week for grass to go from seed to juiceable, so when you start the second cutting of a flat, start sprouting another jar. (see previous volumes of the series for the how-to.)

A lot of these recipes don't start with the end in mind, like most cookbooks. Instead, I encourage you to sprout, ferment, and grow what sounds interesting and then look for something to do with it in these pages. Some things from this series that require multiple steps, like fermented bread (sprouting the grain, fermenting, grinding into raw dough, dehydrating). Best to get comfortable sprouting, then look into what else you can do; in this case fermenting into probiotic water. After you've enjoyed that process, instead of composting out your sprouted, nutrient- and probiotic-rich grains, you may ask "What can I do with these?" That's where the index of this book comes in.

Drinks and Smoothies

As with all raw recipes, smoothies are just a bunch of yummy stuff mixed together with an awareness of nutrition and digestion; whether it's a fruit salad, pudding, or drink just depends on texture. These recipes are, like everything else, just guidelines to get neophytes started (as in "people new to this", not some weird microbial culture, though I wouldn't put it past me). If you have blueberries instead of blackberries, or sunflower sprouts instead of sesame, it'll just be delicious in a different way. I seem to lean a little too heavily on ginger myself, so if you don't like it just take it out. The flavor of ginger exists in its own world, more a mouth feeling than an actual taste, so adding or subtracting it from appropriate recipes won't affect the other tastes, unless you use too much. More importantly, ginger is one if the best digestive aids I know of so I try to throw it in everywhere I can, even though I'd need to plant an acre to keep up with my demand.

Vit-Ali Baba

Middle-eastern fragrances embrace creamy "tahini milk" in this calcium, iron, and protein-rich smoothie.

1 Cup young Coconut Water (or regular water)

3 Tbsp Sesame seeds, sprouted

½ Peach (can be frozen)

½ Inch (10 grams) Ginger

3-5 Dates, pitted

Blend it up!

Grape-Nuts Milk

A simple and wonderfully satisfying drink which is full of probiotics, proteins, carbs, healthy fats, vitamins, and minerals that will benefit every system in the body, even though it's only 4 ingredients. If you have a high-speed blender, look for grapes with seeds, which have heaps of anti-oxidant and polyphenols which have powerful anti-aging effects in the blood vessels, skin, teeth, joints, and immune system. Also a great, easy-to-digest start of a smoothie; throw in a banana, some ginger and berries and lunch is served.

1 Handful Almonds, sprouted

1 Handful Sunflower Seeds, sprouted

1 Handful Grapes

1 Cup Kefir Whey (see "Kitchen Sink Farming Volume 2 - Fermenting"), can be cut with water and/or sweetened with raw honey per preference

Jamaican "A" Lemonade

1 Cup Coconut Water Kefir (see Kitchen Sink Farming Volume 2)

¼ Cup Shelled Hempseeds

¼ Lemon, peel on

½ Banana (can be frozen)

¼ Inch (10 grams) Ginger

Delhi Milk

Raw Milk Kefir, Raw Honey to sweeten Kefir's sour, a small chunk of raw Ginger.

Great on its own, or add sprouted hemp, banana, and/or berries for a protein-packed smoothie

---

Cooking by Freezing:

Freezing fresh food might seem like a way to store it without damaging any of its subtle nutrients and enzymes, but it can be a destructive process. We all know that water expands when it freezes. The water inside of food will also expand, bursting cell walls as it does and damaging the cell's integrity and ability to shelter its vitamins, minerals, and oils. The less water a food has, however, the less damage is done. This can be tested in the dehydrator; if a food doesn't change much in size, like ginger, it doesn't have much liquid to be sucked out or frozen. If it shrinks a lot, like onion or melon, you know that it has inherently has a lot of moisture and will be more damaged by freezing.

Things that have to be thoroughly broken down on the highest speed in the high-speed blender (like wheatgrass) can heat up in a less than delicious way, so blending something previously frozen into it afterwards, like cubes of frozen apples or apple juice, can make it much more palatable.

Raw Honey

Though its production isn't covered in this book, beekeeping is a natural extension of the Kitchen Sink Farming philosophy. Honey that hasn't been cooked into a homogenous syrup contains propolis, pollen, and royal jelly, as well as probiotics, enzymes, and anti-microbial agents. It's the best treatment for allergies, as many allergens that cause symptoms are found in raw honey in non-irritating forms (especially in honey made locally), which don't excite the immune system. It can help fight other kinds of infections as well, especially in the mouth and throat, or when applied topically (you may notice your skin soften as well; honey is immensely moisturizing). Honey is wonderful for digestion, as it's easily absorbed in the intestines and won't ferment like other sugars, while acting as a lubricant and peristaltic agent. Its beneficial bacteria effectively fight colonies of harmful microbes that can lead to anything from gas and indigestion to ulcers to cancer, and many things in between. Living honey fights cancer in other ways, too.

Local, raw, organic honey is my favorite sweetener, not only for its ambrosial taste and texture, but because it's the only sweetener that can actually fight against blood sugar fluctuations and diabetes: raw honey is the ideal "quick fuel" because it contains almost equal amounts of fructose and glucose. Fructose "unlocks" the enzyme from the liver that's necessary for the transformation of glucose into glycogen (the form in which sugar is stored in the liver and muscle cells), so there are no extras sugars sitting around to spike and drop blood sugar, suppress immune functions, leach minerals, and make you fat. An adequate glycogen store in the liver is essential to supply the brain with fuel when we're sleeping and exercising for any length of time. When glycogen stores are insufficient, the brain triggers the release of stress hormones - adrenalin and cortisol - in order to convert muscle protein into glucose. Cheesecake-induced nightmares anyone? Even scarier is that over time, repeated metabolic stresses from cortisol surges lead to impaired glucose metabolism, insulin resistance, diabetes, and increased risk for cardiovascular disease and obesity.

Studies in rats has shown that prolonged exposure to cortisol shrinks the part of the brain associated with goal-setting (the ventral striatum, check it out) and increases the area related to habitual behavior. This is why raw honey is the only non-food sweetener in this book, and keeping bees or creating a relationship with a local organic apiary is a wise move.

Heating raw honey past 110° F kills the beneficial enzymes, probiotics, and many of its perfectly balanced benefits, but there's to another reason not to cook the stuff. When bees go from flower to flower collecting pollen, they sometimes collect plant chemicals that can be toxic to humans. But when the pollen is converted into honey, these malicious substances are bound in a way that renders them inert. Heating honey releases these toxins from their protective bonds, even when raw honey is put into hot tea.

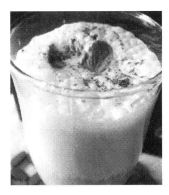

Chaach

A traditional Indian digestive aid of cultured buttermilk and digestive spices, this recipe substitutes "Gheefir" (clarified fermented butter and coconut oil, see Kitchen Sink Farming Vol. 2) for a delicious and savory drink to enjoy with sprouted breads or warm, fluffy quinoa.

½ Cup Gheefir (see Kitchen Sink Farming Vol. 2)

1 Tbsp Fennel, sprouted

1 Inch Ginger, sliced

¼ tsp Turmeric

2 Peppercorns

1 tsp Mint, chopped

¼ tsp Sea Salt

Combine all ingredients in a small jar and stir well. Cover with a sprout bag or coffee filter and infuse for a week on the countertop. Optional: after the week, add coconut oil for warm-weather sweetness or raw honey for dipping raisiny, cakey bread.

Kefir Creamsicle

4 Ripe Oranges, peeled

½ Cup Raw Goat Milk Kefir (see Kitchen Sink Farming Vol. 2)

½ Cup Raspberries

½ Inch (10 grams) Ginger, optional

Put all ingredients in a high-speed blender and blend on high for 30 seconds. Miraculous in the early southern California summer, when citrus tree branches hang low with the weight of sunshine-filled fruit. Using frozen berries or ginger will help to cool this modernized bit of ice cream-truck nostalgia. Sub any berries you like – I like raspberries because the sweetness counters the sour kefir, but cherries and strawberries are also very good.

Any juice can be made into a wonderful popsicle. Pour into an ice cube tray or paper Dixie cups and cover with plastic wrap. Poke thick, natural toothpicks (regular ones are often soaked in formaldehyde), clean twigs, plastic spoons, chopsticks, tongue depressors, (you get the idea) through the plastic, which will hold them up while the liquid is freezing.

Vampire Juice

A beet adds a beautiful living crimson glow to this potent healthy juice. Drink it immediately, as its luminous crimson life force will begin to slip away in a few minutes…

A Red Beet (cut into a few pieces) and its greens (Swiss chard)
A Cucumber (cut into a few pieces)
A Tomato
Handful of spinach or other green
Handful of leafy green sprouts and/or micro-lettuces
Handful of parsley
2 Stalks Celery
¼ inch (10 grams) ginger
8 oz water, kombucha, or kefir

Put all ingredients (pre-chilled in the fridge if not picked fresh) in the high-speed blender in the order given. Blend on high for 30 seconds. Beets and cucumbers float, which is why we put them in first, and push them down with the celery. Adjust the speed until the blender has the most vibration to pull everything down to the blades. When everything liquefies, you'll hear it. Check that everything is thoroughly blended by putting the blender on low and listening for any chunks.

Pour through a sprout bag over a bowl, and by slowly "milking" the bag, drain as much liquid as possible. Save the pulp in the fridge for soup or crackers, feed it to your worms (see "Kitchen Sink Farming Vol. 3: Growing", Vermiculture section), or compost it. The liquid is for you. Add or substitute any veggies from your garden that are ripe or in season. Try not to use fruit, as we use different enzymes to digest them, so it's best not to mix (though tomato and cucumbers are fruit, they are low in sugar and acid and combine easily with vegetables). Carrots and beets have relatively lots of sugar, so use them (and other sugary veggies) in moderation. If you are using a high-speed blender, toss in two carrots and some sprouted flax for body and blend on high for 5 minutes, or until steam starts to rise from the top. Soup!

Lentil-ade

The delicate flavor of red lentils makes a delicious and refreshing lemonade base, and sour kefir is right at home. When life gives you legumes…

½ Cup Sprouted Red Lentils (see "Kitchen Sink Farming Volume 1: Sprouting")
¼ Cup Raw Goat or Cow Milk Kefir
¾ Cup Maple Syrup kefir (see "Kitchen Sink Farming Volume 2: Fermenting")
1 Cup Lemon Juice (about 4 lemons)
½ Cup Raw Honey
8 oz. Filtered Water Ice Cubes

Add some lemon peel for a more intense flavor or a pinch of salt to Thai it up. Try wheatgrass juice in there too: blend it first and strain it through a sprouting bag (or just wait a bit and the pulp will float to the top – you can pour out the clarified juice from underneath.

The formula of lemonade is a ratio of sweet to sour - a good thing to be aware of in all drink concoctions. More complex flavors like salty, savory, and bitter can be used sparingly in drinks, but like mixing primary colors, the basic sweet and sour tastes combine to form a light and refreshing hue. Lemonade is basically 1 part lemon to one part sweetener (though less is more with some types of sweeteners), so start experimenting with your crops as flavoring agents. Funkify your lemonades with the following combos:

Nectarine-Basil

Caesar Salad: romaine, apple cider vinegar, raw honey, perhaps a few mustard sprouts floated on top

Candy-Striped Lemonade, named after the striated yellow beets that are slightly sweet, though any beet will do

Ginger-Lemongrass Limeade

Master Cleanse: Lemon, Maple Syrup, Cayenne

Pineapple Mint

Cucumber

Strawberry Vanilla Bean

Chili Pepper

Seed/Nut Milk

A frothy, delicious vegan milk or cream can be made out of any sprouted nut and many mild tasting seeds. It's also a creamy and versatile base for other drinks, soups, desserts, sauces, and more. Preparing it couldn't be easier – sprout the seeds, blend with water or coconut water, and strain it through a seed bag or mesh coffee filter, saving the high-fiber pulp for crackers, dehydrated cereals, cheese or spreads like Almond Garden Spread (page 496).

1 part seeds to 2 parts water will yield a "whole milk" thickness, and a little vanilla and honey will make it better tasting than any store-bought soy or rice milks. Throw in a banana and drink it straight, or try it in Coconut Pudding (pg 207). Using a nut with a layer between the nutmeat and shell, like an almond, will make a bit of a grainy milk, as the little flecks will be virtually impossible to strain out. It's possible to blanch them in boiling water to remove this coating before blending, but I recommend keeping your seeds alive and choosing a creamier seed, like macadamia, sunflower, or brazil.

Basic Nut Milk

1 Cup Nuts of your choice, soaked and sprouted
2 Cups filtered water
½ Tbsp Raw Honey
Blend all ingredients for 1-2 minutes and strain (or not). Drink or use immediately.

Cocktails

Basil-Grape Mojito

3 Leaves Fresh Basil
6 Red Grapes
½ - 1 tsp Sweetener like Raw Honey or Sugar
½ Lime, cut into 4-8 pieces
1-2 oz Liquor. Traditionally made with rum or cachaca, try it with gin, tequila, absinthe, or vodka (snore)
Ice

> "In my experience, a man with no vices has very few virtues" – Abe Lincoln

Muddle basil, lime, sweetener, and grapes in the bottom of a tall glass or pint jar (use the back of a spoon, tamper from a vita-mix, mortar) until a paste. Add booze and ice, cover with a metal mixing cup and shake, or pour back and forth between 2 glasses until evenly mixed (this is how it used to be done, turn-of-the-century bartenders pouring behind their backs or with the pouring glass over head and the catching glass at waist level.)

Enjoy without guilt. Life is to be lived.

Kefir Ginger Ale

A most refreshing drink as a pick-me-up after working in the sun, or working on a tan.

8 oz Light Rum, Indian gin, or vodka

1 ½ Quarts filtered water

¾ Cup Ginger, peeled and finely chopped or grated

½ Cup Fresh lime juice

¼ C-1/2 C Rapadura (or sugar)

2 tsp Sea Salt

¼ C Kefir Whey ("Kitchen Sink Farming Volume 2: Fermenting")

top with sparkling water, prosecco, or secondary-fermented bubbly mead ("Kitchen Sink Farming Volume 2: Fermenting") mixed with water.

Place all ingredients in a 2qt jug. Stir well and cover with a coffee filter, and leave to brew for 12 hours. Cover tightly, and leave at room temperature for a secondary fermentation for 2-3 days before transferring to the refrigerator to cold-stabilize. Will keep several months.

To serve, strain into a glass. May be mixed with sparkling water, prosecco, or secondary-fermented bubbly mead ("Kitchen Sink Farming Volume 2: Fermenting") mixed with water. Most refreshing sipped room temperature, not gulped down
cold.

Time to Make the Coconuts

Young coconuts are white, squat torpedoes with the hard green shell removed. They're usually wrapped in plastic and sold in natural and Asian markets. In Thailand and India, where they're most commonly from, a machete chops off the point, a straw is inserted, and the sweet, luscious, electrolyte-rich liquid quickly disappears. Every time I see this happen, I half expect a finger to come off with the top of the coconut, so I don't try to copy this technique at home. Instead, I developed an effective and safe way of getting to the coconutty goodness of one of nature's best foods that can't be grown at home.

Tools:

Cleaver, a heavy rectangular knife. Chinese models are available in Asian markets and online for $5.

Rubber Mallet, a hammer with a big rubber cylinder. Hardware store, $8.

Spoon, Kitchen Towel, Blender, 2 Plastic Bags

Instead of whacking off the top of the 'nut while holding it with the other hand, we're going to make 3 downward cuts so that we can remove a triangular cap from the coconut, allowing easy access to its contents. Lay a towel down on your kitchen counter and put the coconut on it, point up, the flat bottom safely keeping it in one spot.

We're going to cut a triangle into the top of the 'nut, so put your cleaver $2/3^{rds}$ down the sloping top, angled in a bit. Holding the cleaver in place with one hand, smack it with the rubber mallet until you strike juice. It will take 2 or 3 solid hits. Turning the coconut, make the other 2 cuts in the top. Juice may splash out of the old cuts when you're whacking, so toss an end of the towel over the top of the 'nut as you hammer.

The triangle cap should now be removable. Take it off and look inside. Because young coconuts are quite perishable as they travel far and wide, they often go bad. The flesh should be bright white; any pink or purple is a sign that the water should be dumped, the 'nut put in one of the plastic bags and returned to the store. I find that usually 1 out of 5 has to be taken back, and every store that sells them is used to a large number of returns. This cap-removal method is superior to drilling holes for this reason, plus it's easier and cleaner.

Pour the liquid into a blender container, if you're making pudding, or right into a jar if you're making coconut kefir or just saving the juice (though it may be easier to pour from a blender into the jar). It's about a pint of juice per 'nut.

Turn the 'nut on its side and, using the cleaver and mallet, cut it in 2 along its equator. Now you can easily scrape out the jelly-like meat with a spoon. You can try to keep the meat whole for easy slicing into coconut noodles, or just toss it into the blender along with the juice and blend it into Coconut Pudding. A little vanilla bean is nice, though it is so sweet and flavorful on its own it really doesn't need anything. It's best right away, and will keep (unfermented) in the fridge for up to a week. Chilling will solidify it, and a spoonful in a smoothie adds an unbelievable rich sweetness.

Mains, Sides, Apps

Any of these dishes can be a main course, or an appetizer or side dish if you're entertaining. As always, start simple, follow the recipe, then get creative. Or if you already know your way around a Vita-Mix, just look at this chapter as "food for thought".

Raw Portobello Mushroom Pizza

This recipe uses a marinated portobello mushroom as the "crust". It's tender, juicy, and slightly chewy, all like a pizza crust should be. The toppings are so amazing you might not notice it's not a traditional crust, but feel free to substitute a flatbread from elsewhere in this book if you prefer or spread some leftover nut cheese on a piece or raw (or otherwise) bread for an accompaniment.

For the "Crust":

4 large Portobello Mushrooms

1 Cup Extra Virgin Olive Oil

1 Cup Apple Cider Vinegar

1/2 Cup Nama Shoyu (Raw Soy Sauce)

For the Pizza Sauce:

3 - 4 small tomatoes, roughly chopped

5-6 sun dried tomatoes, chopped (if not soft, soak in water overnight)

1 Medjool Date, pitted and chopped

1-2 Cloves Garlic, crushed

Handful Fresh Basil, chopped

1 tsp Oregano

Salt and Freshly Ground Black Pepper to taste

Chipotle Pepper to taste

Use a Fermented Seed Cheese from "Kitchen Sink Farming Volume 2" if you like, or…

Quick "Ricotta" Cheese:

1 Cup Raw Macadamia nuts (soaked 1 hour)

Enough water to barely cover nuts in blender

Pinch of Sea Salt and Dash of Ground Pepper (Black or Chipotle)

1/2 Tbsp Light Unpasteurized Miso (optional)

1 Tbsp Basil, finely chopped

1/4 Small Red Onion, chopped

1/2 Clove Garlic, crushed (or more per taste)

For the Toppings:

1/2 Small Zucchini Thinly Sliced, lengthwise using peeler.

6 Baby Bella Mushrooms, thinly sliced and marinated

5-6 Black Olives, thinly sliced

1/4 Small Red Onion, thinly sliced into slivers

1/4 Cup Red and Orange Bell peppers, thinly sliced

1 Small Tomato, thinly sliced

Some Basil Leaves, chopped

Salt, Pepper, Oregano, to taste

Directions for Mushroom "Crusts"

Clean mushrooms. Remove stem. (Peel off skin and scrape out gills gently with a teaspoon)

Massage marinade on both sides mushroom.

Set in marinade, cap side up for 30 min and then flip to other side and massage marinade and seasonings into underside of mushroom. Set 30 min.

Directions for Pizza Sauce

Mix ingredients in a high speed blender or food processor until smooth. Set aside.

Direction For Cheese

Mix macadamia nuts with only enough water to cover and blend in a vita-mix, blender, or food processor until thick, smooth and creamy.

Add salt and pepper, miso, basil, onion, garlic, or whatever additional herbs and spices you like).

Mix well. Return to refrigerator for several hours, or serve immediately.

Directions for Assembly:

1 layer of marinara sauce, spread with spatula.

1 layer of zucchini slices (lengthwise).

Spread a layer of nut cheese using a dull knife or small spatula.

Add toppings: marinated mushroom slices, red and green bell pepper slivers, olive slices, tomatoes, basil, shredded zucchini, red onion, salt, pepper and oregano (to taste).

Dehydrate at 105 degrees for 2-3 hours on a non-stick sheet covered tray.

Zucchini Hummus and Veggie Chips

The following two recipes are good together – sprinkle a few colors of fresh brined olives around the plate.

Hummus is traditionally garbanzo beans (chick peas), sesame tahini (like a nut butter), garlic, lemon, (arguably) olive oil, and salt. It's one of those synergistic culinary miracles when flavors blend together into something brand new, but the left brain can still pick out the individual tastes.

We're adding raw zucchini here for more flavor and a creamier consistency. That'd be enough, but feel free to add one more "flavoring agent", like sun-dried tomato, olive, thyme, jalapeño, etc. I substitute garlic chives for garlic clove because I like the fresher, lighter taste, and whenever I eat garlic I have to sleep exactly one extra hour. Ayurvedic medicine explains the effect of garlic with *tamas* - the lethargy and stagnation that comes from eating something that grows underground. To some people an extra hour in bed would be acceptable, but think about a great hour of your life. Were you kayaking down a raging rapid? Deep in love and connection with an astounding someone? In a flow state creating something amazing with a passionate group of co-workers? Enjoying the minutia of life with a slow and satisfied mind? My sleeping hour could be an hour like that, except… garlic.

It's very important to remove all excess starch from sprouted garbanzo beans, a step many raw folks overlook. Then over fart. Many folks think they can't eat sprouted legumes for this reason. Cooking break starches down into simple sugars, which are much easier to digest. Sprouting does this too, but not as well (starch is energy for a young plant so it keeps some) so we need to take an extra step to remove that starch and it's so very worth it in both taste and digestibility.

The Recipe, Finally:
1 Quart sprouted Garbanzo Beans
1 Quart sprouted Sesame Seeds (start with half a dry cup of each. Garbanzos and Sesame can be sprouted together, just make sure to use a big enough bag as garbanzos double in size or more when sprouted, and you need enough room for rinsing. For sprouting instruction see "Kitchen Sink Farming Volume 1: Sprouting" or use a googler)
2 Zucchinis
1 Cup Garlic Chives
Juice of 2 or 3 Lemons (about 1 Cup)
Handful Dried Tomatoes or other flavoring agent (optional)
Olive Oil, extra virgin and cold-pressed. Because both zucchinis and olives are very high in Omega-6 fats, which are not great in high doses without Omega-3s to balance

them, you may like to substitute a little bit of a high Omega-3 oil like flax, hemp, camelina oil for some of the olive oil.

Pinch of salt

Rinsing Garbanzo Beans

Take your sprouting bag full of garbanzo beans and lay on a large cutting board or clean counter that can take some abuse. Make sure the top of the bag is closed well, tie a slip knot if you like. Use a rubber mallet, bottom of a glass bottle, or some other instrument of destruction and smash the heck out of them. We want each little bean to get smashed, but not so squished that they drain out of the bag when rinsing.

Rinse the garbanzo smush in cool water. It will run cloudy for a while then come clean. Then mix the bag up, it will again get cloudy then clean. Keep doing that until the whole thing is clean. It might take 5-10 minutes. I put the bag in a strainer and run the water over it, coming back every minute or so to massage the puree. Now you've got a sprouted, easy-to-digest hummus base.

Now Then:

In a high-speed blender or processor, blend sprouted sesame, salt, garlic chives, and lemon juice completely, slowly adding the cold-pressed evo until a smooth but not quite pourable consistency is achieved. We add these first because it's easier to homogenize without the garbanzos. Add rinsed garbanzo beans and blend until smooth.

Add the salt, zucchini and chop a little bit (zuke will get watery if too pureed). Toss coarse sea salt over top to diversify bites.

Dip with celery, or cut carrots diagonally into ¼" chips, use fresh or lightly dehydrate.

Also lovely as an open-faced sandwich on a chunk of sprouted bread – use tomato instead of water and add curry powder or garam masala and dates. Spread sunflower-pomegranate cheese and top with sunflower sprouts, or 3-4 inch tender young wheatgrass shoots to kick it old-testament style.

Can be formed into balls or patties as-is and dehydrated to use in wraps or salads. Next time try blending with carrot and sprouted flax seeds, and adding whole peas by hand.

Dolmas

A friend of mine says he grows grape leaves, because his vines are too young to make grapes. It's fine with me though, because fermented grape leaves make wonderfully soft, flavorful wrappers for this simple snack. Soak them in brine or vinegar for a couple of days, laying them flat like the pages of a book on the bottom of a quart jar. Rub them with a little vinegar, if you like, to soften the probiotic taste of fermentation. Collard greens will also work, see pg 462 for preparing them.

8 Fermented Grapes Leaves or 2 Collard Greens

½ Cup Sunflower, Alfalfa, or Clover Sprouts

¼ Cup Pine Nuts, sprouted

¼ Cup Dried Tomato, chopped

2 T Dill, chopped

2 T Raisins (that's dried grapes to you DIYers), soaked in water for a half-hour or more

1 T Coconut Oil, extra virgin and cold-pressed

Pinch sea salt

Mix ingredients with a spoon, plop onto wrappers and roll up, tucking the ends in first. Best served fresh, but can be kept in the fridge for days. Dry the tomato well if dolmas are going to be refrigerated, as osmosis will leach out their liquid.

Pasta

Pasta is all about the al dente texture of noodles and a wonderfully fresh sauce. White flour noodles aren't meant to taste like much of anything, and I think that's just wasted space on the tongue, real estate that's better rented to ingredients with nourishing, living vitality. The next two recipes use spaghetti, fettuccini, even angel hair or lasagna noodles made from raw zucchini, (though noodles can be made from carrots, beets, young coconut meat, or with a little elbow grease, kelp and agar agar), are delicious living examples of traditional marinara and pesto sauces.

Making Noodles

The type of zucchini pasta is determined only by preference and ease, though thinner noodles will leak more juice so need a longer rest before using, losing nutrients as they sit. For wide, flat papardelle noodles, use a vegetable peeler to make thin strips as wide as the veggie itself, turning the zuke until you've shaved it down to the soft, seed filled core, wonderful in a breakfast juice. For fett-zucchini or zucch-guini, line the strips up on top of each other and make lengthwise cuts with a paring knife held like a pencil. Impossibly long strips of spaghetti and capellini are the ultimate veggie noodle, and quite easy to make if you have the right tool: a spiral slicer or saladacco. This is a tool that turns a vegetable against a metal plate with many small cutters, pulling off long thin strands. It's much easier and quicker to make fresh veggie pasta than to boil water for dry, empty-calorie traditional pasta, and also makes great garnishes and additions to vegetable salads, fresh or dried into crispy noodle nests. Zucchini noodles will soften as they sits, so for a more al dente pasta, dehydrate for a hour. They're also great just tossed with olive oil, lemon and salt, and perhaps a little B vitamin-rich nutritional yeast for a light cheesy flavor.

If your zucchinis are fresh-picked they won't cool the sauce down; if they're coming out of the fridge, leave them on the counter to come up to room temperature for 30 minutes or so. I used to try and short-cut that step by floating them in warm water to bring them up to room temperature, but they soak it up lots of liquid and then release it on the plate. Toss the sauce and pasta together immediately before serving. An average zucchini makes a lot of pasta, usually more than enough for one person

Red Lentil Marinara

When tomatoes cook, their starches break down and become sweeter. Since our tomatoes are raw the red bell pepper picks up the slack, and also makes the sauce a vibrant red.

This is a great dish to make for company, as its spectacular appearance and flavor is as well-received as if it had been simmering on the stove for hours. You'll appreciate its quick prep and easy clean up, and your guests will be surprised at how light and energized they feel afterwards.

1 Cup Red Lentils, sprouted

1 Cup Coarsely Chopped Tomatoes, liquid squeezed out for a thicker sauce

1 Cup Red Bell Pepper, chopped

1 Cup Dried Tomatoes, dried for about 24 hours. Store-bought sun dried tomatoes are processed at high temperatures, evident by their brown and lifeless color. You'll be surprised how bright red your tomatoes stay in the dehydrator, even when left in for a week. We want our dried tomatoes to stay slightly soft, but still have the sweetness and meaty texture of traditional sdt's. And along with the red lentil sprouts, they'll also thicken our sauce and add body.

¼ Cup Olive Oil, extra virgin and cold-pressed

A small handful of Garlic Chives, or 1 clove of garlic, pressed

½ Cup Italian herbs: basil, oregano, thyme, parsley

Pinches each of sea salt and ground black pepper

Hint of fresh chili or cayenne, garnish with a swirl of olive oil, extra virgin and cold-pressed

A food processor is the preferred tool for a textured, chunky sauce, as a blender will puree it too smoothly. Process for 30 seconds or so, scraping the sides so it gets evenly blended. Heat up a little bit on the stove for a traditional hot marinara (though it's also delicious cold or room-temp), stirring constantly so no part gets over 110° F. Take it off the burner when it starts to steam.

Pesto

The best home-grown fresh basil, garlic chives, and lemon juice also make the world's best pesto sauce, which just seems happier over zucchini noodles. This recipe improves on the original by using a base of sprouted sunflower seeds and meaty, omega-3 packed walnuts, saving the traditional pine nuts for the garnish.

1 Cup Sunflower Seeds, soaked and sprouted (not micro greens)
½ Cup Walnuts, soaked for 8-12 hours and drained
Double Handful Fresh Basil, chopped, but leave a few leaves whole for garnish
½ Cup Oil (olive is traditional, but flax, sunflower, walnut, or even a combination with coconut are good), extra virgin and cold-pressed
24" Garlic Chives, or 4 cloves, pressed

1 Lemon, peeled and seeds removed

Garnish:

Pine nuts, soaked and sprouted

Diced tomatoes or sliced red plum tomatoes

Basil Flowers and/or Basil Leaf Chiffonade

In a high-speed blender or food processor, combine the main ingredients, reserving half of the basil and nuts, and blend on high until warm, less than 110°. Add rest of basil and nuts and blend on medium, leaving some texture. Toss with the pasta and garnish.

Chiffonade is a cutting technique that makes lovely, delicate strips of an herb leaf or other such veggie. Lay the leaves on top of each other evenly, then roll them up tightly. Use a sharp knife to cut very thin slices perpendicular to the roll, then toss the pile and you will have super cool long thin strips of basil.

Cooking with Science

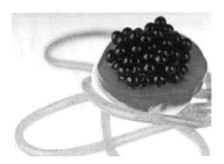

Molecular gastronomy is the whimsical marriage of food preparation and science - the principals of physics, chemistry, and biology are applied in the kitchen for fun and interesting results. These techniques use the chemical properties of natural, sometimes raw foods, like seaweed and soybeans, and can be used to add a wild component to your dishes: caviar made of fruit juices that explode with flavor between the teeth (spherification), impossibly light and ethereal clouds of sauce (foamification), and translucent noodles, sheets, and bowls made of anything from berries to tomato basil soup (gelification). Each of these processes will be presented as a specific recipe but the principals will be self-evident; change the food ingredients as you like and an infinitude of fanciful foods await.

Foamification

Reagent: Soy Lecithin

Foamification, as the name suggests, makes foams or "airs" out of liquids and keeps them that way for a while thanks to the jelling properties of lecithin, which is also necessary for the body to utilize essential fatty acids. The resulting foam is like a cross between cotton candy and snowflakes: dissolving on contact with the tongue and leaving the lingering residue of pure flavor. There are two ways to do this: an immersion (stick) blender foams up liquids to which lecithin has been added so the bubbles stay put, and the foam is scooped off the top with a spoon. The other way is to use a special (and expensive) canister with NO2 cartridges. We'll be doing the former, with a liquid with some fat in it to get the best foam. Any liquid will do, though, and the individual makeup will determine the size, strength, and amount of bubbles.

Steps: (Presented here: Hazelnut Milk Foam)
1 Cup Hazelnuts, sprouted and dehydrated
3 Cup Pure Water
Flavoring agents for your purposes: Raw Honey, Vanilla, etc

In a high-speed blender, blend all ingredients completely, 2-4 minutes. Don't let it heat up too much. Strain well through a sprouting bag, coffee filter, or several layers of cheesecloth.

To resulting nut milk, add 3 g soy lecithin (non-gmo) in a large bowl. The bowl may be covered in plastic wrap to keep the counter clean(er). Put the immersion blender in the milk and turn it on, using the tip of the blender on the surface of the liquid. Experiment with different speeds and angles to produce the most and lightest foam, should be done in about a minute. The foam will last about an hour.

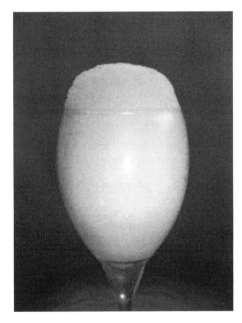

Gelification

Reagent: Agar Agar
Steps (presented here: Arugula Spaghetti, pictured)

This arugula spaghetti recipe makes 6 feet of noodles. Made of arugula water and agar agar, a seaweed-derived jelling agent, it's super easy to do and it only requires a syringe, a rubber tube that fits on the syringe (both of which you can find in medical supply stores) and the agar.

Ingredients
2 Cups Fresh Arugula
2/3 Cup Water
2 or 3 Chives
A pinch of Sea Salt and black or white pepper

Combine ingredients in a high-speed blender or food processor until very smooth.
Wash the tubing well, then suck some olive oil into it and drain, to coat the inside completely.

Per 175 g of arugula puree, combine 25 g water and 3 g agar agar in a saucepan, bring to a boil, stirring constantly with a whisk or egg beater. Remove from heat and skim away any impurities, if desired. Cool to less than 110° F to save the enzymes of the arugula, and mix 2 liquids together. With the tube attached to the syringe, suck the liquid into the tube, filling it. You will have to remove the tube from the syringe, push the plunger down, and reattach to continue sucking. Submerge the tube in ice water until the liquid gels, about 5 minutes. Longer tubes can be rolled and secured with a little tape beforehand.

Reattach the syringe to the tube and push the arugula spaghetti out onto a plate. It can be re-heated in an oven or dehydrator or served cold. Try it with sliced cherry tomatoes, chopped herbs, and balsamic vinegar, or balsamic caviar as in the picture.

Cherry Juice "Ravioli" with Vanilla Cookie

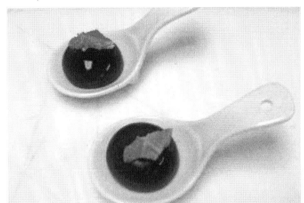

Spherification

Reagents: Sodium Alginate and Calcium Chloride

Spherification is a process that gives liquids a gel-like exterior, while maintaining their drop-like shape and a liquid center. The process happens by heating a liquid with another seaweed-derived substance called Sodium Alginate while in a separate bowl, water is combined with Calcium Chloride. When these two compounds come into contact with each other, a gelling effect is created. The sodium alginate/juice is dropped into the calcium chloride/water bath and the effect happens immediately. It's quite fun to watch a liquid, when dropped into another, hold its circular shape. If your gel is weak, try adding more Calcium Chloride to the bath.

This technique can be used to add another dimension to any liquid in a dish. The "caviar" can be used as a sauce-filled garnish, while the "ravioli" can hold liquids like soup in a precise and novel package.

Steps (presented here: Balsamic Caviar, pictured)
5 grams Sodium Alginate
500 grams Balsamic Vinegar
10 grams Calcium Chloride
1500 grams cold water

Heat Balsamic Vinegar to 110° F, a thermometer is necessary to get the liquid as hot as possible but still keep the enzymes and/or probiotics alive. Turn off the heat and mix in sodium alginate, whisking well. Let liquid reach room temperature.

Whisk together calcium chloride and water until well combined. Place in fridge.

Once room temperature, scoop a little Balsamic Vinegar-Sodium Alginate mixture up with a ¼ teaspoon. Set the bottom of the measuring spoon against the surface of the calcium chloride mixture and fully submerge measure in liquid for about 7 seconds. Then pour the mixture in with a gentle turn of the wrist pulling the measure out of the water as you pour. Leave in solution for 15 seconds.

Gently remove caviar from bath with slotted spoon. Place in another dish filled with cold water to rinse it off. Serve immediately.

Note: the syringe from above can also be used to drop drops of balsamic into a mesh strainer submerged in the CC bath. After 10 seconds (smaller drops need less time), pick the strainer up, rinse off tiny caviar and serve.

Salads and Dressings

What's the one section to be found on every menu in the world, in one version or another in every cuisine in every country? Is the meal more people equate with health, and is the most varied, delicious, and satisfying food in existence? If you haven't guessed by the name of the chapter, it's the salad, and incorporating one into every lunch and dinner or just making a salad's raw awesomeness the entire meal is the surest way to get the most raw nutrition into your life. So why doesn't everyone eat them once or twice a day?

Because they can also seem complicated, intimidating, and time-consuming. This section aims to change that with effortless and cheapo recipes that'll have you whipping up mouthwatering dressings, exciting combinations, and surprising superfluities in no time, and to teach you the principles behind the concepts so you'll never have to look at a recipe again. Salads are the very best way to enjoy your indoor farming efforts, and can be the easiest, as well. Besides having vibrant, fresh ingredients available, dressings are the most important parts of your salad's flavor. Removing one vital ingredient can take a dressing from a delicious treat that brings all contingents of the dish into peaceful harmony, to discordant, mouth-puckering digestive warfare.

My dressings almost always include sprouts, which are an amazing source of natural, flavorful oils. I like to use my explosively vital sprouting seeds in every way possible, but dressings can certainly be made without them if you understand what they were doing in the recipes. Just make sure to include the enormous nutrition of sprouts somewhere in your salad! After all, this book is about growin' food and takin' names and I'm sure that, with a little practice, you'll be using your kitchen's personalized harvest in ways I've never thought of.

Salad dressings are exceptionally easy to make, and once you try some of these recipes I bet you'll never buy one again. They're best when they follow a simple, rough guideline: 1 part acid and 1 to 3 parts base, flavor, and kick. The acid might be vinegar, like one from apple cider brimming with friendly cultures, home-made kombucha that's brewed too long (or just enough if that's what you're going for), or wine vinegars like mirin from fermented rice, and the one that's in that bottle of Trader Joe's red that's been sitting on the coffee table for a couple of days. It can also be a citrus juice like lemon, lime, or tangerine. This is a great use of the fruits of those ridiculous "ornamental" (e.g. "inedible") citrus trees all over apartment complex lawns, which are very acidic. Why anyone would hybridize, sell, buy, or plant something that just "looks" like food is beyond me. Though, I suppose in a way that describes anything that's not grown organically.

"Base" is oil, sprouted seeds or nuts blended into a creamy paste, or preferably a combination of both. When buying oil, make sure it's cold-pressed – the "cold" referring to a gentle process that doesn't cook the oils and turn them carcinogenic, and the "pressing" means not extracted by chemicals for reasons that should be obvious. Fresh oil is also important, because without the protection of a fiber shell or protein sheath, fats can quickly turn rancid, their valuable fat-soluble nutrients like vitamins A and E feasted on by strengthening harmful bacteria. It's very hard to tell if an oil is rotten (including those in flours, nut butters, etc, so look for dark glass and/or refrigeration.

Spice or kick is what dressings need to bring out the flavor of the veggies or fruit they're perched upon; garlic chives, bulbs and sprouts, scallions and onions, radish sprouts, ginger, mustard (jarred or sprouted seeds), a kaleidoscope of peppercorns, wasabi, and fresh chills add different kinds of heat but all succeed in inspiring your taste buds to mine the more subtle richness of a bumpy emerald green spinach leaf or heirloom tomato imploding under the weight of its own juicy sweetness.

Salt is a key in bringing out other flavors, though if you're watching your sodium, salt and sour can be somewhat interchangeable (or raw, intense seaweeds like dulse, wakame, or kombu can be subbed for the same salty character with less sodium). The receptors for sour and salt are right next to each other on your tongue, and are therefore the two flavors most easily confused in the brain - a little science in your salad.

Though not necessary in a well-balanced dressing, another layer of flavor might be hankered for. Flavoring agents can be anything as diverse as fresh herbs, ginger (playing a dual role as kick), raisins, coconut, nutmeg, pomegranate, lemongrass, sundried tomato, sprouted nuts, curry powder, chocolate, or any and all fruits, fungi, or vegetables, fresh or dried. This might be a good place to use peels, cores, or inedible leaves; tomato leaves are not so good in a salad but add a wonderfully garden-fresh tomato suggestion to a dressing. In related news, I once saw a salad dressing recipe that called for bacon grease. Your flavoring might have some sweetness, which many people like, and raw honey will keep the oil and vinegar from separating, in what's called an emulsion. Sweet balances bitter, which is why honey is often combined with mustard, erasing its bitter qualities and uplifting mustard's more delicate flavors. The following dressings are fine on a basic salad of sprouts, greens, and mild vegetables: carrot, tomato, etc. Composed salads come after.

All-Cylinders Creamy Dressing:

(all recipes make enough for 4 small salads or 1 really big one)

½ Cup Neutral Sprouted Seeds like Sunflower, Sesame, Pumpkin, depending on what nutrients and flavor you seek and 2 Tbsp water (optional)

Half a lemon, with or without peel

A piece of chili (I use jalapeño because my plant is prolific, but anything with a little kick will work)

½ Cup Oil, (coconut, hemp, olive, walnut, sunflower, whatever), extra virgin and cold-pressed

4 Tbsp Garlic Chives, or 2 medium-sized cloves of garlic

1 tsp Salt or some Seaweed

Blend in a high-speed blender til creamy. Skip the water and oil and it's a dip for baby carrots or zucchini slices.

Mellifluous Honey-Mustard

Using sultry coconut as the oil reaches into the flavoring category; the mustard is both a kick and flavor, and with the addition of honey this seemingly simple vinaigrette is actually quite robust.

Blend:

½ Cup Coconut Oil, extra virgin and cold-pressed

¼ Cup Rice Wine Vinegar

2 Tbsp Mustard Seeds (yellow and/or brown), sprouted

1 Tbsp Raw Honey

Pinch of Salt

1 Clove Garlic or ¼ Cup Chives

½ Cup Rice Wine Vinegar

Cilantro Dried-Tomato Ranch

Blend:

¼ Cup Sunflower or Olive Oil, extra virgin and cold-pressed

¼ Cup Apple Cider or Kombucha Vinegar (see "Kitchen Sink Farming Vol. 2: Fermenting")

¼ Cup Dried Tomatoes

¼ Cup Sunflower Seeds, sprouted

1 Lemon, peeled

¾ Cup Cilantro (yes, a lot)

Pinch of Sea Salt

6 Whole Black, White, or Pink Peppercorns or 1/4 t ground

4 Cloves Garlic or 1/2 Cup Garlic Chives

3 Green Onions or ¼ of a Small White, Yellow Onion (about 1/8 C)

¼ to ½ Serrano Chile Pepper

1 T Brewer's Yeast (optional) for Cheesiness

¼ C Corn (optional)

If your tomatoes are very dried (or if you're using store-bought), soak them for an hour or two in twice as much filtered water. If you want your dressing super-creamy, throw a ¼ cup of macadamia nuts into the soak water as well.

With 3 Tbsp of the soak water, blend everything but the tomatoes in a high speed blender until smooth. Add the tomatoes and blend at a low setting until they're little red specks. This last step is just for looks, so don't about it if your specks aren't the same size as the neighbor's specks.

Sesame-Garlic Aioli

A natural on hummus in a romaine wrapper with sliced tomato; also great on a salad of greens, bell pepper, cuke and olives with some crumbled seed cheese.

Blend:
½ Cup Sunflower Seeds, sprouted
½ Cup Sesame Seeds, sprouted
½ Cup Sesame Oil, cold-pressed
½ Cup Olive Oil, extra-virgin and cold-pressed
1 ½ Cup Apple Cider Vinegar
4 Tbsp Lemon Juice
4-5 large Garlic Cloves (or a combination of chives and scallions)
1 Tbsp Flax, sprouted (for health benefits, doesn't improve flavor)
½ tsp Black Pepper or more to taste
½ tsp Sea Salt (or 1 Tbsp Nama Shoyu, or ½ Tbsp Dulse Seaweed)
1/8 tsp Mustard Seed, sprouted (or dollop mustard)
Pinch Cayenne or more to taste

Strawberry-Poppy Seed Vin

This naturally sweet dressing is great, especially for sprouts that have grown too long and are starting to get bitter. If you find your sprouted bread has become too bitter in the dehydrator, cut it into croutons and put it in a salad with this vinaigrette. The balance of flavors will delight and the bitter flavors will stimulate digestion, and the fiber from the whole grains croutons will feed the probiotics from the kefir. Everybody wins.

Blend:

¼ Cup Coconut oil, extra virgin and cold-pressed

5 Strawberries

½ of a Lemon, with some peel

Splash of Kefir

Inch of Ginger

Pinch of Sea Salt

Splash of a light Red Wine Vinegar (optional), to deepen flavor

Salt-free Asian Vin

Next time you get sushi, take the extra wasabi and pickled ginger home for this nutty-spicy vinaigrette. I suppose you could also buy them.

Blend:

¼ Cup Olive, Flax, or Hemp oil, extra virgin and cold-pressed

1 Tbsp Coconut oil, extra virgin and cold-pressed

¼ Cup Mirin (Rice Vinegar), or white wine vin

Splash Ume vinegar (from pickled plums - so good, and good for you)

2 Tbsp Sesame Seeds, sprouted

2 Tbsp Kombu or other seaweed

1" Ginger, fresh or pickled

Pinch Wasabi

Dollop of Raw Honey

Scallion, chopped, added afterwards

Cucumber-Clover Vin

As fresh as the hydroponic growing season is long. The cucumber is juicy and mild so will thin the dressing quite a lot; the clover sprouts add a nice zip while advancing the freshness theme. That's why we add a healthy amount of white pepper and sea salt along with a subtle bite of chive and chili, which won't mask the vegetal vitality of the main ingredients.

Blend:

Half a cucumber

Handful of Clover Sprouts

1 Cup White or light Red Wine Vinegar (aka wine left out for a few days)

1 Cup Oil (try a mild mélange of sunflower, avocado, almond, flax, and/or coconut), extra virgin and cold-pressed

2 Tbsp Chives

4 Tbsp or more Whole White Peppercorns

1 tsp Mustard seed, sprouted

Sea salt

Green Salads:

Romaine, fresh corn, "Simple Seed Cheese" made with pepitas (see "Kitchen Sink Farming Volume 2: Fermenting"), , and Cilantro Dried-Tomato Ranch (pg 448), sprinkle with spicy seed mix (pg 487).

Baby Lettuces with Sauerkraut, sliced red pepper and tomato with Mellifluous Honey-Mustard (pg 448), or just some vinegar and coconut oil.

Spinach with Sprouted Sunflower Seeds, a dollop of Kefir Cream Cheese, and Strawberry-Poppy Seed Vin (pg 451).

Raw Slaw

This super-simple slaw is great on its own, next to a wrap or raw taco, or as a condiment for soups, dips, sandwiches, or anything else. Inspired by the tangy German-style cole slaws, this treat is so close to the traditional recipe that everyone will like it, so it's a good choice for a pot luck.

1/2 head Green Cabbage, shredded
1/2 head Purple Cabbage, shredded
2 Carrots, grated
1/3 Cup Apple Cider Vinegar
1 1/2 tsp Mustard Seed, sprouted
1/2 Cup Olive or Flax Seed Oil, extra-virgin and cold-pressed
1/2 tsp Raw Honey
Salt and Pepper to taste
Optional: Spicy Chilies, minced; Apples, cut into matchsticks or chopped; Raisins, soaked in water for 30 minutes.

Combine veggies in a large bowl. Place all other ingredients in a blender and blend until smooth (dressing can also be whisked together if you don't mind whole mustard seeds). Mix veggies and dressing well.

Variation: Coconut-Curry Cole Slaw

Instead of Apple Cider Vinegar, substitute 2 Tbsp Lemon Juice and 4 Tbsp Nama Shoyu (or Soy Sauce).

Instead of mustard, use 3 tbsp sesame seeds (sprouted), 1/3 tsp turmeric, ½ tsp curry, and ½ tsp cumin (sprouted and blended well)

Add 1/3 C raw dried Coconut

Sprout Salads

Apple Pie-laf

Combine:

Legumes like lentil, pea, garbanzo, sprouted, crushed and rinsed (see "Hummus" recipe, pg 425)

Nuts like almond, shelled hemp, pecan, sunflower, sprouted

Diced Apples

Splash Apple Cider Vinegar

Garam Masala (clove, cardamom, ginger, black pepper, cinnamon) to taste

Raw Honey if desired

Top with a dollop of Coconut Cheese or Pudding (pg 206).

Carrot-Pumpkin Salad with Tangerine and Mint

This bright and festive salad, though simple and easy to make, is just bursting with varied and well-balanced flavors. The sprouted seeds are the backup to the headlining carrots. Carrots are available in a rainbow of colors: purple, red, yellow, and white, and this dish can be made even more rock and roll by choosing funky colored varieties to grow. They can then be coarsely grated, mandolined, or cut into matchsticks or quarter moons by slicing the carrot in half long ways, then slicing each half again long ways, then chopping each quarter up the shaft.

4 Large Carrots
½ Cup Sunflower Seeds, sprouted
½ Cup Pumpkin Seeds, sprouted
2 Tbsp Poppy Seeds, sprouted
Pinch Each of: Mint, Cilantro, Chives, all chopped
¼ Cup Light Oil like Olive, Walnut, or Sunflower, Extra Virgin and Cold-Pressed
Juice of ½ of a Lemon
Juice of 1 Tangerine or Sweet Orange
Garnish: ¼ Cup Alfalfa or Clover sprouts, mixed with a pinch of shredded beet for color

Mix all ingredients well in a bowl, add a pinch of finely chopped chili if you like.

Other Salads:
Tantric Kale Salad

Kale is a bright green leafy vegetable that's packed with nutrients and flavor. It's also pretty durn tough, which is why most recipes ask you to steam or sauté it into submission. There's a better way to prep this nutrient-rich veg besides destroying precious vitamins, oils, and enzymes. Keep kale raw *and* sexy by giving it a sensual massage with tenderizing lemon juice and osmosis-inducing salt and oil. Soon your delicious greens will be like soft kisses in your hands.

I often bring this to a party and have people take turns massaging (with very clean hands). Fun for them, all the credit and none of the work for me. Good deal.

2 lb Kale (will shrink a lot), I prefer Lacinato
1/4 Cup oil, (sunflower, olive, or other), extra virgin and cold-pressed
1/3 Cup lemon juice
½ C chopped Scallions

1 t. sea salt

1 Cup Pine nuts, soaked and sprouted (or spicy sunflower-pumpkin mix, pg 486)

1 Cup chopped tomato

¼ Cup Sesame Seeds, sprouted (black is beautiful)

1 Avocado and/or Red Bell Pepper, optional

De-stem the kale by holding the stem and making 1-inch tears at the base of the stem between the it and the leaf. Make a small OK sign with your fingers and pull them stem through it. You should have neatly pulled the stem off of the leaf, leaving it as intact as possible. Don't worry about it if it didn't work this well, a few more chops and you'll be back in business. You can also fold the kale in half and cut around the step. Pile the kale up like the pages of a book and save the tough stems for soup or juice.

Slice the de-stemmed kale into long thin ribbons with the "chiffonade" cut by folding it like a letter, then rolling it along the other axis into a tight tube. With a sharp knife, slice thin strips perpendicular to the roll. You'll be left with long strips which will uncurl into thin ribbons. Put sliced kale in a bowl and make the dressing right on top of it by adding the oil, lemon juice, scallions, salt (and avocado for a fresh creaminess), and reach right in and massaging it for

5-10 minutes. You'll notice the kale reducing in size and becoming much softer in your hands as if it's being cooked. Add the other ingredients and toss well. If you prep everything beforehand, you'll be able to mix it all in without cleaning your hands (again).

Optional: Add crumbled sunflower-corn cheese. Or go Greek by skipping the tomatoes and peppers and add soaked golden raisins and chopped olives. Top with a chunk of kefir laban or Simple Seed Cheese made with pumpkin seed and chopped olives. (see "Kitchen Sink Farming Volume 2: Fermenting" for cheese/laban)

Quinoa-Kimchi Salad

1 Cup Quinoa, sprouted
½ Cup Kimchi (see pg 490)
2 Green Onions, chopped
Splashes of:
Nama Shoyu (or Soy Sauce) or Apple Cider Vinegar
Oil, extra-virgin and cold-pressed (optional)

Kashmiri Karrots

2 Cup Carrots, spirilized (pg 396), matchsticks, or shredded

¼ Cup light Oil (sunflower, olive, avocado, or sesame), extra virgin and cold-pressed

1 tsp Coconut oil (optional), extra virgin and cold-pressed

Juice of 1/2 an Orange

1/8 Cup Fresh Parsley, Chopped

Pinches: Cayenne, Curry Powder, Cinnamon, Cardamom, Clove

Bachelor Pad Thai

1 Cup Leafy Sprout Mix, like onion, clover, sunflower, radish, and alfalfa, for example

½ Cup Tomato, chopped

½ Cup each: quinoa, millet, red lentil, all sprouted of course

For the dressing:

2 Tbsp Kefir (see "Kitchen Sink Farming Volume 2: Fermenting" pgs 244)

Juice of 1/2 a Lime

¼ Cup Peanuts, sprouted

1 tsp each: Fenugreek, Fennel, Flaxseed, all sprouted

1" Ginger, Grated

1 Green Onion (Scallion), chopped

Pinch of Salt

Blend everything, reserving some of the peanut sprouts for garnish

Optional: Add lettuce, mustard greens, chard, avocado. Or kelp noodles (available in well-stocked natural food stores) which are clear and light like Thai rice noodles.

Mung-Cardamom Sundal

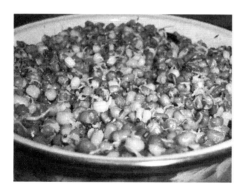

2 Cups Mung Beans, sprouted ("gram dal" in India)
1 tsp Mustard Seeds, sprouted ("urad dal")

1 tsp each, ground: Chana Dal, Asafoetida (Hing), Cumin, Cardamom
1 Tbsp Coconut Oil, extra virgin and cold-pressed
Sea Salt to taste
Garnish with Shredded Coconut

Sammies and Wraps

Burawtos

Wraps are my favorite lunch; they're made of a flavorful pureed filling, a dressing (though being incredibly lazy, I usually just include the dressing ingredients in the filling), and chopped vegetables and sprouts, folded in a dehydrated wrap or collard green. They're almost as versatile as a salad, have a wide range of flavors and textures in one bite, and are, of course, as healthy as it gets. The following recipes use three different types of wrappers: collard green tortillas, romaine tacos, and a dehydrated raw corn crepe though there are other wraps and breads throughout these pages which would also be nice. These recipes each serve 2 as main dishes and 4-6 as sides, and show 1/1 billionth of the possibilities of these hand-held treats.

Garden Wrap

As with most things, simple is best. This quick and easy meal takes a shortcut by relying on the natural scrumminess of fresh vegetables, sprouts, and a handful of container-grown herbs, wrapped in the perfect pocket. Collard greens are packing serious vitamin C, but only when eaten raw, as cooking destroys this immune-system boosting nutrient. Researchers at the University of California at Berkeley have recently discovered that nutrients in collard greens harmonize the immune response system with potent anti-viral, anti-bacterial and anti-cancer activity. When choosing collard greens, look for nice wide leaves without rips, holes or ragged edges.

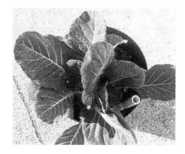

Collards in container with a watering spike

Ingredients:
For the Filling:

About 2 Cups hard fresh veggies as available: bell pepper, carrot, beets, or cauliflower (soft veggies like zucchini and tomato will be too watery when pureed). Apples are great too, but don't overdo it as they're pretty sweet. About half an apple is perfect, seeds removed.

About 2 Cups sprouted grains and seeds: sunflower, quinoa, sesame, pea, garbanzo, amaranth

1 Cup fresh savory herbs like basil, parsley, oregano, thyme, and marjoram

½ - 1 tsp chunky Salt

4 Collard green wrappers, 8-10 inches in diameter
1 Cup dressing, any will do
1 Cup leafy green sprouts: onion, clover, alfalfa etc
Other chopped or shredded veggies as available, like tomato, avocado, cucumber, etc

Method:
Prepare the collard greens first. Rip or cut off the hard stem and put it in with the filling so it doesn't get wasted. Get a nice straight line on the side of the leaf with the stem so it's pretty and even when you go to wrap it, and lay them out on plates. Alternatively, the stem can be completely cut out, and the resulting half leaves cut into half again, so you're

left with 4 equal parts. These are the perfect size for making grape-leaf-less dolmas (pg 420).

In a blender or food processor, puree the veggies and seed or grain sprouts on a medium setting, stopping before the mixture becomes textureless and loses its body. Throw in the herbs and chop a little more. This way each bite will taste different instead of a homogeneous, unrecognizable paste.

Spoon the filling onto the collards along the spine in a strip. Go all the way to the edge that you cut or ripped, and stop a couple of inches away from the other end so it can be folded in. Spoon on a stripe of dressing, top with leafy sprouts, and sprinkle on chopped veggies. Don't overfill or you'll have a hard time folding.

Gently fold the round end of the wrap in towards the middle, perpendicular to the filling. Then fold the sides in, one on top of the other, so that the wrap will stay put when it's turned over and laid down.

Inside-Out Tacos

The mystical combination of hearty and pungent flavors in taco seasoning are something both kids and adults agree on. Add that to crispy lettuce, oily-creamy avocado, and juicy tomato and you have the power to make any mouth water. Taco seasoning is really easy to make, and of course, much better than store-bought versions. This super quick recipe uses the romaine lettuce on the outside, its natural canoe-like shape the perfect vessel for the union of these wonderful flavors. I love finger foods, and often use romaine leaves as fresh chips for scooping up dips.

Ingredients:
For the seasoning (this can also be multiplied, dried, and stored for later use)
2 tsp minced Onion, or half of a Green Onion
1 tsp Salt
fresh Chili to taste, or 1 tsp chili powder
1 medium clove of Garlic, raw or soaked in kombucha to ferment for 3 days to many months (I always have a jar going of peeled garlic in kombucha. Safeway sells small bags of peeled organic garlic, often for cheaper than whole garlic somehow)
1 tsp fresh Oregano

½ tsp Cumin Seed, (can be fresh - sprouted, dried, and ground of course)

Optional: shake of black pepper for more heat, paprika for color

And:

2-3 avocados

1 Tomato, chopped and liquid squeezed out

4 large Romaine Leaves

¼ Cup Sunflower Seed, sprouted

Optional: 2 Tbsp shelled hemp, sprouted

Do:

In a large bowl, mash the avocado with a fork. Add the seasoning and mix well.

Scoop it into the romaine leaves, top with tomatoes and sunflower sprouts for extra crunch.

Inside out Tacos are also great with hummus (pg 425) and Cilantro-Sundried Tomato Ranch dressing (pg 447), or as "ZLT's" – Zucchini Bacon, Lettuce, and Tomato.

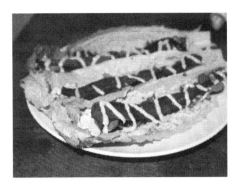

Pictured Here: Smoky Maple Zucchini Bacon with Raw Hummus and Raw Ranch Dressing on a Romaine Leaf

Smoky-Maple Zucchini Bacon

2 Zucchinis, thinly sliced (I use a mandolin slicer set at 2mm)

Marinade:

2 Tbsp each:

Oil of your Choice (Olive is neutral in flavor, Coconut adds a little succulent sweetness and a little white sheen at room temperature just like the "other" bacon)

Maple Syrup

Nama Shoyu (or Bragg's Liquid Aminos, or Soy Sauce)

Apple Cider Vinegar

1/2 – 1 tsp Liquid Smoke

Ground Black Pepper to taste

Cover and marinate zucchini for 12-24 hours. If you need more liquid, you can use water, kombucha, kefir whey (these will of course ferment the zucchini for probiotic goodness) or more vinegar for extra tang.

I like to marinate in a zip-loc freezer bag, close the seal except for a centimeter in the middle, suck all the air out with my mouth, and quickly seal it up. The added negative pressure helps the marinade to penetrate into the zucchini, and less marinade is required.

After marinating for 12-24 hours, lay strips on non-stick dehydrator trays and dry at <110°F for 12-24 hours, then flip them onto the mesh racks and dry for another few hours until they're as crispy as you like. I like to lay the strips down a little wrinkly - a bend here, a hump there – so they look most like fried bacon. At least that's what I tell people who've paid me; it's actually just much easier.

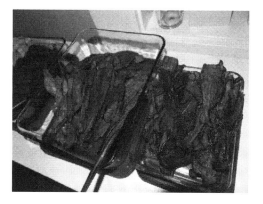

Zucchini Bacon!

Plymouth Rock and Rolls

In the autumn we tend to crave heartier foods, as our ancestors would use this time to store fat to prepare for the coming winter. We don't need to be so primal about our food choices, and with a little awareness we can still feel emotionally satisfied by living foods. These wraps feature higher fiber and essential fatty acid-rich foods (more on EFAs in "Kitchen Sink Farming Volume 1", starting on page 106like corn and hemp, with a comforting dehydrated bread wrapper and traditional fall flavors.

One order of corn-hemp flatbread (pg 510), dehydrated until soft and pliable

For the filling:

1 Cup Hemp Seeds, no shell, soaked and sprouted

1 Cup Corn Kernels, either fresh or dried.

    If fresh: coarsely ground and rinsed to remove the starch

    If dried: sprouted, coarsely ground, and rinsed (see note)

1 Scallion (Green Onion)

1 Clove Garlic

For the Salad:

½ Cup Yams, shredded or spiralized (see pg 396) and soaked overnight in water in the fridge to remove the starch

½ Cup Carrots, shredded

¼ Cup Raisins (soaked with the yams)

2 Tbsp Raw Honey

1 tsp Nama Shoyu or Soy Sauce (ok the Pilgrims probably didn't know about this one but they woulda loved it)

2 Tbsp Apple Cider Vinegar (happy?!)

Pinches Nutmeg, Clove

Filling:

Blend the garlic and onion with half of the hemp seeds until smooth. Add the rest of the hemp and the corn and pulse to mix and keep some texture.

Spoon onto the wrapper, and top with the yam salad. Roll it up and enjoy.

*Note on sprouting corn: corn must be dried very slowly if it's to be re-hydrated and sprouted. I've never been able to do it successfully, though packages of organic seeds sprout beautifully with a subtle sweet corn flavor, but are too expensive to be a viable food. It's best to just use fresh corn, or if you have to dry it, re-hydrate it by soaking it in salt water or salted apple juice to stimulate osmotic

plumping. This will make sprouting impossible, but is a reasonable compromise.

Coconut Tortillas

This is a slightly advanced recipe. A thin, flexible and sturdy wrap is possible raw with the help of flax and the meat of young coconut. There's so much soluble fiber there that the dehydrated wraps will act just like tortillas for a more familiar and gourmet wrap. The beet juice will create a pink color, just for optional fun. Because the wrap is light in color, other natural colorings can be used (turmeric for yellow, parsley juice for green, etc) or none at all.

A close eye must be kept on these to ensure they don't turn into beautiful crackers, so make them when you can stay around the house.

¼ Cup Yellow Flaxseed, unsprouted

1 ½ Cup Young Coconut Meat

1 Tbsp Coriander, sprouted

1 tsp Cumin, sprouted

1 tsp Sea Salt

4 T Beet Juice, optional, for color

½ C Dry Bulk, optional (like Pulp from Juicing Veggies of your choice, or Sprouted Quinoa, etc.)

Grind dry flaxseed into meal in a coffee grinder or Vita mix blender. Add other ingredients and mix thoroughly. Spread evenly onto non-stick dehydrator trays. Start checking after 2 or 3 hours, and flip as soon as they're able to be. Dry until still pliable, cut off edges, and use. They can also be over-dried a little and placed in zip-loc freezer bags for a few days, which will make them even more pliable and strong.

Asian Veggie Nori Wrap

4 Sheets Nori, Sun-Dried is best
For the filling:
2 Cup Sunflower Seeds, sprouted
¼ Cup Poppy Seeds, sprouted
¼ Cup Light Sesame Seeds, sprouted
2 Tbsp Black Sesame Seeds, sprouted
(Sprout the first 3 together if you want; they'll be ground. The black sesame will be sprouted separately so can remain whole for color. Or not.)
16" Garlic Chives, or one Clove Garlic
4" Ginger
3 Tbsp White Miso
2 Tbsp Nama Shoyu or Soy Sauce
¼ of a scrubbed Lemon, peel attached

3 Tbsp Nutritional Yeast

Veggies:
1 Cucumber, a Carrot, handful of Snow Peas, a Green Onion, a few Romaine Leaves, as available. Cut into strips.

Prep, in a food processor or blender:
Grind half the light sesame seed sprouts until they're tahini – a smooth paste. Add the rest of the ingredients (except for the black sesame, poppy seed sprouts and veggies) and blend as smooth as possible. Add black sesame and poppy seeds and mix.

Slice the veggies into long thin strips and assemble sushi roll. Spread the paste all over the sheet of nori except for a ½" or so strip at the top edge. Lay the veggies horizontally near the bottom and with a sushi mat or your hands, fold the bottom end over and roll it up. Wet the exposed strip on the top so it sticks to the outside of the roll. If your roll is fairly tight, you may want to slice it into pretty pieces by making lengthwise cuts with a very sharp knife, or just eat it whole.

Extra Fancy - let some of the veggies stick out a few inches on either end, so when you cut the roll into disks, two of the pieces have veggies sticking out.

Try it with pickled ginger and avocado ponzu sauce.

Raw Pickled Ginger

6" Ginger, thinly sliced with knife or mandolin
2 Tbsp Apple Cider Vinegar
1 Tbsp Lemon Juice
2 tsp Raw Honey

Marinate the ginger for a minimum of 1 day in the refrigerator. Will keep in the refrigerator for a few weeks.

Avocado ponzu

3 Avocados
4 Tbsp Nama Shoyu or Soy Sauce
2 Tbsp Rice Wine Vinegar
1 ½ Tbsp Raw Honey
1 Tbsp Lemon Juice
1 Tbsp Lime Juice
1" Ginger, grated

2 Tbsp finely chopped Garlic Chives

Whisk all liquids with a fork, mash avocados, and then mix in ginger and chives

Soups and Stews

Soups are a snap in a high-speed blender, which can puree and heat by the friction of its whirling blades. Just past a little steam (depending on air temperature, of course) will tell you that your soup is less than 110° F, the optimal temperature for enjoyment that won't destroy enzymes, nutrients, and probiotics. Or use a thermometer for exactness. They can be pureed completely smooth, or a varied and textured stew can be created by blending and heating a base, then throwing in warm veggies, sprouts, or sea vegetables, and lightly chopping in the blender. Ingredients can also be pureed in a food processor, regular blender, or chopped by hand and tossed into a pot, stirred constantly and taking it off the heat at the magic temp.

All-American Chowder

This creamy soup combines sweet white corn, savory herbs, spicy chilies and garlic chives with chunks of rich tomato and blue corn chips, making it red white and blue in color. It's also "all-American" because both corn and tomatoes are native to North America, and can easily be given a Nova Scotian, Midwestern, or Tex-Mex vibe. Also, maybe most importantly, this soup is beloved by all, including the steak-and-potatoes set, which makes it the potage everyone can agree on.

Home-Grown Ingredients:

Nut milk (try hemp), filtered or flavored water for base (pg 415)

1 Cup White Sweet Corn (yellow's fine too)

2 Green Onions (Scallions; or ½ of a white or yellow onion)

12" Garlic Chives

¼-½ Jalapeño (or other hot pepper)

2 Tbsp Apple Cider Vinegar

Salt and Plenty of Black Pepper

1 C Tomatoes; Plum, Cherry, or Chopped

Handful of broken pieces of Raw Crackers (pg 505) or blue corn chip pieces from the bottom of the bag.

Optional: ½ cup fresh complimentary herbs like cilantro and sprouted cumin, French tarragon and basil, or cinnamon, clove, and nutmeg. Save a few particularly nice leaves or flowers for garnish.

Soak tomatoes and a handful of corn on very warm water, so as not to cool the soup when they're added. Combine all remaining ingredients except for crackers/chips in a high-speed blender. Puree on high until 110º F, then add the rest of the ingredients and chop.

Optional 2: reduced balsamic vinegar swirled on top of the soup will add sweetness and is enjoyed by those new or opposed to raw food.

Cream of Mushroom

1 Cup Mushrooms, Crimini or Portobello are preferred. Can be pre-warm marinated (see pg 421) for richer flavor. Note: organic is very important in mushrooms.
1 Cup Sprouted Hemp Milk (pg 415, use less water for a thicker milk and soup)
12" Garlic Chives
1 medium Shallot
½ tsp Fresh Sage (or a pinch if using dried)
¼-½ Jalapeño (or other hot pepper)
Salt
2 Tbsp Mushroom Essence (see below)

Mushroom Essence

1 Part flavorful fresh mushrooms, like chanterelle, trumpet, or oyster (dried can be subbed as well at ½ the amount)

4 Parts Olive Oil, extra virgin and cold-pressed

.5 Parts Black Sesame, Sprouted for 8 hours and dried at 110° F for 12-24 hours

.5 Parts Garlic Chives, Optional

Blend on High for 5 seconds, until just before smooth. Will keep for several weeks in the fridge.

Combine all ingredients (except for mushrooms if they're marinated; drop them in at the end and pulse to break up) in a high-speed blender and puree to 110° F. Garnish with swirl of Mushroom Essence (can be ladled on with a spoon or put into a squirt bottle).

Goulash

A really special creamy tomato soup with a sweet and sour, probiotic-laden snap. see "Kitchen Sink Farming Volume 2: Fermenting" for more on sauerkraut and kefir.

1 Cup Sauerkraut

1 Cup Tomato

½ Cup Raw Milk Kefir

2 Carrots

1 Red Bell Pepper

¼-½ Jalapeño (or other hot pepper)

½ Cup Basil and/or 1 Tbsp Thyme

2 Tbsp Coconut Oil, extra virgin and cold-pressed or MCT oil

½ Beet (for garnish)

Combine all ingredients but kraut in a high-speed blender and blend on high until 110° F. Garnish with a mound of chopped sauerkraut mixed with grated or spiralized beet.

Buddha Belly Soup

They say happiness comes from within. They mean a little down and to the left. It's hard to frown in the presence of this divinely creamy potage, full of dark green kale, contentment-inducing burdock and carrots, three sources of probiotics, fiber, heavenly coconut oil, and deeply nourishing sea vegetables.

1 Cup Water
1 Fermented Leek (or a fresh leek and some sauerkraut. Or, you know, not)

4 large leaves of Kale

3 Carrots

2" Burdock Root

2 Tbsp Flaxseed, sprouted

1 Tbsp Miso (I prefer white and a lot of it, the darker the paste the more intense the flavor)

1 Tbsp Coconut Oil, extra virgin and cold-pressed

¼-½ Jalapeño (or other hot pepper)

1 tsp Cumin, sprouted if possible

Handful Wakame seaweed (it's rich and salty, like the bacon of the sea.)

Handful Quinoa, sprouted

1 Avocado

Combine all ingredients but last 3 in a high-speed blender and blend to 110° F.

Then add wakame, quinoa, avo the blender and mix. So good.

Coconut Corner!

Carrot Coconut Soup with Ginger

A sweet and savory soup that's the perfect marriage of succulent coconut, pungent ginger, fresh parsley, and savory spices.

4 Carrots

Water and Flesh of a Young coconut (about 1 Cup) or substitute a nut milk (macadamia is pricey but nice, hemp and almond are my preferred, both sprouted first of course) and 1/8 Cup dried shredded coconut

2" Ginger

12" Garlic Chives

¼ Cup Parsley (or 1 Tbsp dried)

Pinch of Sea Salt

Garam Masala to taste (or just simple Black Pepper)

Combine all ingredients in a high-speed blender and puree until 110° F. Garnish with shredded coconut and/or chopped parsley.

Chilled Mango Soup with Lime-Macadamia Cream and Coconut Noodles

Luxurious and sexy but still refreshingly light, this cold soup is a wonderful palate-cleanser. It's a lot more involved than most of the recipes in this book, so enjoy it by itself on a summer three-day-weekend, or as part of a multi-course feast. Pineapple can be subbed for the mango.

Soup ingredients:

Flesh from two ripe Mangoes

Water from a young coconut (about 1 cup)

2" Lemongrass (about 1 tsp)

1" Ginger

1 Tbsp Lime Juice

¼ of a Vanilla Bean, seeds scraped

¼-½ Jalapeño (or other hot pepper)

Pinch of Sea Salt

1 Tbsp Raw Honey (optional)

Combine all ingredients in a high-speed blender and blend until smooth. Stick in the fridge.

Coconut Noodles:

Flesh removed from one young Thai coconut and cut into strips (julienned).

Lime-Macadamia Cream:

1 Cup Macadamia Nuts, soaked and sprouted

Zest of one Lime

1-2 tsp Fresh Lime Juice

Small pinch of Sea Salt

Place all ingredients in a high-speed blender and blend until smooth and creamy, like whipped cream. Add coconut water to thin if necessary. Less-expensive sprouted sunflower seeds can be used instead of maces to save some green.

To Compose:
Divide the Coconut Noodles into four bowls. Top with Chilled Mango Soup. Swirl or dollop the Macadamia Cream.

Clover Curry

The varied textures of this quite simple curry make it seem more like a meal than a soup, and the hearty legume and frisky clover sprouts make it both substantial and zinging with life force.

Water and Meat from a Young Thai Coconut
1" Ginger
1/8 C Garlic Chives
¼-½ Jalapeño (or other hot pepper)
2-3 Tbsp Lime Juice
2 Tbsp Cilantro, chopped
1/8 Cup Green Onion (Scallion), diced

1 Banana, chopped (or sliced with a spoon, cereal-style)

1 C Legume Sprouts (like Pea, Lentil, and Garbanzo)

1 C Clover Sprouts

Pinch of Sea Salt

Adzuki Bean Sprouts for garnish, if desired (see "Kitchen Sink Farming Volume 1: Sprouting")

Combine first 5 ingredients in a high-speed blender and blend until 110° F. Combine everything in a bowl or two. Also nice cold.

Snacks and Condiments

Gomasio

A traditional Japanese condiment normally made with toasted sesame seeds, *gomasio* (or *gomasho*) is a healthier alternative to salt. This sprouted, living recipe increased that healthiness by an order of magnitude, using the traditional Japanese ingredients of raw soy sauce and seaweed for the proper saltiness (also making it the same color as toasted seeds), and flax oil for the wonderful rich nuttiness. It's great on everything: raw sushi of course, whole grain or green salads, buttered sprouted loaves, pastas and wraps, and even chocolate desserts.

1 Cup Sesame Seeds, sprouted
2 tsp Flax Oil, Extra-Virgin and Cold-Pressed
1 tsp Nama Shoyu
Pinch ground sea vegetables like dulse, wakame, or nori
Optional: Nutritional Yeast for cheesiness, cayenne, and/or other sprouted seeds or nuts like pumpkin, sunflower, walnut

Combine ingredients in a high-speed blender, food processor, or coffee grinder and blend until a coarse but consistent powder. Place on a dehydrator sheet or wax paper in the dehydrator at 110° F for 2 hours or so, or put in the sun all day, protecting from birds if necessary. When completely dry, put in an airtight jar in a cool cabinet; will keep for several months. Take a bit with you throughout the day and sprinkle some live, salty, nutty goodness on whatever you're having.

Living Parm

The familiar, sharp cheese flavor that's not out-of-place on Zucchini-Tomato Pasta (pg 430) and Raw Pesto (pg 432)

1 Cup Walnuts, sprouted

1 Cup Sunflower Seeds, sprouted

1 Cup Pine Nuts, sprouted (though they add a pleasant dimension, less or none is ok if they're too expensive in your area)

2 Cloves Garlic

2 Tbsp Nutritional Yeast

2 tsp Sea Salt

Combine ingredients in a high-speed blender or food processor and blend until a coarse but consistent powder. Place on a dehydrator sheet or wax paper in the dehydrator at 110° F for 12 hours or so, or place in the sun all day, protecting from birds if necessary. Rake halfway through the drying time with your fingers. Place in an airtight jar in a cool cabinet; will keep for several months.

Spicy Seed Mix

Inspired by the spicy/sour flavor combination specific to Latin American, like chili powder on lemons or unripe guava. An explosively-flavored yet refreshing treat.

1 Cup Sunflower Seeds, sprouted

1 Cup Pumpkin Seeds, sprouted

¼ - ½ Jalapeno or other spicy chili

1 Tbsp Olive or Coconut Oil, Extra-Virgin and Cold-Pressed

Juice of 1 Lime

12" Garlic Chives, chopped

1 Tbsp Cilantro, fresh (use 1 tsp if dry)

¼ Tbsp Cumin, sprouted

Pinch Sea Salt (try smoked sea salt)

Optional: a few Collard Leaves, chopped. I prefer Collard Chips to Kale and they add a rich, fresh flavor here.

Combine all ingredients but seeds in a high-speed blender or food processor and blend well. Stir into seeds and mix with a spoon or hand. Place on a dehydrator sheet or wax paper in the dehydrator at 110° F for 2 hours or so, or place in the sun all day. When completely dry, put in an airtight jar in a cool cabinet; will keep for several months. If your flavors are too intense when it comes out of the dehydrator, lightly mist it with water to re-activate the pumpkin seeds' stickiness, and sprinkle it with sprouted hemp hearts to mellow it out.

Sprinkle over a salad, mix into a flavorful nut or kefir cheese, or even dip a banana into them. Maybe you should triple the recipe – you'll go through them faster than you think and drool at the dehydrator every subsequent batch.

Fall-nuts

With flavors of caramelized, comforting spices, these nuts are great on ripe golden delicious apples, banana ice cream (pg 516), or just by themselves. Pecans are a rich source of mono- and poly-unsaturated fats (the "good" ones), which help fight heart disease and weight loss by helping us feel full. Walnuts are one of the best sources of omega-3's (see pg 106), and provide a rare and beneficial form of vitamin E (gamma-tocopherol), as well as phytonutrients and anti-oxidants that fight cancer, heart disease, and diabetes. Some of these compounds are found in no other foods.

1 Cup Walnuts, sprouted
1 Cup Pecans, sprouted
2 Tbsp Raw Honey
1 tsp Poppy seeds, sprouted
1 tsp Cinnamon
½ tsp Nutmeg
A few Cloves
Pinch of Sea Salt

Combine all ingredients but nuts in a high-speed blender or food processor and blend until a coarse powder. Place on a dehydrator sheet or wax paper in the dehydrator at 110° F for 2 hours or so. Place in an airtight jar in a cool cabinet; will keep for several weeks.

Cultured Kimchi

Sometimes called "Korean Sauerkraut", Kimchi is so much more. Spicy, savory, and great for digestion with ginger and spice, it's a wonderful condiment to grain or green salads and wraps, and adds an explosive but well-balanced flavor to soups and dips.

1 head Cabbage, cored and shredded (I like to combine green, purple, and Napa for variation in taste and texture but any/all are great)
1 bunch Green Onions, chopped
1 Cup Carrot, grated
1 Tbsp fresh Ginger, grated
3 Cloves Garlic, peeled and minced
1/2 tsp ground Red Pepper or fresh Chili to your liking - it's a condiment so make it pretty hot! (Kimchi traditionally gets a pepper called Gochugaru; any spicy chili will do)
1 Tbsp Sea Salt

4 Tbsp Kefir Whey (see "Kitchen Sink Farming Volume 2: Fermenting") or Kombucha

(optional) Juice of 1 Lemon - not traditional in kimchi but I like it

(optional) - 1/2 Cup Daikon or other Radish, grated

(optional)1 Tbsp Black Mustard Seeds, sprouted

Veggies can also be put into a food processor or high-speed blender with the whey and a small amount of water and chopped.

Combine all ingredients in a large bowl and pound with a plastic-wrapped rubber mallet or clean rock to release juices. Separate into 2 quart canning jars and press down with a fist until well-covered with liquid. Close jars tightly and leave at room temp for 3 days, then put in the fridge. Will last for several weeks.

Asian Dip

I started making this delicious and nourishing dip on road trips, mixing the ingredients in an extra empty container. Spread in a romaine leaf with chopped tomato and sprouts, or dip carrots, zucchini, or other veggies.

1 Cup Kimchi

1 Avocado

¼ Cup Sesame Seeds, sprouted

1 Tbsp White Miso

1 Tbsp Dulse

1 Tbsp Mustard, if no mustard seeds in Kimchi

1 Tbsp Flax seeds, sprouted (optional – avocado is high in omega-6's, so it's a good idea to balance them with extra omega-3's from flax or another source)

In a high-speed blender or food processor, grind sesame seeds into a paste (tahini). Stir in all other ingredients.

Summer Sauer Slaw

Two fermented and one fresh = two steps forward, and one more step forward. Fermented cabbage and beets plus fresh shredded carrot make a sweet and sour condiment that enhances the flavors of hearty dehydrated mains, warm savory loaves, and is even wonderful on its own. I discovered this one day when I was craving both a salad and a sweet, the latter of which is often a cry for nourishment from unfriendly bacteria and yeasts. I didn't want to create the difficult-to-digest combination of fruit and vegetables, and sour, fermented foods feed the antecedent to that craving.

A handful of raisins or diced apples may be sewn without judgment to balance your palate or extra-sour fermented veggies. Next to the bright orange carrots, yellow or golden beets create a sunny dish.

1 Cup Fermented cabbage and beets (can be fermented together), chopped
¾ Cup Shredded Carrots (or fermented, then use fresh beets)
½ Cup Pistachios, sprouted (don't skip this part if possible - they're amazing)
1/3 Cup Grapefruit Juice
2 Tbsp Coconut Oil, extra virgin and cold-pressed
Few dashes of Nama Shoyu (or soy sauce)
Mix all ingredients, garnish with chopped garlic chives

Strawberry Ambrosia Leather

This is a dried fruit "roll-up" if I'm allowed to call it that. Combine sweet and sour home-grown strawberries and kefir with hemp and vanilla for a protein and EFA-rich snack.

1 lb Strawberries

½ Cup Kefir

1 Cup Shelled Hemp Seeds, soaked and sprouted (or ground whole sprouted hempseeds for a crunchier texture)

½ of a Vanilla Bean

Put ingredients in blender and blend to desired consistency. I like flecks of berry and the shelled hemp pretty much whole.

Pour 1 cup onto the middle of a dehydrator sheet. With a wide spatula, "paint" the mixture from the middle towards you, turning the sheet as you go so the mixture is even and about an inch from all the edges of the sheet. It's important to keep it fairly flat so it dries consistently.

If you like, your fruit skins can be garnished by making a complimentary-flavored liquid that's a different color. Pour it onto the main mixture in shapes, words, or line art. Get super fancy with a stencil and spray bottle. I like to pour thin parallel stripes then drag a toothpick or chopstick perpendicular to the lines to make webbing. Cool and easy, huh? If you pour small circles and drag through them you'll get hearts. Strawberry Ambrosia Leather with Macadamia-White Chocolate Hearts, anyone?

Dry at 110° F for 6-12 hours, then flip when the top is dry. Slide the teflex sheet off of the tray and mesh screen, turn the tray and screen over and put it on top of the leather. Then flip the whole thing over and carefully peel the sheet off the bottom of the fruit (now the top). Put back in the dehydrator for another 6 hours or so. It will become harder and more brittle the longer it's dried, so play with your desired consistency.

Any fruit or veggies puree can be dried into a sheet, from your leftover raspberry-orange smoothie, to an apple, walnut, and cinnamon puree, to bananas and peanut butter (sprouted, of course). Go crazy, and remember that bitter flavors get more intense when all the water is removed (and sweetness diminishes). The more liquid, the faster it'll dry and the easier it'll crack, so turn down the heat or add some rubbery cohesion with thicker fruit.

Buerre Quotident – "Daily Butter"

I like foods so good that I question what I must have done in past lives to deserve them. Hence: "Daily Butter": a living, protein-packed super-spread. Full RDA of both fiber and EFAs. Minerals, vitamins, blah blah blah... But oh that divine taste!

1 Cup Shelled Hemp Seeds, sprouted
3 Tbsp Golden Flaxseeds, sprouted
1 Tbsp Raw Honey (check out pg 406 for more on raw honey)
¼ of a Vanilla Bean
Pinch Sea Salt

Food process or high-speed blend until warm and smooth. Optional: add sprouted peanuts or almonds at the end of blending to lightly chunk them.

Pitch Black Butter

This nut butter, made with sprouted black sesame seeds, could probably be mistaken for pitch - the thick, dark resin shipbuilders used to seal their hulls, though it's doubtful many people are familiar enough with both substances to make the error. It could also be called "tahini's evil twin", because though they both have the same base, this version is succulent and mysteriously sweet, though still authentically Middle-Eastern.

1 Cup Black Sesame Seeds, soaked and sprouted for at least 12 hours

4 Dates (more if sesame sprouts are more mature and therefore more bitter)

2 Tbsp Coconut Oil, Extra-Virgin and Cold-Pressed, or MCT oil

¼ of Vanilla Bean

Pinch Cinnamon

In a high-speed blender, grinder, or food processor, blend until creamy.

Optional: Stir in ¼ C Cacao Butter (Raw White Chocolate), lightly chopped

Cheeses, Dips, and Spreads

Spreads and dips can be smeared on a romaine leaf with some veggies and dressing, enjoyed with carrots, celery, and chips, or floated atop raw soups for a delicious thickener and garnish.

FYI spread + dressing is a lovely presentation and offers taste variation in each bite. When prepping food for myself I'll often combine the two to skip a step and get to the eating (aka super-lazy). Medium-lazy: make the spread first and don't clean the vita-mix or food processor container before making the dressing, which will not only suck up the residual flavors, it'll clean the blender from the thick spread.

Road Trip Dip

This is the classic lunch I make when travelling in the US; I roll up to the natural food store in town, get the ingredients, grab some utensils and rock it out at a table in their eating area. It can be made in quantity, using all the ingredients and using their containers to store tomorrow's lunch. Nothing is perishable but the avocado and it's usually good for a day at least, and the lemon juice helps preserve it. When we're travelling, we're often tempted to eat unhealthy foods or overspend on healthy ones (both of which can be fun/necessary sometimes so don't feel bad), but this quick, cheap meal is healthier and tastier than what most raw food restaurants offer for $15.

4 Tbsp White Miso
1 Avocado
1 Tbsp Mustard
3 Tbsp Ground Flax Seed (this is usually sold in 1-pound bags, so might be a good idea to buy it at home and bring what you'll need)
Juice of one Lemon

Mix all ingredients to taste – again I just use all of what I get. You can dip veggies in like cherry tomatoes, carrots, and celery (washed in the store's restroom if you want) and/or use romaine leaves as a taco and layer on the veggies and sprouts. So good.

Almond Orchard Spread

Paste needs to stay a little dry to it doesn't run, tomato adds a nice yet obedient juiciness.

2 Cup Almond Pulp (leftover from making almond milk, ("Kitchen Sink Farming Volume 1: Sprouting" pgs 216)
¼ Cup Olive Oil, Extra Virgin and Cold-Pressed
¼ Cup Lemon Juice
1 Cup Dill, fresh
½ Cup Radish Micro greens, chopped
½ Cup Red Bell Pepper, diced
¼ Cup Garlic Chives, chopped
¼ Cup Green Onions, chopped
½ tsp Sea Salt
Tomato for garnish

Mix all ingredients with a spoon or by hand and spread on cracks, sprouted bread, or veggie chips. Garnish with sliced cherry or other tomatoes.

Breads

Though any kind of grain can be made into a raw bread with varying degrees of sponginess, wheat is given here because it's so pervasive. There are a few choices - for straight-up wheat remember that the darker the color the more dense the bread will be. Play with some ancestors of wheat like Spelt for a more buttery texture or Kamut (Khorisan wheat) for a more hearty loaf. Way more than you want to know about these seeds and more in "Kitchen Sink Farming Volume 1: Sprouting".

Basic Sprouted Bread

2 Cup Wheat, sprouted (yields about 3 cups)
1 Cup Raisins
3/4 tsp Sea Salt

The thick dough can bog down a high-speed blender, so bread is best made in a food processor. Process everything, doing small batches if necessary, for 30 seconds to a minute until everything is well blended and you have a sticky dough.

Grease your hands and form the dough into a loaf. In a high-speed blender, the dough can be so well chopped that it loses any loft and becomes very dense. If this is the case, whether by accident or preference, make sure that your loaf isn't more than an inch high so that it will dehydrate evenly. If your dough is still nice and light, you can go up to a few inches, or even use a terracotta (breathable) loaf pan.

Put the loaf on a dryer sheet in your dehydrator, or on wax paper in the oven with the door ajar, and dry at 110° F or so for 3 hrs then 140 ° until dry inside. This can be tested by a toothpick poke, seeing if it's dry when removed. If you're doing a taller loaf, it can be taken out of the pan and laid on its top and dried more, or sliced into pieces and each of those dried to perfection. When your loaf is done, it will have a light-colored, thin, hard outer crust and a cakey, soft interior, like a muffin.

When the loaf is cooled to room temperature you can store it in the fridge in a storage bag to be used within two or three days, or you can wrap it in plastic and store it in a freezer bag in the freezer for a long time.
Breads can be coarsely or finely ground, but I prefer coarse for two reasons - I like to see and crunch whole sprouted seeds; the bright red hull of a quinoa seed with its tail snaking into the meat of a warm loaf is a beautiful thing.

Also, the more coarsely mixed a bread is, one that's just barely holding together by the thought of stickiness, has more loft and flavor. Sprouted bread flours are best gently blended, if they're too blended all the air will go out of them and they'll be bricks. In my opinion they're best half mixed in a food processor, and half left un-ground, especially in the case of smaller seeds like amaranth and quinoa. In a high-speed blender, the dough will be ground into a homogeneous paste rather quickly, so sprout each seed separately and manage their blendedness by the order in which they're added to the machine - whatever's added earlier will be blended more. Food processor owners have a little more freedom to sprout seeds all together.

Follow the same instructions for the following variations:

Date Manna Bread

2 Cups Wheat, sprouted (Kamut for a richer flavor, Spelt for a buttery one)
1/2 lb Dates
1 Cup Raisins
1/4 tsp Clove
1/4 tsp Cinnamon

Apple-Orange Bread

1 Cup Dried Apples, chopped

¼ Cup Orange Juice

1/2 Cup Raisins

1 tsp Cinnamon.

Herbed Multigrain

½ Cup each:

Wheat, sprouted

Quinoa, sprouted

Amaranth, sprouted

Oats, sprouted

1 Cup Golden Raisins, soaked in a little water overnight

then drained and ground with the rosemary

4 Tbsp Rosemary, fresh

1 tsp Salt

Basil Dried Tomato

To basic wheat or multigrain dough add:

1 Cup Dried Tomato

½ Cup Golden Raisins

¼ Cup Basil, fresh

1 tsp Sea Salt

Cinnamon Almond Bread

2 Cup Almond Pulp (leftover from making almond milk, pg 216)
½ Cup Raisins
¼ Cup Olive or Almond Oil, Extra Virgin and Cold-Pressed
¼ Cup Coconut Oil, Extra Virgin and Cold-Pressed
¾ Cup Flaxseed, sprouted
¼ Cup Raw Honey
1 tsp Cinnamon
1 tsp Sea Salt

Grind flaxseeds to a smooth paste. Mix almond pulp and flax paste together in a large mixing bowl with a spoon. Add the remaining ingredients and mix well.
Scoop onto a dehydrator tray lined with Teflon sheets or Parchment paper. The dough should be about ¼" thick. Use a large spatula or your hand to smooth it flat.

Dry at 110° F for 2-4 hours, until it can be flipped. Slide the teflex sheet off of the tray and mesh screen, turn the tray and screen over and put it on top of the bread. Then flip the whole thing over and carefully peel the sheet off the bottom (now the top). Put back in the dehydrator for another 2 hours or so.

> **Easy Crackers**
>
> If you're making a thick paste like hummus or dip, leave some of it in the blender or food processor. Add some soaked flaxseeds and re-blend, then spread it out on dehydrator sheets and dry at 110 for 12-24 hours, flipping halfway through. With just a couple of minutes' extra effort you'll soon have a pantry full of living, delicious crackers for when you're craving something crunchy and substantial.

Onion Bread

1 Cup Golden Flaxseeds, sprouted

1 Cup Sunflower Seeds, sprouted

1-3 Jalapenos

2 Cloves Garlic

½ Cup Fresh Savory Herbs: Thyme, Tarragon, Basil, Rosemary, Marjoram, you get the idea

½ Cup Nama Shoyu (or soy sauce)

¼ Cup Olive or Sunflower Oil, Extra Virgin and Cold-Pressed

3 large Yellow Onions, chopped and soaked in water for 15 minutes to remove the starch and unleash their natural sweetness. Chopping them *in* running water will stop the tears.

3 Tomatoes, chopped

1 Bell Pepper (yellow for color), chopped

In a high-speed blender or food processor, grind flaxseeds to a smooth paste and remove to a bowl. Blend rest of ingredients but last 3 and remove to bowl. Mix well with flaxseed paste. Add chopped veggies and mix by hand. Spread dough on Teflon sheet or parchment paper and put in the dehydrator at 110° F for about 24 hours, flipping halfway through.

Mediterranean Almond Bread

2 Cup Almond Pulp (leftover from making almond milk, pg 216)

½ Cup Flaxseed, sprouted

½ Cup Olive Oil, Extra Virgin and Cold-Pressed

¾ Cup Dehydrated Tomatoes, chopped

2 Tbsp Lemon Juice

1 tsp Sea Salt

½ Cup Fresh Savory Herbs

2 Zucchini, chopped

1-2 Apples, cored and chopped

In a high-speed blender or food processor, grind flaxseeds to a smooth paste and remove to a bowl. Blend rest of ingredients but last 2 and remove to bowl. Add zuke and apple and mix well by hand.

Spread dough on Teflon sheet or parchment paper and put in the dehydrator at 110° F for about 12 hours, flipping halfway through.

Ginger Snap Bread

1 ½ Cup Kamut, sprouted

1 ½ Cup Sesame, sprouted

1 Cup Dates

2" Ginger

¼ Cup Dried Coconut

In a high-speed blender or food processor, combine all ingredients and blend until consistent.

Spread dough on Teflon sheet or parchment paper and put in the dehydrator at 110° F for about 12 hours, flipping halfway through.

Aztec Warrior Bread

Quinoa and chia make a power-packed combination for battling on the dessert hills of Mexico, or for fighting a cold in a frosty London flat. Try it with pepita-chili cheese and mashed avocado.

1 1/2 Cup each:
Spelt, sprouted
Quinoa, sprouted
Amaranth, sprouted
½ Cup Chia Seeds, sprouted
1 ½ Cup Raisins, soaked in water overnight, drained and ground
1 tsp smoked Sea Salt

Follow basic bread directions. The chia will make this loaf quite dense, so will need a day and a half or so to dehydrate. Temp can be turned up by 10-15° every 8 hours or so until 160 ° is reached.

Lentil-Millet Bread

1 Cup Lentils, sprouted

1 Cup Quinoa, sprouted

1 Cup Brown Rice, germinated (See "Kitchen Sink Farming Volume 1: Sprouting")

3/4 Cup Millet, sprouted

3/4 Cup Sunflower Seeds, sprouted

2 Tbsp Golden Flax, sprouted (soaked)

4 Tbsp Coconut Oil

3 Tbsp Raw Honey

3 Tbsp Chia Seed (soaked)

1 1/2 tsp Sea Salt

Corn-Hemp Flatbread

2 Cups Fresh Corn

1 Cup Shelled Hemp Seeds, sprouted

1 Cup Almonds, sprouted

½ Cup Golden Flaxseed, sprouted

1 Clove Garlic

2 Tbsp Coconut Oil

½ tsp Turmeric for color (and detoxifying)

Grind with a high-speed blender until smooth and pourable.

Add water, kombucha, or other liquid if needed.

Prepare to dehydrate! With a spatula, spread batter ½ inch thick (or ¼ for chips) on teflex sheets, push the mixture to the edge of the sheet and run a thumb around the edges to clean them up.

Or make 4" tortillas or chips (dry well) by dropping about ¼ cup and spreading with spatula.

Dry a little for soft and roll-able, or a lot for crispy crunchy. Another great thing about living foods is that you can eat them at any stage of preparation; it's not like cookie dough with raw egg and processed white flour. Eat your raw and dehydrated foods at any and every stage of the process to find what you like. Once you've gotten the loaf thing down, all of the ingredients and amounts in these recipes come down to personal preference, as they're just as nutritious (and probably better-tasting to you) with your own variations and experimentations.

Try:
Rye-Fennel Bread with Jicama and Triticale
Oatmeal-Raisin Bread
Chocolate-Almond
Try substituting fig or papaya for raisins in previous recipes

Breakfasts!

Simple Cereal

½ Cup Sunflower Seed, Sprouted

½ Cup Shelled Hemp Seed. Sprouted

¼ Cup Fruit, fresh or dried: grapes, diced apples, bananas, etc

½ Cup Kefir

1 Tbsp Raw honey

1 Tbsp Whey-Fermented Apple Butter (pg "Kitchen Sink Farming Volume 2: Fermenting")

Optional: ½ tsp Ginger, grated, or cinnamon, or vanilla

Gently blend kefir, honey, and spices, and pour over sprouted seeds and fruits. Top with a dollop of kefired ginger-apple butter. Good morning.

Spanish Scramble

This easy scramble subs living nuts for eggs, giving the comforting flavors and colors of a farm-fresh brunch without the cholesterol, hormones, or vitality-sapping qualities of a traditional American breakfast.

Nut Scramble:

1 Cup Almonds, sprouted

½ Cup Sunflower Seed, sprouted

¼ tsp Sea Salt

½ tsp Turmeric (for color and an anti-inflammatory balance to the nuts and nightshades)

½ Cup Water or Kombucha

Veggies:

2 Tbsp Scallions (Green Onions), diced

½ Cup Tomatoes, diced

¼ Cup Cilantro, chopped

Pinch Black Pepper

Few Spinach Leaves or a Sliced Tomato

Smoothly puree sprouted almonds with a little water, salt and turmeric. Add sprouted sunflower seeds to coarsely chop, adding water to make a loose paste. Fold in chopped veggies.
Serve lightly packed with hands or ice cream scoop on spinach leaves or tomato slices, and sprinkle with black pepper.

Spr-oatmeal

1 Cup Whole Oats (not groats), sprouted

½ Cup Shelled Hemp Seed, sprouted

½ Cup Raisins (or dates for more sweetness); raisins may be soaked in kefir for a couple of hours to soften them and to awesomely turn the kefir purple.

2 T Coconut oil, extra virgin and cold-pressed

¼ Cup Raw Milk Kefir

Handful Walnuts, sprouted and chopped

Optional: Maple syrup, Raw Honey or Palm Sugar for a different sweet than dried fruit; a vanilla bean can be added to the first step.

In a high-speed blender, blend all ingredients but walnuts and half of the raisins until less than 110°. (Or puree in a food processor and warm in a dehydrator or pan.) Add raisins and mix, then transfer to a bowl, add kefir and top with chopped sprouted walnuts.
See "Kitchen Sink Farming Volume 1: Sprouting" pg 124 for a rant about raw oatmeal.

Coconut Muesli

Mix:
Grated fresh coconut or chopped young coconut meat with:
Fresh or dried fruit - raisins, chopped figs, banana, papaya
2 Tbsp Coconut Pudding ("Kitchen Sink Farming Volume 2: Fermenting" pg 217)

Desserts

The longer I eat simple, living food, the more I'm satisfied with whole, pure treats. Maybe it's the same gradual phenomenon of simplification that makes elderly people think hot water is delicious, or maybe it's my plodding acceptance that it's easy to lose the natural creamy sweetness of a banana with freezing, pureeing and drying, then mixing it with 15 other ingredients. It took me dozens of attempts at a grape-walnut torte for a girlfriend before I could swallow the fact that a shell of soaked and dried walnuts, blended with a little bit of raisins to make it sticky, filled with pureed whole red grapes and a little sea salt, was best.

I no longer try to divide whole foods and bring their disparate parts back together like an alchemist trying (and failing) to make gold out of incongruent ingredients and a complicated procedure. Now, I humbly try to bring out the best in whole foods, by drawing back the curtain on the stage of my plate, letting a light shine on the diva of a grape or a walnut. The shocking sweetness of a couple of plump dates is better than candy, and I prefer a tangerine picked from the tree in my mom's backyard to the key lime pie she's "slaved over for hours" (but don't tell her that).

But that doesn't make for a very interesting dinner party, so the following recipes, attempting to showcase naturally-occurring flavors are a little more fun and elaborate than picking a peach or peeling an orange. The recipes in the chapter are certainly less spectacular than they could be, but they are examples of the way that I've come to cooperate with sweets after years of trying to exert my will over them.

Most of these recipes involve drying in one way or another, and so while a suggestion of a shape will be given (cookie, torte, etc), the finished product can be made into any form you like, whether pressed with the bottom of a glass or between the palms in disks for cookies or mini cake layers, spread a half inch high and cut into rectangles when dry for bars, or spread very thickly and dried at a low temperature for several days to make a loaf or cake. Some recipes will lend themselves better to one shape or another, whether for technical reasons (a naturally wet batter, such as the fruit leathers, are better thinner so they can dry more evenly), or for aesthetics (oat-real-raisin seems decadent as a cookie, but make it into a bar and it seems like a trail snack. I prefer naughty. Or don't blend it so well and fling spoonfuls with abandon onto a dehydrator sheet and you've got granola, great with sprouted almond milk or enjoyed with the contents of a young coconut, eaten right out of the shell. I actually first discovered granola when making cookie dough and my electricity went out mid-blend.

Banana Ice Cream

This is the easiest dessert in the world and starts with inherently creamy bananas, frozen and blended into a smooth treat in a blender or food processor. More than 30 seconds in a high-speed blender will start to liquefy them, so make sure to keep them blending evenly, stopping at first sign of thaw. The cream can be scooped and shaped just like ice cream, and may be even better than plain bananas.

The science behind banana ice cream is this: a high-speed blender breaks the bonds between frozen banana molecules (Ba-Na2) so though they're still frozen they're now independent and can slide around each other.

A universe of flavors can be added to the whole bananas, like coconut pudding, cacao powder and maple syrup, mint, or vanilla bean. Or they (or other frozen or dried fruit like mango, berries, raisins, dried banana, nuts, or cacao nibs) can be chopped and stirred into the blended ice cream, giving a varied, chunky texture.

2-3 Bananas, frozen

If using a high-speed blender, put bananas in and add anything else you like that will be completely pureed. Quickly turn it up to high and vigorously push it down with the tamper for 10-20 seconds, until it's completely smooth. Add optional ingredients and pulse, or just chop and toss them on top in the bowl. If using a regular blender or food processor, you'll have to pulse and mix by hand a few times.

Oatmeal-Raisin Cookies

1 Cup Whole Oats, sprouted
1 Cup Shelled Hemp Seeds, sprouted
1 Cup Raisins, soaked in water overnight to soften, and drained
Zest of 4 Lemons or 2 Oranges
½ of a Vanilla Bean
5 Dates, seeded
1 tsp Cinnamon

Combine everything in a food processor or high-speed blender, reserving half of the hemp, zest, and most of the raisins. Be careful in the high-speed blender to stop blending before they're a generic homogeneous mess. Blend until smooth, then add the reserved ingredients and mix. Spoon onto a non-stick dehydrator sheet and press into cookies with the oiled bottom of a glass. Dehydrate for 12-24 hours, flip cookies and dehydrate for another 6-12 hours, until desired crunchiness is achieved.

Vanilla-Poppy seed Horns with Cashew-Lemon Frosting

Dehydrator Baking Tip

A banana will add chewiness and some sweetness, nuts will add crunch (these are opposite things). So if when you were a kid you lusted after those impossibly soft cookies that were 90% mono and diglycerides, throw in a banana. If, on the other hand, you're making a batch for the old folks home where they prefer to be reminded of their depression-era hockey puck biscuits, add some sprouted peanuts or macadamia nuts, or, if you're doing something heavy on the cacao, hazelnuts.

Chocolate Peanut Butter Tarts

(makes 4 single-serving tarts)

2 Cups Peanuts, sprouted

1 Cup Almonds, sprouted

½ - ¾ Cup Cacao Powder, depending on intensity

½ Cup Raw Honey (or Maple Syrup, or Dates)

2 Tbsp Whole Oats, sprouted and dried

1 tsp Almond or Vanilla Extract

Pinch of Sea Salt

Blend almonds, oats, salt, and ¼ Cup of the honey until medium smooth, and press into oiled 4" tart pans with removable bottoms or spring-forms. Freeze for 4 hours and remove from tart pan by gently pressing up on the bottom to remove ring piece, then sliding bottom off, or unhook spring-form ring and remove bottom.

Coarsely chop remaining ingredients in a blender or food processor and fold into tart shells. Decorate with fresh sliced strawberries and a spring of mint and serve within half an hour.

Smoky Apple Butter Bars

2 C Whey-Fermented Apple Butter ("Kitchen Sink Farming Volume 2: Fermenting")

½ C Apples, chopped

½ C Wheat, sprouted (or a variety of, like Spelt or Kamut)

¼ C Sunflower Seeds, sprouted

¼ C Peanuts, sprouted

¼ C Raisins (or Maple Syrup, not actually raw, but a nice flavor here)

1" Ginger, grated

¼ tsp Clove (about 2 cloves)

¼ tsp Paprika

Pinch Sea Salt

In a high-speed blender, combine sprouted wheat and raisins with enough apple butter to blend until smooth. Add rest of ingredients, except chopped apples, and blend coarsely. Add chopped apples and stir.

Spread ½" high on dehydrator sheets and dry at 110° F for 12-24 hours, until it can be flipped. Slide the sheet off of the tray and mesh screen, turn the tray and screen over and put it on top of the bars. Then flip the whole thing over and carefully peel the sheet off the bottom (now the top). Dry for another 6-12 hours, then remove from sheets and cut into bars. Depending on how dry, bars can be stored in a in the fridge for 2-3 weeks, or in a sealed container in a pantry for 1 week.

Strawberry-Tomato Ice Cream

Strawberry ice cream is the classic high-speed blender dessert, because the frozen strawberries and seeds blend up into a creamy scoopable dessert, somewhere between ice cream and sorbet. This recipe adds tomato, which is not necessary a companion plant to strawberries, but they have similar needs and will probably show up near each other in a vertical wall garden or small-scale hydro set-up. As far as being at-home in a dessert, tomato is a fruit after all, and sugary sun-ripened plum, grape, and cherry tomatoes (especially the "black cherry" variety) are often as sweet as actual plums, grapes, and cherries. In this luscious ice cream tomatoes add a nice base note that will be hard for your guests to put their finger on.

Great as-is, or add any number of coarsely-chopped flavorings: mint, coconut, golden raisins plumped in orange juice, nuts, hempseeds, or blend cashews completely for a nutty oiliness. Sweetener is optional, though raw honey's floral flavor blends well with this dessert. Raspberries and cherries can also be added for sweetness, and will make a nice swirl of color if blended for just for a second on two at the end. Raw goat milk kefir will add a nice creamy texture and sharp sour cream-like flavor which is wonderful, though I recommend sweetening it up a bit. To get the ultimate creaminess, scoop out some solid kefir that has separated from the whey.

1 Cup Strawberries, frozen
½ Cup Tomatoes, frozen
Optional: 2 T Kefir and 2 T Raw Honey

Put all ingredients in a high-speed blender, adding anything else you like that will be completely pureed. Quickly turn it up to high and vigorously push it down with the tamper for 15-30 seconds, until it's completely smooth. Add optional ingredients and pulse, or just chop and toss them on top in the bowl.

Banana-Hemp Cookies

Most of the desserts in this book can also be considered healthy snacks, and these cookies are no exception. They can double as high-protein energy bars, road food, or dried nut-butter honey receptacles. Or eat un-dried as a fruit-and-nut butter, spread on an apple or right off your (or someone else's) fingers.

2 Cup Shelled Hemp Seeds, sprouted
2 Bananas

Half pinch of sea salt

Juice of ¼ lemon

Optional: Cinnamon, Ginger, Raw Honey and/or Vanilla

Put all ingredients into a high-speed blender and blend until almost smooth. Scoop them out with a tablespoon and drop them onto non-stick dehydrator sheets with the help or another spoon or your finger. With the back of the spoon, press them into disks and dehydrate at 110° F for 6-12 hours, then flip them onto the dehydrator's mesh screen and dry 3-6 hours more.

Optional: add a dried fruit like cherries or dates. Use half shelled and half unshelled hemp seeds (both sprouted) for a crunchy texture.

Tahini Halava with Candied Cherry Frosting

2 Cups Sesame Seeds, sprouted

4 medium-sized Dates, seeds removed and finely chopped

1 Cup Cherries, dehydrated for 12 hours (add raw honey if the cherries aren't so sweet)

1 Vanilla Bean or 1 tsp Vanilla Extract

Pinch Sea Salt

In a high-speed blender or food processor, process sesame seeds, salt, and vanilla until an even paste. Add chopped dates and mix by hand. Press into an approx 8" by 12" food storage container (should be 1"-2" high) and chill in the fridge for at least 2 hours. Tip out of container and onto a plate. Wrap a plastic or other porous container with plastic wrap beforehand.

Put semi-dried cherries into a high-speed blender or food processor and blend until sticky and chunky. Scoop out with a spatula and frost the halava, then cut into squares and serve immediately.

Macaroons

So simple to make, I first "discovered" this format when I was in a hotel down the street from a Whole Foods and craving a sweet snack to watch a movie with. I've since made them several times while travelling and am reminded how good they are every few years by one of those friends. The coconut oil solidifies in the fridge to give the macs a firm-yet-light texture, and adds that traditional coconut flavor.

The directions are all the same...

Mix all ingredients well with a spoon or hand and form into golf ball-sized macaroons. Refrigerate for at least 30 minutes

… only the ingredients change

Hemp Cacao-Nut Macaroons

Hemp seed is quick to sprout and supplies unparalleled protein and essential fatty acids. Maple syrup is the most aligned sweetener to the flavor profile, but I like to use raw, local honey whenever I'm travelling to safeguard against new allergens. The dessert connoisseur will appreciate the way sea salt teases out the sweetness of the other ingredients.

½ Cup Shelled Hemp Seed, sprouted
½ Cup Coconut, Shredded (usually bought this way (look for organic and unsulfured), but try grating fresh coconut yourself sometime. Sublime.)
½ Cup Cacao Powder
½ Cup Maple syrup or Raw Honey
¼ Cup Coconut oil, (liquefied, soak the jar in warm water if necessary), Extra Virgin and Cold-Pressed
1 T Vanilla powder, paste, or (last choice) extract
¼ tsp Sea Salt

Sunflower-Orange Macaroons

Another quick sprouter, sunflower's complex nuttiness is complimented by the uplifting zing of citrus. Raw honey is directly sweet without a lot of meandering, so there's room to play with bitter flavors like orange zest, and the bitter almond drives the whole thing home. The ease of sprouting sunflower, and the raw honey and bee pollen make this a great travel snack and allergy-fighter. You could start the seeds soaking in the morning and enjoy this dessert the same night.

1 Cup Sunflower Seed, sprouted and coarsely ground or chopped

Juice and Zest from ½ an Orange

½ Cup Raw honey

½ Cup Coconut oil, Extra Virgin and Cold-Pressed

½ tsp Bitter Almond Extract

1 Tbsp Bee pollen (optional)

Berry Tart with Almond Crust and Sweet Kefir Cream

Because of the three step process of sprouting almonds and two steps of dehydration (assuming your kefir is ready to go), this recipe takes a little while, but in a week you'll wish you'd taken the few minutes now to rock these out! Making a seed and nut tart shell is surprisingly easy, though a small "spring-form", like the ones used for cheesecake, or tart pan with a removable bottom, will help chefs with less than nimble fingers. If all else fails, a flat dried bottom, like a home-done graham cracker, is just as good.

Silky Chocolate Tart, Sprouted Almond-Maple Kefir Crust
Prepare the filling first, set aside, and use the unwashed food processor to make the crust.

For the Chocolate Filling:
2 barely ripe Avocados, at room temperature
½ Cup Cocoa or Cacao powder
¾ Cup Maple Syrup Kefir (see "Kitchen Sink Farming Volume 2: Fermenting")
1 Tbsp Vanilla Extract or half a Vanilla Bean
Pinch of Sea Salt
2 Tbsp Coconut Oil, room temperature

Tart Crust:
4 Cups Almonds, sprouted and dehydrated (see "Kitchen Sink Farming Volume 1: Sprouting")
½ cup cocoa or cacao powder

1 Tbsp Vanilla Extract or half a Vanilla Bean
Pinch of Sea Salt
¾ Cup Maple Syrup Kefir

Instructions:
Line a 9" removable bottom tart pan with saran wrap.

Place the ingredients for the chocolate filling in a food processor fitted with chopping blade and process until smooth. Scrape the filling into a bowl and set it aside.

Fit the bowl and blade back onto the food processor (no need to clean the bowl in between). Place all ingredients for tart crust except maple syrup into food processor. Process until fine textured with small bits of almonds. Measure out a ¼ cup of the crumbs and sprinkle them across the bottom of the tart pan. Add the maple syrup to the remaining crumbs and process 1-2 minutes until the tart crust becomes as thick as cookie dough. Pat crust into tart pan. Spread the chocolate filling over the crust, cover and refrigerate overnight.

Putting It All Together

I think my breakfast is a good example of producing an array of nutritive and delicious foods, alive in many senses of the word, from a small urban space.

JP's morning juice:

1 Cup Kombucha

1 Cup Probiotic Water (see "Kitchen Sink Farming Volume 2: Fermenting")

1 Meyer Lemon (peeled, but a little washed peel still attached), from a tree in a pot on my outside stairs

Handful Mint, from a window pot

Big handful Wheatgrass, a transient neighbor of the mint

(Last three ingredients are in "Kitchen Sink Farming Volume 3: Growing")

Some Parsley, Kale, or other healthy stuff

1" fresh Ginger Root, grown in container for the sake of this sentence

Everything thrown into a high-speed blender for about 30 seconds. Picked or poured fresh, each ingredient is at room temperature, so some ice cubes can be blended in to chill down the drink. When I'm making it for someone for the first time, I add some apple juice ice cubes I have in a zip-loc at the bottom of my freezer for just such an occasion. Personally, I try to avoid sugar in the morning and fruit juice in general, but this juice is pretty durn acidic without a little sweetness. Maybe start by adding some apple juice, or just drop in half an apple if you don't mind it a little sludgy, and slowly wean yourself.

I like to drink it immediately, while the fiber is still in suspension. If you like more liquid juice, just wait a minute and the indigestible plant matter ("cellulose" or insoluble fiber, mostly from the cell walls of the wheatgrass) will float to the top. Then, the bright green liquid will easily pour out from underneath the floating cellulose, and can be drunk straight from the blender pitcher as though it was painstakingly strained. It can also be painstaking strained.

The probiotic water stimulates metabolism and supplants millions of beneficial organisms. Ginger is a big "Good Morning!" to the digestion, increasing the digestive fire, regulating hormones and boosting the immune system, and the many benefits of kombucha and wheatgrass have been extolled ad naseum elsewhere in this series. The lemon adds an alkalizingly sweet tanginess, and its anti-oxidant and liver-cleansing properties help get rid of toxins that have been pulled out of the cells and deposited in the blood for removal during sleep. And one lemon supplies double the recommended daily allowance of vitamin C – first thing in the morning is as good a time as any to combat free radicals and (again) boost the immune system. Mint is both energizing and calming. It's a strong diuretic and therefore further helps in eliminating toxins; it also whitens the teeth and adds a delicious zip to this already delightful potion. With fermented, sprouted, and container-grown ingredients, this simple juice is the epitome of Pajama Permaculture, and a detailed list of its benefits could fill many books. How much are these nutritional and medicinal virtues worth? With pharmaceuticals as the measuring stick, certainly hundreds of times more than it costs us to enjoy them, with the added benefit of building health instead of masking symptoms and further aggravating the root cause of the imbalance.

As you can see, a page has gone into describing something that takes less than a minute to execute. This is a good metaphor for everything in this book, where the learning effort far overshadows the actual work; where like an iceberg the few necessary practical facts are held in view by a mass of primal wisdom.

Recommended Reading

Fermentation:

The Art of Fermentation: An In-Depth Exploration of Essential Concepts and Processes from Around the World by Sandor Ellix Katz and Michael Pollan

Wild Fermentation by Sandor Ellix Katz *with an incredible recommended reading list

Understanding: Bacteria Discovery Education School (DVD, and on YouTube)

Sprouting:

Sprouts: The Miracle Food: The Complete Guide to Sprouting by Steve Meyerowitz and Michael Parman

The Sprouting Book: How to Grow and Use Sprouts to Maximize Your Health and Vitality by Ann Wigmore

The Wheatgrass Book: How to Grow and Use Wheatgrass to Maximize Your Health and Vitality by Ann Wigmore

Gardening:

Fresh Food from Small Spaces: The Square-Inch Gardener's Guide to Year-Round Growing, Fermenting, and Sprouting by R.J. Ruppenthal

Dirt: the Ecstatic Skin of the Earth by William Bryant Logan

Vegetarianism, Veganism, and Raw Food Prep:

Eating Animals by Jonathan Safran-Foer.

Diet for a New America and The Food Revolution by John Robbins.

Beyond Beef: The Rise and fall of the Cattle Culture by Jeremy Rifkin

RAW by Charlie Trotter

Ani's Raw Food Kitchen: Easy, Delectable Living Foods Recipes by Ani Phyo

Environment, GMOs, and Agribusiness:

The Power of Community: How Cuba Survived Peak Oil (DVD and on YouTube)

The Weather of the Future by Heidi Cullen

Stolen Harvest: The Hijacking of the Global Food Supply by Dr. Vandana Shiva

The World According to Monsanto (DVD)

Evolution and Pleasure

Stumbling on Happiness by Daniel Gilbert

How Pleasure Works by Paul Bloom

Supernormal Stimuli: How Primal Urges Overran Their Evolutionary Purpose by Deidre Barrett

Resources:

Seeds, Grains and Nuts:

NutsOnline.com - A family business with great prices, customer service, and a touch of whimsy in everything they do. They once sent a stuffed elephant with my order. Sold.

Wheatgrasskits.com - A great source for certain seeds as well as sprouting supplies

Nutiva - The best hemp seeds and coconut oil. I get the 3-lb bag of organic shelled hempseeds and double pack of 54-oz jars of organic coconut oil, and I buy them through amazon.com to get free shipping and a "Subscribe and Save" discount. They also make a raw coconut oil which comes in glass and is great, and more expensive.

Sprouting Bags – available from great companies like Pure Joy Planet, but I use reusable mesh produce bags that are about 20 times cheaper and might last longer, but have a slightly wider mesh so the tiniest seeds like amaranth need the real deal. Or panty hose.

Probiotic Cultures

Dairy Kefir - kefirlady.com – a great source for dairy kefir grains grown in organic raw goat milk, and at the time of this writing she sells a ¼ cup for $20 with shipping; top-quality grains at the best price on the net for the quantity. Is also very available to answer questions and share the enthusiasm.

Kombucha, Juice Kefir, Apple Cider Vinegar – try your local craigslist first, then eBay. Can also be started from a raw and unflavored product from your local natural foods store.

Index

"The Worst Mistake in the History of the Human Race" article, 51
"open air" compost bin, 359
"The Flowing Bowl", 215
acetaminophen, 146
acetic acid, 203- 206, 235
achylia gastrica, 242
ADD, 68
ADM, 37
Adzuki, 89
aging, 68, 97, 118, 125, 127
airlock, 204, 251
alcohol, 117, 152, 160, 204-217, 228, 239, 256
Alexander Fleming, 181
Alexander Solzhenitsyn, 237
alfalfa, 59, 74, 79, 84, 89-90, 97-99
algae, 317, 319, 354
alkalinity, 116, 117, 235, 267, 280
alkaloids, 117, 155
allergies, 15, 65, 114, 124
allium, 155
almonds, 70, 104, 157-163
Alpha Linolenic Acid, 102
Alzheimer's, 131, 269
amaranth, 77, 91
amasake, 131

Amazon, 124
amino acids, 20, 21, 61, 65, 68, 91, 97, 100, 106, 113, 126, 247
ammonium nitrate, 39
analgesic, 236
androgens, 235
anemia, 236
Anheuser-Busch, 34
anise, 143, 144
Ann Wigmore, 264, 527
antibiotics, 181
anti-coagulants, 135
antioxidants, 236, 270
anti-parasitic, 128
antiseptic, 128
antispasmodic, 144, 147, 236
anxiety, 236, 241
apple butter, 247
apple cider vinegar, 203
artheriosclerosis, 157
arthritis, 93, 146, 203, 236, 270
artificial light, 284, 63
arugula, 94
asthma, 116
athlete's foot, 269
Aurora Organic Dairy, 35
automatic sprouter, 80
avocados, 104
Ayurvedic medicine, 133, 254
Aztecs, 91, 98
B vitamins, 67, 120, 126, 130

B1, 22, 93
B12, 93, 135, 266, 271
bacteria, 25, 27, 28, 61, 62, 177-252
barley, 86, 93, 132
basal ganglia, 56
bat guano, 94
bean sprouting, 82
bedding materials for worms, 367
beef, 38, 106, 125
bergamot oil, 233
Bible, 143
black beans, 91
Blandov Brothers, 243
blood pressure, 115, 131, 267
blood sugar, 99, 115, 131, 150, 256
body odor, 269
bone loss, 68
BPA, 76
brain, 24, 54-57, 100, 117, 120, 129, 131, 164
Brassica Protection Products, inc, 95
bread, 59, 76, 101, 114, 132-136, 150, 195, 197, 221-224, 247
breast size, 147
broccoli, 79, 90, 94, 95, 96, 97, 146, 153
BroccoSprouts, 96
buckwheat, 94
burns, 269
Bush administration, 48
butter, 15, 18, 221, 226, 247, 252-254, 259, 261

butyric acid, 235
buzz words, 35
c. diphtheriae, 242
cabbage, 96-98, 128, 153
cadmium, 268
caffeine, 117, 233
calcium, 21, 63, 67, 89, 91, 93, 96, 98, 105, 109, 115, 120, 121, 126, 133, 138, 140, 159, 163
cancer, 15, 23, 26, 33, 52, 64, 94-97, 107, 109, 116, 127, 131, 146, 154, 160, 236-237, 242, 257, 258, 264, 270, 289
candida, 128, 166, 235, 236, 270
candidiasis, 235
caraway, 143-144
carbon dioxide, *see CO2*
carcinogen, 97, 146, 236, 241
cardamom, 85, 138, 145
carminative, 144, 147
carotene, 93
cars, 39, 41
casein, 254
cashews, 104, 162
Cato the Elder, 97
Caucus Mountains, 240, 243
cauliflower, 94, 96, 97
celery, 90, 93, 103, 146
celibacy, 147
cell regeneration, 236
cellular degeneration, 118
cellulose, 161, 165

cereal, 120
Charile Bell, 52
cheese, 61, 68, 163, 177, 184, 197-202, 226, 246-249, 259
chelated, 72
chia, 81, 98, 103, 108
chick peas, 104
children, 27, 29, 41, 52, 53, 54, 100-102, 120-125, 134, 135, 152
China, 13, 33, 37, 41, 94, 116, 145
Chinese cuisine, 118
chives, 151
chloramine, 232
chlorine, 73, 74, 78, 218, 232
chlorophyll, 79, 80, 84, 121, 133, 263, 267, 270, 271, 283, 286, 303, 373, 374, 375
cholecystitis, 242
cholesterol, 52, 108-109, 115-116, 138, 142, 146, 157, 166
cigarettes, 117
cilantro, 147
Claude Levi-Strauss, 211
cleansing, 272
clogged arteries, 118
clover, 79, 84, 90, 98, 99
CO2, 204, 210, 214, 216, 217, 220
cocaine, 117
coconut, 64, 94, 101
coconut oil, 255, 256
cold stabilization, 187

colic, 147
colitis, 242, 267
collagen, 236
colloidal silver, 195
colon cancer, 52, 131
complete protein, 106, 126
composting, 355, 357, 359, 360, 364
ConAgra, 37
continuous fermentation, 206, , 230244, 245
copper, 67, 99, 127, 135, 138, 159, 164, 165, 166
coriander, 142, 143, 147
corn, 25, 27, 51, 54, 120
corticoids, 235
cow manure, 94
cow milk, 244, 253, 261
crucifer, 94, 128
Cuba, 41-46
cumin, 142, 143, 144, 147, 148
curry, 147-148
daikon, 90, 148
dandruff, 247
Darjeeling, 233
Dead Sea Scrolls, 264
depression, 236, 258
detoxification, 235, 237
diabetes, 45, 52, 116, 126, 150
diarrhea, 242, 267
dill, 143, 148
distilled water, 72
DNA, 25-27, 48, 179-182
dog chews, 88
dog food, 88

Dole, 37
Dr. Alexis Carrel, 272
Dr. Bernard Jensen, 269
Dr. Jared Diamond, 51
Dr. Johannes Kuhl, 242
Dr. Rajendra Pachauri, 49
Dr. Watson, 49
Dr. Yoshihide Hagiwara, 264, 267
drugs, 33, 56, 152
dysentery, 242
e. coli, 242
earl grey, 233
earthworm castings, 275
Easter Island, 46
ECDC [European Centre for Disease Control], 182
eczema, 102
edestin, 110
Edmond Bordeaux Szekely, 264
enzyme inhibitors, 4, 67
EFAs. *See* Essential Fatty Acids
effects of artificial light on pumpkins, 284
effects of different kinds of light on animals, 284
egg vinegar, 203
EI's. *See* Enzyme Inhibitors
eisenia foetida, 367
Eli Metchnikoff, 235, 241
embargo of Cuba, 42
emmenagogic, 147
Environmental Choice Program, 36

enzyme inhibitors, 65, 67, 71, 72, 111, 123, 129, 158, 160, 165
Enzyme Inhibitors, 20
enzymes, 18, 20, 51, 60-69, 75, 84, 90, 100, 107, 111, 121, 127, 129, 146, 154, 161, 162, 197, 221, 222, 237, 257, 266, 268, 271, 375-376
ephedra, 211
epileptics, 129
Essene Gospels of Peace, 264
Essenes, 221
essential fatty acids, 64, 100-101, 108
estrogens, 235
Eubie Blake, 273
evaporated cane juice. *See* sugar
evolution, 57, 179, 180, 182, 212, 259
excess mucus, 150
expectorant, 144, 150
Exxon, 49
fast food, 13, 50, 51-54, 152
fat burning, 102
FDA, 32, 35
fennel, 85, 142, 143, 145, 149
fenugreek, 85, 142,, 150
fertility, 269
fertilizer, 24, 33, 35, 39, 43, 44, 93, 140, 276, 280, 286, 288, 294,

306, 316, 354, 364, 366, 369
feta, 197, 249
fiber, 20, 43, 64, 78, 80, 81, 98, 100, 115, 119, 120, 125, 130, 133, 135, 137, 138, 161, 165, 166
fibromyalgia, 236, 258
fish oil, 105
flax, 14, 81, 85, 87, 88, 98, 100-104, 108
fluorine, 232
forest, 19, 26, 47, 355, 357
free radicals, 60, 94, 127, 152, 270
GABA, 129
gall bladder, 256
gamma-aminobutyric acid, *see* GABA
garbanzo, 104, 142
garlic, 77, 105, 142, 151, 155
garlic chives, 151
garlic sprouts, 142
gas, 24, 39, 40, 43, 45, 66, 73, 88, 144, 147
gastroenteritis, 242
GBR. *See* Germinated Brown Rice
genetic modification, *see* GMOs
genetic Promiscuity, 179
George Washington Carver, 123
Gerber's, 37

germ, 77, 119, 132, 137, 141
Germany, 58, 132, 136, 145
germinated brown rice, 129
ghee, 15, 133, 254, 255, 257, 260
ginger beer, 210, 217, 218
globular proteins, 104, 106, 107
gluconic acid, 235
glucoraphanin, 94
glucoronic acid, 235
glucosamines, 189, 236
glucosinolates, 96
glucuronidase, 236
gluten, 86, 101, 114, 126, 132, 137
GMOs, 25, 27, 30, 32
GMO labelling, 15, 24, 25, 32
goat milk, 18, 214, 244, 246, 253, 261, 529
GOP, 46
grapefruit seed extract, 319
gray hair, 269
Great Depression, 134
Green Giant Fresh Inc.,, 95
halitosis, 269
Harmony Farms, 95
hazelnuts, 163
heart disease, 45, 52, 53, 107, 126, 157, 160
heavy metals, 269, 355

Heinz, 37
hematinics, 236
hemoglobin, 236, 267
hemp, 78, 87, 88, 103, 105, 106, 107, 109, 110, 111, 112, 138, 155
hemp oil, 108
Henry Ford, 134
hepatotoxins, 236
herbs, 142
high blood pressure, 52, 146
Hippocrates, 265
Hokkaido University, 237
honey, 178, 195, 204, 205, 208-217, 234, 239, 244, 249, 251
honeybush, 233
hormone regulation, 129
hormones, 52, 104, 107, 109
hunter-gathererers, 50, 117
Hunzas, 115
hyaluronidase, 236
hydrogen peroxide, 195, 289
hyper-maturation, 50
immune system, 18, 87, 107-109, 137, 159, 183, 226, 235, 236, 261
immunoglobulins, 107
inductively coupled plasma spectometer, 274
infant mortality, 45
infants, 149
infections, 142
inflammation, 100, 102, 142, 146, 150, 166
injera bread, 101
inositol, 108
insulin, 107, 115, 127, 150, 256, 258
iron, 22, 67, 84, 89, 93, 98, 105, 109, 118, 120, 126, 135, 138, 140, 164, 166, 267, 270, 271, 374, 375
iron deficiency. *See* anemia
Ito Shoichi, 130
John Ott, 284
Johns Hopkins University, 55, 94
jun, 226, 239, 240
kale, 94, 97, 153
Kamut, 18, 101, 112, 113, 114, 137
kefir, 15, 18, 86, 188, 192, 206, 209, 214, 226, 240-260, 529
Khorasan wheat, *see* Kaumt
kid's menus, 52
kidney diseases, 256
kimchi, 97, 195
kombucha, 17, 188, 194, 203, 206, 209, 226-250
kombucha vinegar, 203
laban, 247-249
lactation, 269
lactic acid, 235
lactobacillius, 185
lactobacillus, 97
lactose, 15, 241, 254

lactose intolerance, 15
leafy greens, 79, 84, 94
legumes, 104, 119, 122
lentils, 70, 85, 104, 114
leukemia, 131
licorice, 143, 149
life expectancy, 45
lifespan, 51, 117
lignans, 100, 132
linoleic acid, 104, 120, 138
lipase, 16, 189, 214, 217, 227, 241, 256, 257
liver, 105, 146, 151, 152, 226, 235, 237, 256, 258-262, 268, 272, 310
livestock feed, 134
living foods, 59
Louis Pasteur, 184
lumbricus rubella, 367
lung congestion, 150
lust, 56, 143, 147
lysine, 91, 126
macadamia nut, 163
magnesium, 91, 96, 99, 109, 113, 115, 116, 121, 125, 126, 130, 133, 135, 138, 140, 159, 164, 166, 267, 271, 373
malic acid, 235
manganese, 99, 127, 135, 164, 165, 166
manure, 43, 275, 288, 358, 367, 369, 373
maple syrup, 204, 244, 250, 251
Marco Polo, 242

Marcus Aurelius, 148
marijuana, 110
master cleanse, 250
Mayans, 98
McDonald's, 50, 52, 54
McDonalds, 52
mead, 210-213
menopause, 131, 132
menstruation, 147
mental health, 102
mercury, 31, 268
methonine, 91
micro lettuces, 64, 139, 263, 295, 296
microgreens, 122, 139, 146, 151
migraines, 116
milk, 15, 18, 37, 51, 52, 91, 93, 96, 98, 120, 125, 126, 128, 133, 135, 138, 158, 159, 161
milk thistle, 151
millet, 116, 138
mineral deposits, 235
miso, 61, 135
mold, 275, 276, 282, 283, 308
monoamine oxidase, 236
monoculture, 93
Monsanto, 26, 27, 30, 31, 34, 134
mosquito repellent, 146
mucilages, 81, 153
mung beans, 21, 66, 118
muscle spasms, 144, 146, 147

mustard, 24, 81, 83, 89, 96, 97, 128, 142, 153, 154
Myriad Genetics, 33
natto, 135
negative ions, 269
nerve cells, 55, 56
Nestle, 36
niacin, 99, 113, 116, 125, 164
nicotine, 268
nitrogen, 21, 23, 24, 94, 97, 122, 134
Nobel Prize, 235, 241, 272
nomadic man, 211
nori, 101
NPK, 23, 24
nucleic acid, 235
nut butter, 18, 64, 112, 133
nut cheese, 66, 149, 158
nut milk, 78
nutrient absorption, 102
oat groats, 119
oats, 67, 87, 119, 120, 137
obesity, 53, 268
oleic acid, 104, 162
oligosaccharides, 233
olives, 104
omega-3s, 98, 101, 102, 103, 108, 162, 166
onion, 79, 155
osmosis, 190, 193, 232
overweight children, 52
oxalic acid, 235

oxygen, 74, 77, 83, 86, 87, 101, 102, 121, 150, 267, 269, 270, 289, 290, 291, 308, 311, 317, 319, 357, 359
Paleolithic period, 50
panic attacks, 129
parallel gene transfer. *See* Genetic Promiscuity
parrot food, 88
passive composting, 360
pasteurization, 159
peak oil, 39, 41
peanuts, 65, 70, 104, 122, 123, 124, 125, 157
peas, 18, 37, 70, 85, 104, 121, 158
pecans, 164, 166
penicillin, 181, 182
pepitas, 165, 166
peptic ulcers, 242, 267
permaculture, 356
pesticides, 23, 24, 26, 27, 32, 35, 37, 39, 40, 43, 44, 93, 97, 134, 137, 140, 152, 189, 232
Peter Fitzgerald, 53
pH, 116, 117, 118, 203, 209, 235
phosphorus, 23, 89, 96, 99, 115, 116, 119, 125, 126, 133, 138, 140, 159, 162, 163, 164, 165, 166
phytic acid, 67, 129
phytoestrogens, 109
phytoserols, 157
pickle, 190, 238

pickles, 149
pine nuts, 164
pistachios, 70, 158, 165
plasma, 107
plastic water bottles, 76
pleasure, 14, 57
PMS, 129, 147
poison ivy, 104, 162, 269
pollutants, 235
polyunsaturated oils, 108
polyvinyl chloride, 268
poop, 369
poppy, 89, 155
potassium, 21, 23, 89, 105, 109, 115, 118, 130, 133, 135, 138, 159, 162, 163, 164
pre-biotic, 115
pre-frontal cortex, 56
pregnancy, 242
probiotic water, 184, 185, 187, 197, 199, 200, 201, 224
produce bags, 77
protein, 21, 25, 61, 64, 85, 89, 91, 93, 100, 105, 106, 107, 110, 111, 113, 115, 118, 119, 120, 121, 125, 126, 134, 137, 138, 140, 155, 157, 159, 165, 166, 197, 199, 236, 252, 253, 254
PSRAST, 28
psyllium, 81
Pump N Seal, 77
pumpkin, 14, 138, 158, 165, 166

Pure Joy Planet, 77
QAI, 37
Quaker Oats, 119
quinoa, 66, 70, 85, 125, 126, 127, 186, 197, 222, 224
radish, 79, 84, 90, 96, 128, 148
recycling, 289, 310, 319
red wigglers, 367
rejuvelac. *See* probiotic water
resveratrol, 160
retinoids, 235
reverse osmosis, 72
rice, 37, 51, 54, 107, 129, 130, 131, 140, 144, 145
Ronald Reagan, 237
rooibos, 233
s. paratyphi, 242
sagging skin, 268
salmonella, 242
salt, 51, 189, 190, 191, 193, 199, 221, 223, 248, 249
Samurai, 203
saponin, 127
saturated fat, 52, 117, 256
sauerkraut, 18, 77, 97, 98, 190
SCOBY, 206, 227, 229, 230, 238, 250
secondary fermentation, 231
seed cheese, 197
seed factories, 70
seed hibernation, 222
seed milk, 64

Seed/Nut Digestibility
    Chart, 60
selenium, 150, 162
Sencha tea, 233
serotonin, 116, 138
sesame, 105, 133, 142
sexual maturity, 52
sexual vitality, 129
SGS, 94
Sholl Group, 95
shoots, 294, 297
silicon, 91, 120, 126
sinigrin, 153
skin, 63, 67, 92, 99, 100,
    102, 107, 151, 152,
    160, 161
sleep, 269, 273, 356
soap, 126
SOD, 269
sodium, 21, 93, 109, 159
soilless media, 279
soma, 211
sour cream, 246, 247
Soviet Union, 41, 45
soy oil as fuel, 134
soy sauce, 135
soybeans, 134, 135
spelt, 136, 137
spleen, 146
squash, 158, 165, 166
St. Hildegard, 136
staphylococcus, 181, 183
star anise, 144
starch, fat, and salt, 51
sterilization, 194
sterilizing soil, 276
Steve Meyerowitz, 264,
    527

stimulant, 147
straying husband, 144
stress, 69, 125, 129, 138,
    152
strokes, 45, 67
strontium, 268
structural protein, 107
sugar, 53, 177, 203, 204,
    205, 208, 212, 218,
    219, 220, 228, 229,
    231, 233, 234, 239,
    244, 249, 251, 256,
    258, 259
sugar mills, 45
sulforaphane, 94
sulfur, 109, 247
sunflower, 63, 64, 65, 82,
    85, 87, 122, 125, 138,
    139, 163, 164, 222
sunflower lettuce, 298,
    299
sunlight, 284, 323
sunshine, 121
synovial fluid, 236
tahini, 133
Taiitiriya Upanishad, 365
tamago-su, 203
tamari, 135
tannins, 233
Target, 35, 37, 360
teeth, 72, 109, 132
tempeh, 135
terminator gene, 30
TerraChoice, 36
thanklemesien, 183
"The Future of Food"
    movie, 29
thrush, 235

thyroid, 268
Tibet, 94
Time Lapse Research Laboratory, 284
topsoil, 33, 48
tortillas, 101
trans-fats, 52, 108
travelling, 23, 63, 84, 85
Triticale, 139
tryptophan, 27, 28, 116, 135, 138
tuberculosis, 110
tumors, 268, 269
Tylenol, 146
ulcers, 269
United Nations Intergovernmental Panel on Climate Change, 48
urushiol, 104, 162
USDA, 34
Vampire Juice, 407
vegan diet, 266
vermiculture, 357, 364, 367
vinegar, 203, 204, 205, 206, 207, 208, 209, 213, 226, 230, 235, 237, 238, 260
vinegar flies, 207, 237
Vishnu, 133
Vit-Ali Baba, 399
vitamin A, 105, 128, 133, 164

vitamin C, 66, 93, 97, 118, 128
vitamin E, 64, 125, 126, 159, 262, 484
Wal-mart, 35
walnuts, 138, 164, 166
water heaters, 45
weight loss, 130, 149, 257
Wendy's, 36
wheat, 18, 51, 70, 76, 77, 86, 93, 94, 112, 113, 114, 120, 126, 132, 136, 137, 139, 140, 184, 203, 222, 223
wheatgrass, 264, 266, 267, 268, 270, 527
whey, 198, 247, 249
WHO. *See* World Health Organization
whole Foods, 18, 37
wild rice, 140
Willpower, 55
World Health Organization, 53
World War 2, 93
worms, 43, 355, 357, 364, 365, 366, 367, 368, 369, 371
yeast infections, 235
yoga, 14, 50
yogurt, 177, 188, 226, 246
zinc, 67, 99, 109, 113, 130, 138, 159, 164

Stay Connected!

Visit

www.KitchenSinkFarming.org

for tips, recipes, news, giveaways, and general delicious nerdiness.

Printed in Poland
by Amazon Fulfillment
Poland Sp. z o.o., Wrocław